Psychiatric Diagnosis and Management in Primary Care

Editor

GENEVIEVE L. PAGALILAUAN

MEDICAL CLINICS
OF NORTH AMERICA

www.medical.theclinics.com

Consulting Editors
DOUGLAS S. PAAUW
EDWARD R. BOLLARD

September 2014 • Volume 98 • Number 5

ELSEVIER

1600 John F. Kennedy Boulevard • Suite 1800 • Philadelphia, Pennsylvania, 19103-2899

http://www.theclinics.com

MEDICAL CLINICS OF NORTH AMERICA Volume 98, Number 5
September 2014 ISSN 0025-7125, ISBN-13: 978-0-323-32331-4

Editor: Jessica McCool
Developmental Editor: Yonah Korngold

Medical Clinics of North America (ISSN 0025-7125) is published bimonthly by Elsevier Inc., 360 Park Avenue South, New York, NY 10010-1710. Months of publication are January, March, May, July, September, and November. Business and editorial offices: 1600 John F. Kennedy Boulevard, Suite 1800, Philadelphia, PA 19103-2899. Periodicals postage paid at New York, NY, and additional mailing offices. Subscription prices are USD $255.00 per year (US individuals), $471.00 per year (US institutions), $125.00 per year (US Students), $320.00 per year (Canadian individuals), $612.00 per year (Canadian institutions), $200.00 per year (Canadian and foreign students), $390.00 per year (foreign individuals), and $612.00 per year (foreign institutions). To receive student/resident rate, orders must be accompanied by name of affiliated institution, date of term, and the signature of program/residency coordinator on institution letterhead. Orders will be billed at individual rate until proof of status is received. Foreign air speed delivery is included in all Clinics' subscription prices. All prices are subject to change without notice. **POSTMASTER:** Send address changes to *Medical Clinics of North America*, Elsevier Health Sciences Division, Subscription Customer Service, 3251 Riverport Lane, Maryland Heights, MO 63043. **Customer Service: Telephone: 1-800-654-2452** (U.S. and Canada); **1-314-447-8871** (outside U.S. and Canada). **Fax: 314-447-8029. E-mail:** journalscustomerserviceusa@elsevier.com (for print support); journalsonlinesupport-usa@elsevier.com (for online support).

Reprints. For copies of 100 or more of articles in this publication, please contact the Commercial Reprints Department, Elsevier Inc., 360 Park Avenue South, New York, NY 10010-1710. Tel.: 212-633-3874; Fax: 212-633-3820; E-mail: reprints@elsevier.com.

Medical Clinics of North America is also published in Spanish by McGraw-Hill Interamericana Editores S. A., P.O. Box 5-237, 06500 Mexico, D.F., Mexico.

Medical Clinics of North America is covered in *MEDLINE/PubMed (Index Medicus), Current Contents, ASCA, Excerpta Medica, Science Citation Index, and ISI/BIOMED.*

Printed in the United States of America.

PROGRAM OBJECTIVE
The goal of the *Medical Clinics of North America* is to keep practicing physicians up to date with current clinical practice by providing timely articles reviewing the state of the art in patient care.

LEARNING OBJECTIVES
Upon completion of this activity, participants will be able to:
1. Discuss anxiety disorders, addiction disorders, bipolar disorders, and seasonal affective disorders in the primary care setting.
2. Review psychopharmacology in the primary care setting.
3. Describe the relationship between psychiatric disorders and sleep issues.

ACCREDITATION
The Elsevier Office of Continuing Medical Education (EOCME) is accredited by the Accreditation Council for Continuing Medical Education (ACCME) to provide continuing medical education for physicians.

The EOCME designates this enduring material for a maximum of 15 *AMA PRA Category 1 Credit*(s)™. Physicians should claim only the credit commensurate with the extent of their participation in the activity.

All other health care professionals requesting continuing education credit for this enduring material will be issued a certificate of participation.

DISCLOSURE OF CONFLICTS OF INTEREST
The EOCME assesses conflict of interest with its instructors, faculty, planners, and other individuals who are in a position to control the content of CME activities. All relevant conflicts of interest that are identified are thoroughly vetted by EOCME for fair balance, scientific objectivity, and patient care recommendations. EOCME is committed to providing its learners with CME activities that promote improvements or quality in healthcare and not a specific proprietary business or a commercial interest.

The planning committee, staff, authors and editors listed below have identified no financial relationships or relationships to products or devices they or their spouse/life partner have with commercial interest related to the content of this CME activity:
Susan M. Bentley, DO; Edward R. Bollard, MD, DDS, FACP; Carolyn J. Brenner, MD; Whitney Carlson, MD; Lydia Chwastiak, MD, MPH; Heidi Combs, MD, MS; Carmen Croicu, MD; Shaune DeMers, MD; Kyl Dinsio, MD; Amelia N. Dubovsky, MD; Mark H. Duncan, MD; Brynne Hunter; Margaret L. Isaac, MD; Wayne Katon, MD; Meghan M. Kiefer, MD; Amanda Kost, MD; Yonah Korngold; Clarissa Calliope Kripke, MD, FAAFP; Sandy Lavery; Jesse Markman, MD, MBA; Jessica McCool; Jill McNair; Joseph O. Merrill, MD, MPH; Sirisha Narayana, MD; Christina Nicolaidis, MD, MPH; Justin Osborn, MD; Lindsay Parnell; Douglas S. Paauw, MD, MACP; Santha Priya; Jacqueline Raetz, MD; Dora Raymaker, MS; Scott A. Simpson, MD, MPH; Stanley I. Shyn, MD, PhD; Eliza L. Sutton, MD; L. Renata Thronson, MD; Christopher J. Wong, MD.

The planning committee, staff, authors and editors listed below have identified financial relationships or relationships to products or devices they or their spouse/life partner have with commercial interest related to the content of this CME activity:
Eric B. Larson, MD, MPH has royalties/patents with UpToDate, Inc.
Genevieve L. Pagalilauan, MD has an employment affiliation with Johns Hopkins Practical Reviews in Internal Medicine.

UNAPPROVED/OFF-LABEL USE DISCLOSURE
The EOCME requires CME faculty to disclose to the participants:
1. When products or procedures being discussed are off-label, unlabelled, experimental, and/or investigational (not US Food and Drug Administration (FDA) approved); and
2. Any limitations on the information presented, such as data that are preliminary or that represent ongoing research, interim analyses, and/or unsupported opinions. Faculty may discuss information about pharmaceutical agents that is outside of FDA-approved labelling. This information is intended solely for CME and is not intended to promote off-label use of these medications. If you have any questions, contact the medical affairs department of the manufacturer for the most recent prescribing information.

TO ENROLL
To enroll in the *Medical Clinics of North America* Continuing Medical Education program, call customer service at 1-800-654-2452 or sign up online at http://www.theclinics.com/home/cme. The CME program is available to subscribers for an additional annual fee of USD $267.

METHOD OF PARTICIPATION

In order to claim credit, participants must complete the following:

1. Complete enrolment as indicated above.
2. Read the activity.
3. Complete the CME Test and Evaluation. Participants must achieve a score of 70% on the test. All CME Tests and Evaluations must be completed online.

CME INQUIRIES/SPECIAL NEEDS

For all CME inquiries or special needs, please contact elsevierCME@elsevier.com.

MEDICAL CLINICS OF NORTH AMERICA

RELATED INTEREST

Psychiatric Clinics of North America, March 2013, (Vol 36, No. 1)
Complementary and Integrative Therapies for Psychiatric Disorders
Philip R. Muskin, Patricia L. Gerbarg, and Richard P. Brown, *Editors*
http://www.psych.theclinics.com/

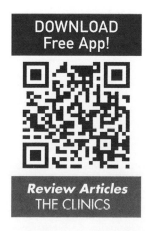

**DOWNLOAD
Free App!**

Review Articles
THE CLINICS

NOW AVAILABLE FOR YOUR iPhone and iPad

Contributors

CONSULTING EDITORS

DOUGLAS S. PAAUW, MD, MACP
Professor of Medicine, Division of General Internal Medicine, Rathmann Family Foundation Endowed Chair for Patient-Centered Clinical Education; Medicine Student Programs, Professor of Medicine, University of Washington School of Medicine, Seattle, Washington

EDWARD R. BOLLARD, MD, DDS, FACP
Professor of Medicine; Associate Dean for Graduate Medical Education; Designated Institutional Official (DIO), Penn State–Milton S. Hershey Medical Center, Hershey, Pennsylvania

EDITOR

GENEVIEVE L. PAGALILAUAN, MD, FACP
Associate Professor, Department of Medicine, Division of General Internal Medicine, Roosevelt General Internal Medicine Clinic, University of Washington Medical Center, Seattle, Washington

AUTHORS

SUSAN M. BENTLEY, DO
Assistant Professor, Department of Psychiatry and Behavioral Sciences, Harborview Medical Center, Seattle, Washington

CAROLYN J. BRENNER, MD
Assistant Professor, Department of Psychiatry and Behavioral Sciences, Harborview Medical Center, University of Washington, Seattle, Washington

WHITNEY CARLSON, MD
Clinical Assistant Professor, Division of Geriatric Psychiatry, Harborview Medical Center, University of Washington, Seattle, Washington

LYDIA CHWASTIAK, MD, MPH
Associate Professor, Department of Psychiatry and Behavioral Sciences, University of Washington School of Medicine, Seattle, Washington

HEIDI COMBS, MD, MS
Associate Professor, Department of Psychiatry and Behavioral Sciences, Harborview Medical Center, University of Washington, Seattle, Washington

CARMEN CROICU, MD
Assistant Professor, Department of Psychiatry and Behavioral Sciences, University of Washington School of Medicine, Seattle, Washington

SHAUNE DeMERS, MD
Assistant Professor, Division of Geriatric Psychiatry, Harborview Medical Center, University of Washington, Seattle, Washington

KYL DINSIO, MD
Acting Assistant Professor, Division of Geriatric Psychiatry, Harborview Medical Center, University of Washington, Seattle, Washington

AMELIA N. DUBOVSKY, MD
Department of Psychiatry and Behavioral Sciences, Harborview Medical Center, University of Washington School of Medicine, Seattle, Washington

MARK H. DUNCAN, MD
Acting Assistant Professor, Department of Psychiatry and Behavioral Sciences, University of Washington, Seattle, Washington

MARGARET L. ISAAC, MD
Assistant Professor, Medicine; Attending Physician, Harborview Medical Center, University of Washington School of Medicine, Seattle, Washington

WAYNE KATON, MD
Professor; Vice-Chair; Director of Division of Health Services and Psychiatric Epidemiology, Department of Psychiatry and Behavioral Sciences, University of Washington School of Medicine, Seattle, Washington

MEGHAN M. KIEFER, MD
Acting Instructor, Division of General Internal Medicine, University of Washington General Internal Medicine Center, University of Washington School of Medicine, Seattle, Washington

AMANDA KOST, MD
Assistant Professor, Department of Family Medicine, University of Washington, Seattle, Washington

CLARISSA CALLIOPE KRIPKE, MD, FAAFP
Health Sciences Clinical Professor; Director of Developmental Primary Care, Family and Community Medicine, University of California, San Francisco, San Francisco, California

ERIC B. LARSON, MD, MPH
Clinical Professor, Medicine; Vice President for Research and Executive Director, Group Health Research Institute, University of Washington School of Medicine, Seattle, Washington

JESSE MARKMAN, MD, MBA
Acting Assistant Professor, Department of Psychiatry and Behavioral Sciences, Harborview Medical Center, University of Washington, Seattle, Washington

JOSEPH O. MERRILL, MD, MPH
Associate Professor, Department of Medicine, Harborview Medical Center, University of Washington School of Medicine, Seattle, Washington

SIRISHA NARAYANA, MD
Acting Instructor, Division of General Internal Medicine, Department of Medicine, VA Puget Sound Health Care System, University of Washington, Seattle, Washington

CHRISTINA NICOLAIDIS, MD, MPH
Professor, Regional Research Institute, School of Social Work, Portland State University; Associate Professor, Departments of Medicine and Public Health & Preventive Medicine, Oregon Health and Science University; Co-Director, Academic Autism Spectrum Partnership in Research and Education, Portland, Oregon

JUSTIN OSBORN, MD
Assistant Professor, Department of Family Medicine, University of Washington, Seattle, Washington

GENEVIEVE L. PAGALILAUAN, MD, FACP
Associate Professor, Department of Medicine, Division of General Internal Medicine, Roosevelt General Internal Medicine Clinic, University of Washington Medical Center, Seattle, Washington

JACQUELINE RAETZ, MD
Assistant Professor, Department of Family Medicine, University of Washington, Seattle, Washington

DORA RAYMAKER, MS
Co-Director, Academic Autism Spectrum Partnership in Research and Education; Research Associate, Regional Research Institute, School of Social Work, Portland State University, Portland, Oregon

STANLEY I. SHYN, MD, PhD
Acting Assistant Professor, Department of Psychiatry and Behavioral Sciences, Harborview Medical Center, University of Washington, Seattle, Washington

SCOTT A. SIMPSON, MD, MPH
Psychosomatic Medicine Fellow, Department of Psychiatry and Behavioral Sciences, Harborview Medical Center, Seattle, Washington

ELIZA L. SUTTON, MD
Associate Professor, Department of Medicine, University of Washington, Seattle, Washington

L. RENATA THRONSON, MD
Clinical Instructor, Division of General Internal Medicine, Department of Medicine; Adult Medicine Clinic, Harborview Medical Center, Snake River College Faculty, University of Washington School of Medicine, Seattle, Washington

CHRISTOPHER J. WONG, MD
Assistant Professor, Division of General Internal Medicine, Department of Medicine, University of Washington, Seattle, Washington

Contents

xii   Contents

number of somatic symptoms and the persistence of symptoms are associated with co-occurring depression or anxiety disorders. It can be challenging to simultaneously address possible medical causes for physical symptoms while also considering an associated psychiatric diagnosis. In this article, strategies to improve the care and outcomes among these patients are described, including collaboration, education about the interaction between psychosocial stressors and somatic symptoms, regularly scheduled visits, focus on improving functional status, and evidence-based treatment of depression and anxiety.

Substance use disorders are common in primary care settings, but detection, assessment, and management are seldom undertaken. Substantial evidence supports that alcohol screening and brief intervention for risky drinking and pharmacotherapy are effective for alcohol use disorders. Substance use disorders can complicate the management of chronic non cancer pain, making routine monitoring and assessment for substance use disorders an important aspect of long-term opioid prescribing. Patients with opioid use disorders can be effectively treated with methadone in opioid treatment programs or with buprenorphine in the primary care setting.

Sleep issues are common in people with psychiatric disorders, and the interaction is complex. Sleep disorders, particularly insomnia, can precede and predispose to psychiatric disorders, can be comorbid with and exacerbate psychiatric disorders, and can occur as part of psychiatric disorders. Sleep disorders can mimic psychiatric disorders or result from medication given for psychiatric disorders. Impairment of sleep and of mental health may be different manifestations of the same underlying neurobiological processes. For the primary care physician, key tools include recognition of potential sleep effects of psychiatric medications and familiarity with treatment approaches for insomnia in depression and anxiety.

As the population ages, primary care providers will be frequently called on to manage psychiatric disorders suffered by their older patients. This overview of delirium, dementia, depression, and alcohol and substance misuse highlights the common presentations and suggests initial approaches to treatment. The challenges facing caregivers are also discussed.

Autism spectrum disorder (ASD) is defined by differences in social communication and restricted, repetitive patterns of behavior, interests, or activities. Skills and challenges can change depending on environmental stimuli, supports, and stressors. Quality of life can be improved by the use of accommodations, assistive technologies, therapies to improve adaptive function or communication, caregiver training, acceptance, access, and inclusion. This article focuses on the identification of ASD in adults, referrals for services, the recognition of associated conditions, strategies and accommodations to facilitate effective primary care services, and ethical issues related to caring for autistic adults.

Margaret L. Isaac and Eric B. Larson

Medical disease sometimes affects patients through neuropsychiatric manifestations. When neuropsychiatric symptoms are predominant, identifying medical disease early in the illness course is imperative because many of these conditions are reversible with appropriate treatment. A high index of suspicion is required on the part of clinicians, particularly when patients also present with physical signs or unexplained symptoms that might suggest a broader, systemic process. The processes that most commonly cause neuropsychiatric symptoms include infectious, autoimmune, endocrinologic, metabolic, and neoplastic diseases. This article focuses on the most common of these conditions, and conditions for which early diagnosis and treatment are particularly important.

Foreword

Psychiatric Diagnosis and Management in Primary Care

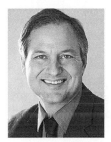

Douglas S. Paauw, MD, MACP
Consulting Editor

Mental illness is extremely common in the United States, with about 25% of the US population suffering from a diagnosable mental illness annually. Primary care physicians provide the majority of care for patients with mental illness in the Unites States and make the majority of psychiatric diagnoses. This issue of *Medical Clinics of North America* covers this important topic. Dr Pagalilauan has put together an issue that covers the common and challenging mental illness problems seen in primary care. Also included are articles on the ubiquitous problems of sleep disorders and addiction. I know that you will find this issue extremely valuable and informative.

Douglas S. Paauw, MD, MACP
Division of General Internal Medicine
Department of Medicine
University of Washington School of Medicine
Seattle, WA 98195, USA

E-mail address:
DPaauw@medicine.washington.edu

Med Clin N Am 98 (2014) xv
http://dx.doi.org/10.1016/j.mcna.2014.07.002
0025-7125/14/$ – see front matter © 2014 Published by Elsevier Inc.

medical.theclinics.com

Preface

Psychiatric Diagnosis and Management in Primary Care

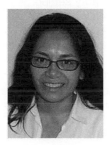

Genevieve L. Pagalilauan, MD, FACP
Editor

This issue focuses on common psychiatric issues encountered in the primary care setting. Increasingly, patients are seeking care for psychiatric disorders from ambulatory primary care providers.[1] In turn, there has been a marked increase in the number of prescriptions for antidepressants, anxiolytics, and antipsychotic medications by nonpsychiatrist primary care providers.[2] However, based on a survey of accredited family medicine, internal medicine, obstetrics, and pediatric residency directors, the majority of program directors are dissatisfied with the psychiatric training in their programs (64% in family practice and 31% in non-family practice programs).[3]

Primary care providers need to be facile with not only basic but also more complex presentations of common mood disorders. This issue reviews depression, anxiety, and bipolar disorders, but also the more subtle gradations of grief reaction, dysthymia, and seasonal affective disorder. The first step in the process of excellent care is understanding the screening and diagnostic options, including testing accuracy and limitations. The article on screening primary care patients for psychiatric conditions emphasizes the crossover in symptoms and signs among common conditions like depression, dysthymia, anxiety, bipolar, and PTSD. Fortunately, there are validated, time-efficient tools for accurately screening for the most commonly encountered psychiatric conditions in primary care.

The advent of DSM-5 (Diagnostic and Statistical Manual of Mental Disorders–5) has changed the diagnostic criteria for many psychiatric conditions. The most notable changes are for autism. DSM-5 unifies under the condition of autism spectrum disorders four different conditions that were separate in DSM-IV (autistic disorder, Asperger disorder, childhood disintegrative disorder, and pervasive developmental disorder not otherwise specified). The very thoughtful article on the care of primary care patients on the autism spectrum incorporates an evidence-based, expert-based,

Med Clin N Am 98 (2014) xvii–xix
http://dx.doi.org/10.1016/j.mcna.2014.07.001
0025-7125/14/$ – see front matter © 2014 Published by Elsevier Inc.

medical.theclinics.com

and patient-centered approach to help primary care providers recognize adults that may have gone previously undiagnosed and care for those patients who carry the diagnosis from childhood and transition into adult care. This review article is rich with practical advice on this heterogeneous condition, including recommendations for communication with patients and their families, connection to services and resources, identification of associated conditions, and practical management recommendations for common presenting concerns in the ambulatory setting.

While many primary care providers are increasingly comfortable with caring for patients with psychiatric conditions, some conditions remain an area of significant angst for providers. This angst is often driven by a lack of understanding of the condition, inadequate training in the identification and management of these conditions, and subsequently, a feeling of failure and lack of efficacy in caring for patients with these troubles. Hence, this compendium of review articles includes thoughtful reviews on the approach to caring for patients with borderline personality disorder, somatoform disorders, and addiction disorders.

This compendium of reviews also highlights issues in the care of geriatric populations, insomnia, pharmacotherapy, and psychiatric manifestations of medical conditions. The growing geriatric population requires primary care doctors to consider unique presentations of common psychiatric conditions, comorbid memory disorders, and behavioral manifestations, as well as vulnerabilities and harms to medication management. It is estimated that up to 50 to 70 million Americans suffer from insomnia. The insomnia review article highlights the complex relationship between insomnia and other primary psychiatric conditions and reviews both pharmacologic and nonpharmacologic approaches to care. The psychopharmacology review addresses common questions about dosing, indication, side effects, toxicity, and medication interactions related to psychotropic medications. The intriguing review on psychiatric manifestations of medical conditions reminds providers to broaden the differential and consider other medical systemic illness as possible explanations for apparent psychiatric symptoms. Other possible explanations include infectious, endocrine, autoimmune, metabolic, and neoplastic conditions.

Caring for patients with psychiatric conditions is part of our charge as primary care providers. Many of us received inadequate training in this area, and yet we are responsible for the empathic, ethical, and efficacious treatment of these conditions for our patients. Much has changed in the evidence for and against approaches we may have learned in our "in-the-trenches" training on these conditions. Updating and refining our knowledge base and skills in this area is imperative for the excellent care of our patients who suffer from morbidity and mortality that is as devastating yet as treatable as other conditions that we encounter in our primary care practices.

Genevieve L. Pagalilauan, MD, FACP
Department of Medicine
Division of General Internal Medicine
Roosevelt General Internal Medicine Clinic
University of Washington Medical Center
4245 Roosevelt Way NE
Seattle, WA 98105, USA

E-mail address:
jadepag@uw.edu

REFERENCES

1. Olfson M, Kroenke K, Wang S, et al. Trends in office-based mental health care provided by psychiatrists and primary care physicians. J Clin Psychiatry 2014;75(3): 247–53.
2. Olfson M, Blanco C, Wang S, et al. National trends in the mental health care of children, adolescents, and adults by office-based physicians. JAMA Psychiatry 2014; 71(1):81–90.
3. Leigh H, Stewart D, Mallios R. Mental health and psychiatry training in primary care residency programs. Part II. What skills and diagnoses are taught, how adequate, and what affects training directors' satisfaction? Gen Hosp Psychiatry 2006;28(3): 195–204.

Erratum

Please note that in Hong E, Kraft MC. Evaluating Anterior Knee Pain. *Med Clin North Am.* 2014;98(4):697-717, author Eugene Hong's name was misspelled on the article's title page. The corrected listing is Eugene Hong, MD, CAQSM, FAAFP.

medical.theclinics.com

Psychopharmacology

L. Renata Thronson, MD[a],*, Genevieve L. Pagalilauan, MD[b]

KEYWORDS

- Psychopharmacology • Antidepressant • Mood stabilizer • Antipsychotic
- Primary care • Depression • Anxiety • Bipolar

KEY POINTS

- Primary care providers (PCPs) are prescribing more psychotropic medications.
- Medication side effects are a major barrier to adherence and successful treatment. When PCPs understand both class and individual drug effects, they can better tailor medication recommendations for individual patients.
- Psychotropic medications have significant medication interactions with commonly prescribed medications, such as antibiotics, antihypertensives, and other psychotropic medications.

INTRODUCTION

The use of medications to treat psychiatric conditions is a mainstay of treatment in primary care practices. This article reviews the major classes of antidepressants, anxiolytics, mood stabilizers, and antipsychotic agents and focuses mainly on issues pertinent to the adult ambulatory population.

GENERAL APPROACH TO TREATMENT

- Pharmacotherapy (with or without psychotherapy) is effective for a range of psychiatric conditions and, in general, confers a moderate treatment effect size.
- Nonpsychiatrists are increasingly responsible for the initiation and management of pharmacotherapy in the ambulatory setting.
- Primary care providers (PCPs) must familiarize themselves with the indications, risks, and benefits of medications used to treat common mental health conditions.

Funding Sources: None.
Conflict of Interest: None (L.R. Thronson); reviewer Johns Hopkins *Practical Reviews in Internal Medicine* (G.L. Pagalilauan).
[a] Division of General Internal Medicine, Department of Medicine, Adult Medicine Clinic, Harborview Medical Center, University of Washington School of Medicine, 325 9th Avenue, Seattle, WA 98104, USA; [b] Department of Medicine, Division of General Internal Medicine, Roosevelt General Internal Medicine Clinic, University of Washington Medical Center, 4245 Roosevelt Way North East, Seattle, WA 98105
* Corresponding author.
E-mail address: lrenata@uw.edu

Psychiatric conditions that cause functional impairment or reduction in quality of life can be approached by several modalities. Nonpharmacologic treatment is conventionally used as monotherapy for less severe manifestations of psychiatric disease and is combined with pharmacotherapy to treat more severe disease. Nonpharmacologic therapy includes behavioral interventions; self-care, such as exercise and dietary interventions; and, importantly, psychotherapy in its many forms. Pharmacotherapy is typically reserved for moderate to severe manifestations of psychiatric disease.[1] In practice, many clinicians use pharmacotherapy monotherapy because access to psychotherapy and other supported nonpharmacologic approaches may not be readily available.

The efficacy of psychotherapy and pharmacotherapy for various psychiatric conditions has been questioned and continues to be a source of controversy. A 2014 large and well-done meta-analysis found that for most psychiatric conditions, pharmacotherapy and psychotherapy had a moderate beneficial effect size (0.5 confidence interval, 0.41–0.59) in comparison with placebo.[2] The study's analysis of head-to-head trials showed psychotherapy and pharmacotherapy were similar in efficacy across conditions, though pharmacotherapy was a superior treatment of dysthymia and schizophrenia, and psychotherapy was superior for the treatment of bulimia and major depression relapse. The meta-analysis supported the use of combination therapy, showing an improved efficacy of treatment with a combination of psychotherapy and pharmacotherapy (vs either alone) for most psychiatric conditions with the exceptions of schizophrenia and posttraumatic stress disorder (PTSD).

Increasingly, PCPs are responsible for initiation and titration of pharmacotherapy. A 2014 study that looked at trends in US mental health care between 1995 and 2010 found that nonpsychiatrist providers diagnosed mental health disorders and prescribed psychotropic medications more commonly than psychiatrists for children (72% nonpsychiatrist), adolescents (52%), and adults (64%).[3] The study, based on the National Ambulatory Medical Care Survey, found the prevalence of mental health–related visits was higher for adults than children, and the number of visits for psychotropic medication management increased equally for those older and younger than 21 years. However, the study found a near doubling of the diagnosis of mental health disorders and referrals to psychiatrists in people younger than 21 years, whereas those older than 21 years had minimal increases. Largely, the increased diagnosis and pharmacologic management of attention-deficit/hyperactivity disorder and other behavioral disorders in children and adolescents drove the trend. Similar trends have been seen in Canadian and European populations (**Box 1**).

Before initiating pharmacotherapy, providers should make a concerted effort to determine the accurate psychiatric diagnosis and exclude common mimics of psychiatric disease that may present with similar symptoms. Failure to identify bipolar depression as the cause of depressive symptoms can lead to inadvertent triggering of a manic event with the initiation of an antidepressant instead of a mood stabilizer.[4,5] Failure to recognize Lewy body dementia as the cause of visual hallucinations can lead to empirical treatment with a neuroleptic agent, resulting in confusion, worsening movement disorder, autonomic dysfunction, and an increased risk for mortality.[6]

Disease-Specific Considerations

Antidepressants

PCPs who manage mood disorders should have a working understanding of 2 to 3 antidepressants per class. Side effects are the number one reason for discontinuation of anxiety and depression medications.[1] Hence, providers must be aware of common

---

Box 1
Approach to psychopharmacologic medication selection

- Consider patients' experience with specific psychotropic medications or classes of medications (side effects/efficacy).

- Understand and review with patients the risk for common or severe side effects.

   o Try to harness a side effect in a positive way (example: using sertraline, which commonly causes looser stools, in a patient with chronic constipation).

   o Identify the unacceptable side effects and make them a top priority over other considerations.

- Consider the costs.

- Look for and discuss medication interactions.

- Be aware of the variable efficacy of medications for population subsets.

- Solicit patients' preferences and concerns.

Data from Qaseem A. Using second-generation antidepressants to treat depressive disorders: a clinical practice guideline from the American College of Physicians. Ann Int Med 2008;149(10):725–33.

---

medication side effects and engage patients in shared decision making when selecting a medication. Side effects typically occur within the first 2 weeks of medication initiation and with dose increases. Helping patients understand the temporal lag between the onset of side effects (within days) and efficacy (often 3–6 weeks or more) is also important for adherence.[1,7] Equally important is the risk for medication interactions.[8] Psychotropic medications are potential cytochrome P450 inhibitors and activators; hence, a full medication interaction review should be conducted before initiating these medications.

Antianxiety medications

Most antidepressants are effective anxiolytic medications, except bupropion, which commonly exacerbates anxiety when used alone for treatment. Guidelines recommend antidepressants as the first-line therapy for anxiety disorders.[9,10] Selective serotonin reuptake inhibitors (SSRIs) and serotonin-norepinephrine reuptake inhibitors (SNRIs) effectively prevent anxiety symptoms, reduce the risk for relapse, and have a better safety profile in comparison with benzodiazepines, which confer no long-term preventive benefit.[11] However, benzodiazepines remain an important option in the clinical toolbox for treating acute anxiety and panic disorder; a 2014 systematic review calls into question why benzodiazepines are not used as the first-line therapy for some.[12] The risks for habituation, withdrawal, and the contraindication of use of benzodiazepine use in people with addiction disorders are important considerations to discuss with patients during shared decision making.

Mood stabilizers

Mood stabilizer are less commonly initiated or managed by PCPs. However, because most mood stabilizers are antiseizure medications, PCPs have a level of familiarity and comfort with them. Because of the narrow therapeutic index and risk for drug interactions and adverse events with mood stabilizer use, the biggest pharmacotherapy responsibility for most PCPs is the monitoring and management of mood disorder medications to avoid harms and ensure ongoing efficacy.[13,14]

Antipsychotics

Antipsychotic medications are used broadly to treat delirium by nonpsychiatrists in the inpatient setting. However, ambulatory providers have less call to initiate antipsychotic agents. In the ambulatory setting, antipsychotics are used more often as an adjunct in treatment-resistant depression or in an off-label fashion to treat neuropsychiatric symptoms (hallucinations, agitation, and other unwanted behaviors) in dementia than for the primary treatment of psychosis in schizophrenic individuals or mania in people with bipolar. Ironically, antipsychotic agents confer a greater danger with the off-label use in geriatric populations; a 2013 Cochrane review addressed several concerns.[15] The review emphasized the lack of evidence for efficacy especially beyond short-term use and highlighted that the use of antipsychotic medications in this population is associated with excess mortality and an absolute risk for death of 1%. The US Food and Drug Administration (FDA) has issued a black box warning against the use of typical (2008) and atypical antipsychotics (2005) for dementia-related psychosis.[16] However, a risk for increased mortality is not seen with the use of these medications in patients who are schizophrenic and bipolar.

MOOD DISORDER MEDICATIONS

Case 1: A 27-year-old woman presents to the clinic with depression, anhedonia, and insomnia of 3 weeks duration. She has a no features of mania, a normal thyroid-stimulating hormone (TSH), and no substance use. Her Patient Health Questionnaire-9 score is 18 out of 27, which is consistent with moderate/severe depression. She is interested in starting a medication but is concerned about the sexual side effects and the risk for worsening insomnia. Which of the following medications do you recommend?

1. Sertraline
2. Bupropion
3. Mirtazapine
4. Paroxetine
5. Venlafaxine
   (Answer 3)

Discussion

All the presented antidepressants are theoretically efficacious for her depression. The clinician should tailor the choice of medications to reduce the risk of unwanted side effects and possibly improve current symptoms. In this case, the patient has insomnia and wants no sexual side effects. Although both bupropion and mirtazapine are reasonable to avoid sexual side effects, bupropion is activating and may worsen her insomnia. Mirtazapine dosed at night should help with sleep and minimize sexual dysfunction. In practice, the most likely roadblock to using mirtazapine is the risk for weight gain and that should be discussed overtly before initiating the medication.

All classes of antidepressant medications are equally efficacious for first-time episodes of major depression and confer a 60% to 70% response rate.[7,17] Nonetheless, SSRIs are most widely used. The popularity of second-generation antidepressants like SSRIs, SNRIs, and novel antidepressants (bupropion and mirtazapine) is because of their perceived safety benefit and lower side-effect risk in contrast to first-generation antidepressants, such as tricyclic antidepressants (TCAs) and monoamine oxidase inhibitors (MAOIs).[18] A British study showed TCAs to have the highest case fatality rate in the setting of medication overdose (13.8), followed by venlafaxine (2.5), mirtazapine (1.9), and then SSRIs (0.5). Citalopram carried the highest risk among SSRIs with a case fatality rate of 1.1 in overdose situations (**Table 1**).[19]

SSRIs

SSRIs increase serotonin levels in the synapses almost immediately, but a therapeutic response takes weeks to months to achieve. Some postulate this is because of downstream effects of the increased serotonin levels.[20] Because SSRIs bind selectively to serotonin receptors, side effects mediated by histamine, dopamine, and acetylcholine receptor blockage are avoided. However, the side-effect frequency within the class varies considerably. Common SSRI side effects include nausea, diarrhea, sleep disturbance, dizziness, sexual dysfunction, headache, dizziness, and weight changes (**Table 2**).[7]

More serious complications of SSRIs have recently come to light. SSRIs (and SNRIs) have been associated with an increased risk of falls and fractures.[21,22] The most problematic time frame is during initiation and dose titration. Upper gastrointestinal (GI) bleeds are a serious risk when SSRIs are combined with nonsteroidal antiinflammatory drugs (NSAIDs). This risk is especially so in those on medications like corticosteroids that predispose to upper GI ulceration or bleeding, but that risk is mitigated by concurrent use of proton pump inhibitors.[23,24] SSRIs have long been thought to be a safe haven against arrhythmia compared with TCAs. However, the FDA released a black box warning for citalopram causing QT prolongation and increased risk for torsade de pointes in 2011; the FDA recommends that citalopram not be used in conditions that increase the risk for prolonged QT.[25] This risk may also apply to escitalopram, its racemic enantiomer, though data are lacking. Syndrome of inappropriate antidiuretic hormone secretion (SIADH) has been described with SSRI use leading to symptomatic hyponatremia in some.[7] The highest-risk patients for SIADH caused by SSRIs are elderly women on diuretics, and vigilance during the first 6 weeks of initiation is prudent (**Box 2**).[26]

Table 1	
Risk of fatality from mood disorder medication overdose	
Medication	**Relative Toxicity Index**
TCAs	
Lowest risk: amitriptyline	1.0
Highest risk: doxepin	2.6
Average of 7 studied TCAs	1.6
SNRIs	
Venlafaxine	0.29
NaSSA	
Mirtazapine	0.22
SSRIs	
Lowest risk: fluvoxamine	0
Highest risk: citalopram	0.12
Average of 5 studied SSRIs	0.06

Abbreviation: NaSSA, noradernergic and specific serotonergic antidepressant.

Data from Hawton K, Bergen H, Simkin S, et al. Toxicity of antidepressants: rates of suicide relative to prescribing and non-fatal overdose. Br J Psychiatry 2010;196:354–8.

Table 2
Antidepressant side-effect frequency %

Drug	Diarrhea	Dizziness	Headache	Insomnia	Nausea
Bupropion	8.7	12.5	27.2	11–40	9–24
Citalopram	8	Up to 14	Up to 18	Up to 15	21
Duloxetine	7–13	6–17	NR	8–16	11
Escitalopram	6–14	4–7	24	7–14	15–18
Fluoxetine	12	2–11	16.6	9–26	20–30
Fluvoxamine	NR	NR	14.5	NR	22.2
Mirtazapine	8.8	12	12	8	↑ Appetite 17
Paroxetine	18	4–6	17–27	Up to 24	26
Sertraline	13–24	6–17	25	12–28	13–30
Venlafaxine	5.5	11–24	25–38	14–24	22–58

Abbreviation: NR, not reported.

Data from Hansen RA, Gartlehner G, Lohr KN, et al. Efficacy and safety of second-generation antidepressants in the treatment of major depressive disorder. Ann Intern Med 2005;143(6):415–26.

SSRIs are FDA approved for a broad range of psychiatric conditions, including major depression, generalized anxiety disorder (GAD), panic disorder (PD), obsessive-compulsive disorder, PTSD, premenstrual dysphoria disorder, social anxiety disorder, and bulimia nervosa.[27] Many SSRIs are used in an off-label fashion for conditions for which other SSRIs are FDA approved but also for conditions for which no SSRIs are approved. Off-label conditions include premature ejaculation, urinary incontinence, migraine prophylaxis, and fibromyalgia.[28] Notably, fluoxetine, paroxetine, and sertraline are approved for PD; escitalopram and paroxetine for GAD; and paroxetine and sertraline for PTSD (**Tables 3** and **4**).[27]

Medication interactions are important considerations when prescribing and monitoring antidepressants. Some antidepressants are metabolized by hepatic

Box 2
Antidepressants' side effects and harms

- Sexual dysfunction
  - Sertraline>venlafaxine>citalopram>paroxetine
  - No effect with bupropion, mirtazapine
- Weight gain
  - Highest with mirtazapine and paroxetine
- Upper GI bleed
- Falls
- Fracture
- Stroke
- Arrhythmia
- SIADH

Data from Gartlehner G, Gaynes BN, Hansen RA, et al. Comparative benefits and harms of second-generation antidepressants: background paper for the American College of Physicians. Ann Intern Med 2008;149(10):734–50; and Serretti A, Chiesa A. Treatment-emergent sexual dysfunction related to antidepressants: a meta-analysis. J Clin Psychopharmacol 2009;29(3):259–66.

Table 3
FDA-approved indications for second-generation antidepressant medications

Medication Name	FDA-Approved Indication
Bupropion	Depression
Bupropion SR	Depression
Bupropion ER	Depression Seasonal affect dis
Citalopram	Depression
Cymbalta	Depression GAD DPNP
Desvenlafaxine	Depression
Escitalopram	Depression GAD
Fluoxetine	Depression OCD PD Bulimia
Fluvoxamine	OCD
Fluvoxamine ER	OCD Social anxiety disorder
Maprotiline	Depression
Mirtazapine	Depression
Paroxetine	Depression OCD PD GAD Social anxiety disorder PTSD
Paroxetine CR	Depression PD Social anxiety disorder PMDD
Paroxetine mesylate	Depression OCD Panic GAD
Sertraline	Depression OCD Panic disorder Social anxiety disorder PMDD PTSD
Venlafaxine	Depression
Venlafaxine ER	Depression Panic disorder GAD Social anxiety disorder

Abbreviations: DPNP, diabetic peripheral neuropathic pain; OCD, obsessive compulsive disorder; PMDD, premenstrual dysphoric disorder; Seasonal affect dis, seasonal affective disorder.

Data from Illinois BBo. Antidepressant agents step therapy criteria with medical diagnoses option. Chicago (IL): Blue Cross and Blue Shield of Illinois; 2010.

Table 4
Dosing of second-generation antidepressants

Drug	Initiation Dose	Therapeutic Dose	Maximum Dose
Bupropion (ER)	100–150 mg qAM	150 mg BID	200 mg BID
Citalopram	20 mg qd	40 mg	40 mg
Desvenlafaxine	50 mg qd	50 mg qd	100 mg qd[a]
Duloxetine	20–30 mg qd	60 mg	120 mg qd (60 BID)
Escitalopram	10 mg qd	10–20 mg qd	20 mg qd
Fluoxetine	20 mg qd	40–60 mg qd	80 mg qd
Mirtazapine	15 mg qhs	30–45 mg	45 mg
Paroxetine	20 mg qd	20–50 mg qd	50 mg qd
Sertraline	50 mg qd	50–200 mg	200 mg
Venlafaxine (ER)	37.5–75.0 mg qd	75–225 mg qd	225 mg qd

[a] No additional efficacy.

Adapted from CMS Medicaid Integrity Program (MIP). Antidepressant medications: U.S. Food and Drug Administration-approved indications and dosages for use in adults. Available at: http://www.cms.gov/Medicare-Medicaid-Coordination/Fraud-Prevention/Medicaid-Integrity-Education/Pharmacy-Education-Materials/Downloads/ad-adult-dosingchart.pdf; Accessed July 21, 2014.

cytochrome P450 isoenzymes (citalopram and paroxetine), whereas others are important inhibitors (fluoxetine and paroxetine).[29] A significant manifestation of the risks of this inhibition is paroxetine's effect on tamoxifen via inhibition of cytochrome P450 2D6 (CYP2D6). Tamoxifen is a prodrug whose metabolites are responsible for beneficial effects against breast cancer recurrence. A retrospective study in Canada found women concurrently prescribed tamoxifen and paroxetine had a increased risk of breast cancer specific death, with a number needed to harm of only 7 if there was a 100% overlap between the medications.[30]

A cannot-miss medication interaction risk for SSRIs (and many other classes of psychotropic medications) is serotonin syndrome. Made famous by the case of Libby Zion, serotonin syndrome is characterized by the alarming symptom conglomeration of hyperthermia, altered mental status, and tremor or clonus. Serotonin syndrome manifestations can include diarrhea and vomiting as well as telltale physical examination findings of rigidity, hyperreflexia, and ocular clonus.[31] Failure to recognize this syndrome and stop the offending agents can lead to death. The risk for serotonin syndrome is theoretic for most standard dosing of a singular SSRI and another serotonergically mediated medication (SNRI, TCA, trazodone, mirtazapine, triptans, lithium, buspirone, antiemetics, drugs of abuse including ecstasy, and the opiates methadone, fentanyl, meperidine).[32] The most worrisome interactions occur with psychotropic medications, opiates, and linezolid (chemically a MAOI); this combination has been associated with severe cases of serotonin syndrome.[31] Importantly, the interaction can occur in medications that have been discontinued. Medications like fluoxetine and MAOIs can remain in the system for up to 6 weeks after discontinuation and have been described to be causative of serotonin syndrome in that setting.[31]

SNRIs

Like SSRIs, SNRIs prevent the reuptake of serotonin in the central nervous system (CNS) synapses but also increase the presence of norepinephrine. This mechanism is similar to the mechanism of action of TCAs but with less binding to other neurotransmitter receptors, such as acetylcholine and histamine; hence, SNRIs are thought to have a similar efficacy as TCAs but with fewer side effects. An additional benefit of

SNRIs is the modulation of pain; the selective norepinephrine reuptake inhibition is postulated to affect the descending inhibitory pathway that reduces pain perception.[33]

SNRIs are FDA approved for depression (venlafaxine, venlafaxine ER, desvenlafaxine, duloxetine), GAD (duloxetine, venlafaxine ER), PD (venlafaxine ER), and social anxiety disorder (venlafaxine ER).[27] Additionally, several SNRIs are FDA approved for pain modulation in conditions like neuropathic pain (duloxetine), fibromyalgia (duloxetine, milnacipran), and chronic musculoskeletal pain (duloxetine).[27] Non–FDA-approved conditions wherein SNRIs are used in an off-label fashion include migraine prophylaxis and treatment of hot flashes (see **Table 2** for indications and **Table 3** for SNRI dosing information).[30]

In general, SNRIs have very similar side effects as SSRIs, though they tend to have less sexual side effects.[7] However, the higher amounts of norepinephrine can elevate blood pressure; SNRIs should be used with caution in patients with hypertension, congestive heart failure, or a recent myocardial infarction. (See **Table 1** for a comparison of side effects among antidepressants and **Box 2** for additional information on SNRI side effects.)

Notably, SNRIs (especially venlafaxine) and the SSRI paroxetine are associated with a discontinuation syndrome.[17] Discontinuation syndrome is characterized by anxiety, irritability, dizziness, confusion, sweating, tremor, nausea, palpitations, and headache.[34] Hence, SNRIs and paroxetine should be slowly tapered before discontinuation to avoid these symptoms.

The risk for medication interactions is similar for SNRIs and SSRIs. Duloxetine and venlafaxine are metabolized by the liver (CYP1A2 and CYP2D6, respectively); duloxetine is a moderately potent inhibitor of CYP2D6, increasing its risk for causing toxic levels of other antidepressants, antipsychotics, and beta-blocker antihypertensives.[35] Providers should consider SNRIs and SSRIs similar in their risk for serotonin syndrome in combination with serotonergic medications and GI bleeding in combination with NSAIDs.

SNRIs are considered a first-line therapy for both anxiety and depression.[7] A 2013 meta-analysis of 22 meta-analyses found some evidence that SNRIs, particularly venlafaxine and to a lesser degree duloxetine, have higher response and remission rates in comparison with SSRIs, especially in patients with more severe depression.[36] Clinicians should consider the unique benefits of SNRIs on pain modulation as well as the unique side-effects profile when tailoring medication selection for specific patients.

Unique Mechanism Antidepressants

Bupropion and mirtazapine are 2 unique mechanism antidepressants that should be familiar to all clinicians who treat mood disorders. Both are FDA approved for the treatment of depression, and bupropion ER has additional indications for the treatment of seasonal affective disorder and smoking cessation (see **Table 2**).[27]

The mechanism of action for bupropion is not fully known. It is thought to work via presynaptic dopamine and norepinephrine reuptake transporters; it is a weak reuptake inhibitor of noradrenaline, serotonin, and dopamine.[17] In addition to its use in major depression and seasonal affective disorder, bupropion is prescribed in an off-label fashion as an augmentation agent for treatment-resistant depression.[18] Notably, bupropion has a strong noradrenergic effect and has very little serotonergic effects. Clinicians should warn patients about the activating side effects cause by the unopposed noradrenergic action, including insomnia, tremor, anorexia, palpitations, diaphoresis, and agitation. Importantly, bupropion is thought to lower the seizure threshold and should not be used in patients with a history of seizure.[18] However, because bupropion minimally affects serotonin receptors, it avoids problematic sexual side effects caused by SSRIs and SNRIs. Unlike most antidepressants that, regardless of FDA labeling, are successfully used in both anxiety and depression, bupropion should not be used as a solo agent for anxiety.

Mirtazapine has a unique mechanism of antagonizing presynaptic alpha 2 adrenergic receptors and effectively increasing serotonin neurotransmission.[34] It also blocks histamine receptors at lower doses, and astute clinicians prescribe it for use at night to address insomnia.[34] The same histamine receptor blockade can stimulate weight gain, an unwanted side effect for most patients; but again, the savvy provider will use mirtazapine in lower-weight patients or those who experience anorexia with their mood disorder. Because mirtazapine selectively blocks the 2C serotonin receptor, it uniquely avoids sexual dysfunction side effects common in both SSRIs and SNRIs and should be considered an alternative agent when those symptoms arise.[34]

Bupropion deserves special mention when considering medication interactions. It is a potent cytochrome P450 2D6 inhibitor. Hence, it is like duloxetine but more problematic in its risk for causing toxic levels of the beta-blockers, antidepressants, and antipsychotics that are metabolized through that specific cytochrome.[35] Several other medications are also metabolized through CYP2D6, and clinicians should check for medication interactions any time there are changes to the medication list of patients treated with bupropion.

TCAs

TCAs, like SSRIs and SNRIs, inhibit the reuptake of serotonin and norepinephrine; but they also inhibit histamine, muscarinic, and alpha-1 adrenergic receptors.[34] Clinicians should think about TCA side effects as similar to SSRIs and SNRIs but with the addition of antihistamine and anticholinergic symptoms. As a result, they can be more difficult to tolerate because of drowsiness and weight gain mediated by histamine blockade, constipation, dry eye, dry mouth, urinary retention, tachycardia caused by the anticholinergic effects, and orthostatic hypotension and dizziness brought on by alpha-1 receptor blockade.[34]

Most guidelines consider TCAs a second-line therapy for major depression despite similar efficacy as SSRIs and SNRIs because of the high side-effect burden and concern for the higher risk of fatality in overdose situations with TCAs caused by fatal arrhythmia.[19] TCAs have a quinidinelike effect, and an electrocardiogram should be checked if TCAs are used in patients with cardiac disease to assess for QRS prolongation and the risk for ventricular tachycardia.[37] Nonetheless, guidelines are more supportive of the use of TCAs, namely, imipramine for GAD and as a second-line agent for PD.[27] Clomipramine is endorsed as a first-line agent in 3 guidelines and as a second-line agent in 2 guidelines for obsessive-compulsive disorder (OCD).[27] TCAs are also used in an off-label fashion as an adjunct for treatment-resistant depression, neuropathic pain control, insomnia, enuresis, and headache prophylaxis.

TCAs, like all the major categories of antidepressants, are metabolized through the liver. Clomipramine and doxepin are at risk for inhibiting CYP2D6, increasing their risk for increasing the toxicity of many antidepressants and antipsychotic agents metabolized through that cytochrome. The most practical consideration for most providers is the risk for TCA toxicity in combination with most SSRIs or SNRIs. Doses greater than 30 mg of a TCA in combination with an SSRI or SNRI can rapidly cause TCA toxicity, and TCA levels should be check when combining more than 30 mg (**Table 5**).

MAOIs

Briefly, MAOIs have limited application in the primary care setting. Mechanistically, they are like TCAs increasing the effects of serotonin, norepinephrine, and dopamine, with the addition of tyramine. However, many MAOIs act by irreversibly inhibiting the

Table 5
TCA dosing

Drug	Indication	Starting Dose (mg)	Therapeutic Dose (mg)
Amitriptyline	Depression	25–75	50–150
	Neuropathic pain*	25	25–100
	Postherpetic neuralgia*	25	75–150
Amoxapine	Depression	25–50	200–300
Clomipramine	OCD	25	150–250
Desipramine	Depression	25–75	100–200
Doxepin	Depression	25–75	150–300
	Anxiety	25–75	150–300
	Insomnia*	10	10–50
Imipramine	Depression	25–75	150–300
	Chronic pain*	0.2–0.4 mg/kg	100–300
Nortriptyline	Depression	25–50	50–150
Protriptyline	Depression	5–10 TID	5–10 TID–QID
Trimipramine	Depression	75	50–150

* indicates off-label use.
Adapted from CMS Medicaid Integrity Program (MIP). Antidepressant medications: U.S. Food and Drug Administration-approved indications and dosages for use in adults. Available at: http://www.cms.gov/Medicare-Medicaid-Coordination/Fraud-Prevention/Medicaid-Integrity-Education/Pharmacy-Education-Materials/Downloads/ad-adult-dosingchart.pdf; Accessed July 21, 2014.

enzyme monoamine oxidase.[38] It takes weeks for the body to make more enzymes, so the physiologic affects of the MAOI last much longer than other antidepressants after discontinuation.[38] The side effects are similar to TCAs and can be difficult to tolerate. Like TCAs, MAOI overdose can be fatal because of arrhythmias. They are hepatically metabolized, so the same cautions for interactions as with other antidepressant medications hold true. The broader concern is for serotonin syndrome in combination with other antidepressants and medications that increase serotonin.[31] Furthermore, patients must be wary of foods that increase tyramine, as there have been reports of hypertensive crisis-like events (sudden pulsatile headache, hypertension, palpitations, nausea) associated with certain foods (aged cheeses and meats, beer, soy products, sauerkraut, and fava beans; older diets were likely overly strict) while taking MAOIs.[38] The role of PCPs is to be aware that MAOIs may still be used in rare patients and to know the implications for medication and dietary management.

Benzodiazepines

Benzodiazepines work through the gamma-amino-butyric (GABA) receptor. The GABA receptor modulation is thought to inhibit reuptake of neurotransmitters, like serotonin, norepinephrine, and dopamine.[39] Benzodiazepines are helpful for short-term treatment of anxiety, as they help to abort anxiety symptoms quickly.[10] However, they do not prevent anxiety and yet confer a risk for dependence. Furthermore, benzodiazepines are not effective for depressive symptoms and have not been shown to be effective for people with anxiety plus comorbid depression or OCD.[10] Hence, guidelines recommend benzodiazepines should be considered a second-line therapy for anxiety disorders. There is a paucity of studies that directly compare benzodiazepines against antidepressants for anxiety.[12]

Typical side effects include sedation, memory or cognitive impairment, and psychomotor impairment.[11] PCPs should be aware that there are important differences among benzodiazepines based on their rapidity of onset and duration of action. In order to reduce the risk for habituation, benzodiazepines should be prescribed at the lowest effective dose for the shortest duration possible.[40]

Benzodiazepines are sedative hypnotics and should not be used in conjunction with other sedatives, including sleep medication, narcotics, and alcohol. Abrupt discontinuation of benzodiazepines after higher dose, longer duration use can cause a withdrawal, and in rare instances seizure and even death.[39]

Benzodiazepines are metabolized via cytochrome P450 3A4/5/7 and have significant medication interactions. St John's Wort decreases benzodiazepine blood levels and macrolides (except azithromycin), protease inhibitors, azole antifungals, as well as diltiazem and verapamil, which increase blood levels.[35]

MOOD STABILIZER MEDICATIONS

Several classes of medications are used successfully as mood stabilizers to treat bipolar affective disorder. These medications include lithium and anticonvulsant and antipsychotic medications. Severely ill patients may be initiated on combination therapy with lithium or valproate plus an atypical antipsychotic.[41]

Lithium

Lithium is indicated for both induction therapy in acute mania and for maintenance therapy in bipolar disorder.[41] It is shown to reduce suicidality, self-harm, and all-cause mortality in patients with mood disorders.[42]

Lithium is typically dosed 2 to 3 times per day at a lower dose and titrated to an optimal therapeutic level as noted in **Table 6**.[43] In geriatric populations, the starting dosage is 150 mg twice daily, and total doses should not exceed 900 mg daily. The optimal serum levels in both younger adults and geriatric patients are 0.6 to 1.2 mEq/L.[44]

Lithium has both acute and long-term side effects relating to multiple organ systems (**Table 7**). In the short-term, GI and neurologic side effects (nausea, weight gain, and a

Table 6				
Mood stabilizer dosing and monitoring				
Medication	Initial	Dose Titration	Therapeutic Total Daily Dose	Monitoring
Lithium	300 mg BID or TID	↑ By 300–600 mg every 2–3 d (acute mania) or every 7 d	900–1800 mg	0.6–1.2 mEq/L Check 5–7 d after reaching therapeutic dose
Valproate	250 mg BID or TID	↑ By 250–500 mg every 1–3 d	1500–2500 mg	50–125 mcg/mL Check 2–5 d after dose change and every 6–12 mo
Carbamazepine	100–200 mg qd–BID	↑ By 200 mg every 1–4 d	800–1000 mg	4–12 mcg/dL
Lamotrigine	25 mg qd × 2 wk	↑ To 25 mg 2 × per d for 2 wk, then by 25–50 mg qwk	200–400 mg	No blood level monitoring

Data from Refs.[51,55,56,113,114]

Table 7
Nonantipsychotic mood stabilizer side effects and monitoring

Medication	Acute	Chronic	Monitoring

Lithium	GI
	  Nausea
	  Weight gain
	Neuro
	  Cognitive slowing
		Neuro
		• Tremor
		Renal
		• ↓ Ability to concentrate urine → polyuria, polydipsia
		• Nephrogenic diabetes insipidus uncommon
		• Rare renal failure
		Endocrine
		• Hypothyroidism
		• Goiter
		• Autoimmune thyroiditis
		• ↑ Parathyroid hormone levels → hypercalcemia
		Cardiac
		• ECG repolarization changes
		• Rare arrhythmia
			Baseline
			• Renal, thyroid function, calcium, parathyroid hormone, pregnancy test, ECG
			Periodic
			• Renal and thyroid function every 3 mo for 6 mo then every 6–12 mo
			• Cr >1.6 should be comanaged with nephrologist
			• Lithium levels

Valproate		Neuro • Tremor • Sedation GI • Nausea • Diarrhea • Weight gain • Mild LFT abnormalities • Rare hepatic failure • Rare pancreatitis Heme • Rare thrombocytopenia	Baseline • CBC 2 × per month × 2 mo • LFTs 2 × per month × 2 mo Periodic • CBC and LFTs 1–2 times per year • Valproate levels
Carbamazepine	Derm • Rarely Stevens-Johnson syndrome • Rarely toxic epidermal necrolysis	Neuro • Headache • Nystagmus • Ataxia • Sedation Derm • Rash GI • Abnormal LFTs	Baseline • CBC 2 × per month × 2 mo • LFTs 2 × per month × 2 mo Periodic • CBC and LFTs 1–2 times per year
Lamotrigine	Derm • Rarely Stevens-Johnson syndrome • Rarely toxic epidermal necrolysis	Neuro • Headache • Dizziness/vertigo • Ataxia • Sedation • Tremor • Visual disturbances Derm • Rash GI • Nausea/vomiting • Diarrhea	Baseline • Creatinine Periodic • Eye examinations

Abbreviations: CBC, complete blood count; Derm, dermatologic; ECG, electrocardiogram; Neuro, neurologic.
  Data from Refs.[27,43,45–48,50,115–117]

small degree of persistent cognitive dulling) most frequently lead to intolerance and discontinuation.[45–48]

Tremor can also be problematic for patients early in the treatment course. There is wide variation in estimates of tremor frequency among lithium users, but it is one of the drug's most common side effects.[49] Clinically, lithium tremor can be distinguished from other causes of tremor by its onset on initiation of the drug or upward titration of the dose and by its typically symmetric involvement of the upper extremities.[49] Lithium-induced tremor is exacerbated by many of the same factors that worsen essential or physiologic tremors, such as caffeine, physical stress or anxiety, fatigue, and medications. Lithium tremor frequently resolves with time; but for disabling or disturbing symptoms, treatment involves decreasing the dose of lithium (if possible), modulation of concurrent aggravating factors, or pharmacotherapy such as is used in essential tremor.[49]

In the long-term, renal and thyroid toxicities are the most important clinical considerations (see **Table 7**).[45] Serum creatinine should be monitored every 6 to 12 months and more frequently if other risk factors for kidney disease are present.[48] Lithium impacts thyroid function in multiple ways. Most notably is the inhibition of thyroid hormone release from the gland, resulting in hypothyroidism or the development of goiter.[47,50] The resulting hypothyroidism can be treated with levothyroxine while lithium therapy is continued.

There is very weak evidence that lithium is teratogenic. Current recommendations are to avoid lithium during pregnancy, but some suggest that the benefit of mood stability during pregnancy outweighs the very small risk.[47]

Because lithium levels are influenced by renal function and salt and water balance, it is no surprise that many antihypertensive classes affect serum lithium concentrations. Because lithium has a narrow therapeutic index, PCPs must be aware that antibiotics, NSAIDs, theophylline, and low-sodium diets can affect lithium levels.[43,48,51]

Movig and colleagues[52] found that polyuria was strongly associated with concomitant use of serotonergic agents. The lithium medication interactions reviewed in this section are not absolute contraindication; however, lithium levels should be monitored closely when combined with these drugs (**Table 8**).

It is difficult for patients to adhere to and continue on lithium because of its side-effect profile. PCPs must thoughtfully titrate this medication and communicate effectively with patients about the side effects in order to successfully have patients benefit and adhere to this medication. Providers and patients must remain vigilant of medication interactions and signs of lithium toxicity. Serum lithium levels should be checked to assess for efficacy and toxicity (**Box 3**).

Anticonvulsants

Valproate, carbamazepine, and lamotrigine are commonly used as mood stabilizers. Valproate and carbamazepine, alone or in combination with an antipsychotic, are efficacious in the treatment of acute mania.[41,53] Both of these, as well as lamotrigine, may be used as monotherapy or in combination with other medications for maintenance therapy in bipolar disorder.[41,54]

Dosing is variable for each anticonvulsant medication, though the approach of an initial lower dose, rapid titration to a therapeutic dose, and serum monitoring of levels is similar for valproate and carbamazepine (see **Table 6**).[51] The notable exception is for lamotrigine, which does not have a mechanism for reliable serologic monitoring and requires careful titration.

PCPs should be especially wary of lamotrigine during the initiation stage given the risk for Stevens-Johnson. Early epilepsy trials showed cases were rare, largely

Table 8
Medication interactions with mood stabilizers

Mood Stabilizer	Medication ↑ Blood Level	Medication ↓ Blood Level	Other Interactions
Lithium	• Thiazide diuretics • ACE inhibitors • Potassium-sparing diuretics • Calcium channel blockers • Tetracyclines • Metronidazole • NSAIDs • Low-sodium diets	• Potassium-sparing diuretics • Calcium channel blockers • Theophylline	↑ Polyuria • Serotonergic medications
Valproate P450 inhibitor	• Aspirin • Naproxen • Magnesium- and aluminum-containing antacids	• Carbamazepine • Sex hormone therapy/oral contraceptives	↑ Medication levels • Phenobarbital • Clonazepam • Multiple other medications
Carbamazepine P450 inducer	• Valproate • Fluoxetine • Macrolide antibiotics • Metronidazole • Isoniazid • Diltiazem/verapamil	• Phenytoin • Phenobarbital • Primidone	↓ Medication levels • Valproic acid • Clonazepam • Lamotrigine • Topiramate • Multiple medications, including TCAs, antipsychotics, oral contraceptives, chemotherapy agents, cyclosporine, glucocorticoids
Lamotrigine	• Valproate	• Sex hormone therapy/oral contraceptives • Carbamazepine	

Abbreviation: ACE, angiotensin-converting enzyme.
  Data from Refs.[43,48,51,52,56,118–120]

Box 3
Lithium clinical pearls

• Lithium is contraindicated in patients with significant renal impairment, sodium or volume depletion, and significant cardiovascular disease.

• The likelihood of lithium toxicity increases when its excretion is impaired, as in volume depletion, renal impairment, or in geriatric patients. Severe or sudden worsening of side effects should prompt consideration of lithium toxicity.

• Although a common side effect of lithium even at therapeutic drug levels, tremor is also one of the most common signs of lithium toxicity, so the appearance or worsening of a tremor should prompt the clinician to check drug levels and consider causes of impaired lithium excretion.

• Acute onset of nocturia may be the first clue of nephrogenic diabetes insipidus. The normal kidney concentrates urine at night when no fluid is ingested; when tubular concentration is impaired, the presenting complaint may be nocturia.

• Lithium can exacerbate psoriasis.[48]

confined to the first few weeks of initiation of lamotrigine,[55] and were possibly associated with high initial doses of the drug.[56] To reduce the risk of a life-threatening skin rash, lamotrigine must be titrated slowly[55,56] and should not be use as the first-line therapy in acute mania (as practical medications for mania must be titrated quickly to effect).

For maintenance therapy in bipolar disorder, the initial dosage of lamotrigine is 25 mg/d for 2 weeks. Subsequently, the dosage is increased to 25 mg twice daily for 2 more weeks. Finally, the dosage is increased by 25 to 50 mg/d each week thereafter, until the final therapeutic dose is reached (up to 200–400 mg daily in 2 divided doses).[51,56]

In 2008, the FDA determined a positive association between anticonvulsants and suicidality.[57] Subsequently, however, 2 large analyses of medical claims and clinical trials data showed no increase in suicidality among patients treated with anticonvulsants for bipolar disorder.[57,58] In fact, treatment with anticonvulsants seems protective against suicide attempts, compared with no treatment, in patients with bipolar disorder.[58]

Common side effects and recommended monitoring for the anticonvulsant mood stabilizers are summarized in **Table 7**. Although rare, clinicians should remain alert to the clinical cues to pancreatitis when prescribing valproate.[43] Divalproex can be substituted for valproate to minimize common GI distress side effects. Despite the rare but serious risk for Stevens-Johnson, lamotrigine was similar to placebo for common side effects, including serologic derangements in some clinical studies.[56] Carbamazepine and valproate use require monitoring for blood derangements and liver abnormalities, and a baseline kidney function should be checked before lamotrigine use.

Serious medication interactions occur with the use of anticonvulsant mood stabilizers because valproate is a potent cytochrome P450 inhibitor and carbamazepine a significant P450 inducer.[43,56] Complicating matters, all of the anticonvulsant mood stabilizers are themselves metabolized via cytochrome P450 pathways. **Table 8** summarizes the important medication mood stabilizer medication interactions. PCPs should check for medication interactions whenever initiating or titrating anticonvulsant mood stabilizer medications or whenever a new medication is added to a regimen containing them (**Box 4**).

Antipsychotics

A more detailed account of antipsychotics is reviewed in the section on non–mood stabilizer uses of antipsychotics, and the specific considerations for using antipsychotics in mood stabilization are covered here. Although most PCPs will not be initiating antipsychotics for mania or maintenance of bipolar disorder without the direct guidance of a psychiatrist, they should be aware of the indications, general dosing, and basic management considerations. Both first- and second-generation antipsychotics are used in the treatment of acute mania[53] and have been found effective not only for psychotic symptoms but for general symptoms of mania. Second-generation

---

Box 4
Anticonvulsant mood stabilizer clinical pearls

- The immune tolerance to lamotrigine is lost after a dosage interruption greater than 1 week. Therefore, patients with lapses in therapy should resume lamotrigine according to the slow upward titration described earlier.[56]

- Carbamazepine is a potent P450 inducer, so it has many medication interactions.

antipsychotics are commonly used for maintenance therapy in bipolar disorder and have been seen to prevent both mania and bipolar depression.[41,54,59,60]

There is positive evidence for 2 atypical antipsychotics in the treatment of bipolar depression. Quetiapine monotherapy has been shown to be efficacious in the treatment of depression in bipolar disorder,[61] comparable with lithium monotherapy[62] and better than paroxetine monotherapy.[63] Combined with fluoxetine and as monotherapy, olanzapine is also an effective therapy for bipolar depression. (**Table 9** includes details of dosing for the various affective disorder indications.)[64]

The strong antipsychotic effect of haloperidol and other typical antipsychotics is attributable to dopaminergic antagonism; this mechanism also results in some of the well-known side effects of this medication class: extrapyramidal symptoms, tardive dyskinesia, and hyperprolactinemia. Typical antipsychotics are more likely than atypicals to cause extrapyramidal symptoms (EPS). EPS symptoms include akathisia (a sensation of motor restlessness with or without actual movement), secondary parkinsonism, acute dystonia, and tardive dyskinesia.[65,66] Unlike in schizophrenia, the use of antipsychotics in bipolar disease and other affective disorders rarely results in tardive dyskinesia because typical antipsychotics are rarely used long-term for mood stabilization and atypical antipsychotics are much less likely to cause tardive dyskinesia as a side effect.

Atypical antipsychotics are more apt than typical antipsychotics to cause metabolic derangements, including weight gain, dyslipidemia, glucose intolerance, and diabetes.[67] Atypical antipsychotics can also cause anticholinergic side effects and orthostatic hypotension. There is substantial variation among medications in all of these side effects. Of those used to treat acute mania and bipolar disorder, aripiprazole and ziprasidone have the fewest metabolic side effects. Quetiapine and olanzapine, followed by risperidone, have the worst metabolic side-effect profiles. Among these 5 atypical antipsychotics, risperidone is the most likely to cause hyperprolactinemia and sexual side effects.[66,68] **Table 10** reviews antipsychotic side effects and their clinical management.

Because of metabolism through the cytochrome P450 system, multiple antipsychotic medications have significant medication interaction risks.[69] Providers must be wary not only about starting or changing doses of the antipsychotics but also about how other medications may interact with antipsychotics: sometimes by increasing or decreasing the antipsychotic blood levels, and sometimes by potentiating a different unique side effect. Medications as common as antihypertensives and antibiotics may cause serious medication interactions with antipsychotics. Although the use of antidepressants in bipolar affective disorder is of questionable efficacy, it is encountered frequently in practice. Clinicians should be aware that many antidepressants (some SSRIs, SNRIs, and bupropion) are inhibitors of the cytochrome P450 hepatic metabolism system.[35] When these antidepressants are used in combination with some antipsychotics (examples: risperidone and haloperidol), they may significantly increase the serum level of the antipsychotic agent leading to toxicity symptoms.[35] See **Table 11** for details about antipsychotic medication interactions. Additional discussion on antipsychotic medication interactions is also found in the section next (**Box 5**).

ANTIPSYCHOTIC MEDICATIONS

Antipsychotic medications are FDA approved for a broad array of indications. First generation antipsychotics are approved (with variable FDA indication dependent on the specific medication) for schizophrenia, bipolar, agitation, severe behavioral

Table 9
Antipsychotic medication dosing in mood-related disorders

Medication	Indication	Initial Dose	Titration	Therapeutic Dose
Typical				
Haloperidol	Acute mania	0.2 mg/kg/d	—	5–15 mg qd
Atypical				
Aripiprazole	Acute mania	10–30 mg daily	—	15–45 mg daily
	Treatment-resistant depression (augmentation)			2–15 mg daily
Olanzapine	Acute mania	10–15 mg QHS		10–30 mg daily or in divided doses
	Maintenance of bipolar	5 mg QHS	↑ By 5 mg daily	5–20 mg daily
	Psychotic depression	5 mg QHS	↑ By 5 mg daily	10–20 mg daily
Quetiapine	Acute mania	100–200 mg QHS	—	400–800 mg daily or in divided doses
	Maintenance for bipolar	50 mg QHS	↑ 50–100 mg daily	300–600 mg daily
Risperidone (PO)	Acute mania	1–2 mg daily	—	4–8 mg daily
Risperidone (IM)	Maintenance of bipolar	—	—	12.5–25.0 mg every 2 wk
Ziprasidone	Acute mania	40 mg BID	—	80–160 mg daily or in divided doses

Abbreviation: IM, intramuscularly.
Data from Refs. [41,51,53,54,59,60,64,78,79,83,87,88,121–124]

Table 10
Antipsychotic medication side effects and side-effect management

Antipsychotic Side Effects	Clinical Manifestations	Management
Akathisia	• Sensation of motor restlessness with or without actual movement • Most common EPS	• ↓ Antipsychotic dose • Add benzodiazepines • Add propranolol • Add benztropine
Secondary parkinsonism	• Masked facies • Resting tremor • Cogwheel rigidity • Shuffling gait • Bradykinesia	• Add benztropine

Acute dystonia	• Involuntary contractions of major muscle groups
	  ○ Torticollis
	  ○ Laryngospasm
		• Add anticholinergics
		  ○ Benztropine
		  ○ Diphenhydramine
		• Add benzodiazepine
		• Change antipsychotic medication

Tardive dyskinesia	• Consequence of long-term high-dose use • Involuntary movements frequently involving the lips, tongue, jaw, face, trunk, and extremities	• Discontinue offending antipsychotic medication • Consider switch to a lower risk antipsychotic
QT prolongation	• Rare but serious risk of sudden death	• Use with caution in any condition with prolonged QT • Consider avoidance or dose ↓
Neuroleptic malignant syndrome	• Rare but serious risk • Hyperthermia • Muscle rigidity • Altered mental status • Autonomic dysfunction • Death	• Discontinue offending antipsychotic agent • Supportive care
Metabolic side effects	• Weight gain • Dyslipidemia • Glucose intolerance • Diabetes	• Disease-specific intervention • Statins • Metformin
Anticholinergic symptoms	• ↓ Salivation, bronchial secretions, sweating, GI motility • ↑ Heart rate • Impaired concentration • Confusion • Memory impairment	• ↓ Antipsychotic dose • Change to a different antipsychotic with lower anticholinergic effects • ↓ Or eliminate other medications with anticholinergic effects • Atropine for anticholinergic delirium once offending agent is discontinued

Data from Refs.[65–68,71,72,125,126]

problems, agitation, psychosis, Tourette syndrome, and generalized nonpsychotic anxiety.[70] Second-generation antipsychotics are approved (with variable indication dependent on the specific medication) for schizophrenia (acute, general, treatment resistant, reduction of suicidality in schizophrenia), bipolar (acute mania, maintenance

Table 11
Antipsychotic medication interactions

Cytochrome Metabolism/ Antipsychotic Agent	↑ Antipsychotic Level	↓ Antipsychotic Level	Other Effect
CYP2D6 and CYP3A4 metabolized • Haloperidol • Aripiprazole[a] • Risperidone[a] • Clozapine	• Fluoxetine • Duloxetine • Paroxetine • Bupropion • Amiodarone • Azole antifungals • Diltiazem verapamil • Macrolide antibiotics except azithromycin	• Carbamazepine • Rifampin • Phenytoin • St Johns Wort	• Avoid/caution use in medications that cause prolonged QT
CYP2D6 metabolized • Fluphenazine[a] • Thioridazine	• Fluoxetine • Paroxetine • Bupropion • Duloxetine • Sertraline • Amiodarone	• Rifampin	• Avoid/caution use in medications that cause prolonged QT
CYP3A4 metabolized • Ziprasidone • Quetiapine	• Many antimicrobial agents	• Carbamazepine • Rifampin • Phenytoin • St John's wort • Efavirenz	• Avoid/caution use in medications that cause prolonged QT
CYP1A2 metabolized • Clozapine • Olanzapine[a]	• Fluvoxamine • Diltiazem • Verapamil • Azole antifungals • Macrolides except azithromycin	• Carbamazepine • Barbiturates • Phenytoin • Tobacco smoke	• Modify/monitor use with hypertension medications because of additive effect
Minimal (<50%) hepatic metabolism • Paliperidone	—	—	• Renally excreted so dose ↓ in the setting of renal impairment • Avoid/caution use in medications that cause prolonged QT • Monitor for hypotension with use of antihypertensives

[a] No listed contraindication for prolonged QT.
Data from Refs.[66,69,71,127]

therapy, mixed manic states, bipolar depression, monotherapy, or as an adjunctive agent), depression (adjunct), and irritability in autistic disorder in children.[70] The breadth of these indications is beyond the scope of this review, though the indications for bipolar (reviewed earlier), schizophrenia, depression, and off-label uses in geriatrics are covered.

First-generation antipsychotics modulate their effects, both efficacious and unwanted, by blocking dopamine receptors. Second-generation antipsychotics antagonize D2 dopamine receptors as well as serotonin receptors.[14] The difference in

---

Box 5
Clinical pearls for the use of antipsychotic medications in bipolar disorder

- Neuroleptic-induced akathisia is a common and commonly overlooked side effect of both typical and atypical antipsychotic medications. Intensely unpleasant for some patients, akathisia can influence medication adherence; but if recognized by clinicians, it can be treated. The first-line therapy for akathisia from antipsychotics is anticholinergic therapy. Benztropine, 1 to 2 mg twice daily, can be easily and relatively safely prescribed in the primary care setting.[128]

- Patients taking antipsychotics should be monitored for extrapyramidal symptoms weekly for 2 weeks on initiation of the medication and after every dose increase.[129]

- All antipsychotic medications have multiple drug interactions because of the hepatic metabolism via the CYP pathways. Clinicians should be alert to potential interactions when initiating antipsychotics or increasing their dose or when adding a new medication to a regimen including an antipsychotic drug.

- Although atypical antipsychotics share many side effects as a class, there is substantial variation within the group of drugs. Clinicians can select from among the atypical antipsychotics according to relative importance of different side effects to the individual patient.

- Levels of olanzapine and clozapine, metabolized via the CYP1A2 pathway, may be decreased by cigarette smoking.[71] Clinicians may notice a slightly decreased drug effect when patients are transitioned from a nonsmoking hospital unit to the outpatient setting.

- Classifying antipsychotics into 2 distinct classes (typical and atypical) may be somewhat misleading in that the indications and side-effect profiles both overlap and are heterogeneous within the classes. One valid distinction, however, is that the atypical class carries less risk of extrapyramidal side effects, including tardive dyskinesia.[68]

---

mechanisms account for differences in the side-effect profiles of first- and second-generation antipsychotics. See the section on antipsychotics for mood stabilization discussed earlier and **Table 10** for details on antipsychotic side effects. Specific considerations based on the indication of antipsychotic use are reviewed in the later sections.

The dangers of antipsychotics being metabolized through the hepatic cytochrome P450 system are addressed in the mood stabilizer section and are summarized in **Table 11**. Even for providers who rarely initiate or adjust antipsychotic medications, they should take note of several important medication interactions. First, almost all antipsychotics prolong the QT segment and increase the risk for fatal dysrhythmias when used in people prone to prolonged QT or when given in conjunction with medications that prolong QT (examples: antiarrhythmics, methadone, and prochlorperazine [also a D2 receptor antagonist]).[66,68,71,72] Second, all antipsychotics cause orthostatic hypotension to a degree[14] because they block alpha 1 receptors like blood pressure medications, such as doxazosin and prazosin. High-risk patients for this side effect are those already on antihypertensives, elderly individuals, and those with cardiovascular diseases. Slower titration of the antipsychotics and, often, proactive dose reduction of antihypertensives are necessary to avoid syncope, falls, transient ischemic attacks, and other adverse events related to orthostatic hypotension. Lastly, first-generation antipsychotics and risperidone, a second-generation antipsychotic, can cause hyperprolactinemia.[14] Although some patients will present with classic symptoms of galactorrhea, acne, and menstrual irregularities, others will be apparently asymptomatic. Recent studies suggest that long-term antipsychotic-related hyperprolactinemia may cause osteoporosis and increased risks of hip fracture.[14]

Use in Schizophrenia

Antipsychotic medications are the first-line therapy for schizophrenia in the settings of both acute psychosis and chronic disease maintenance. There is a paucity of strong evidence to support the use of one antipsychotic (typical or atypical) over any other. The exceptions are that clozapine seems more effective in treatment-refractory disease[67] and that second-generation antipsychotics may show greater long-term benefit than first-generation drugs for maintenance therapy in schizophrenia.[73] Therefore, drug selection is individualized and based not on relative efficacy but rather on prior treatment response, drug tolerability, side-effect profile, and available formulation.

In addition to haloperidol, discussed for alternate indications earlier (see the mood stabilizers: antipsychotics section), phenothiazines (fluphenazine, trifluoperazine, perphenazine, chlorpromazine and thioridazine) and other fist-generation antipsychotics (thiothixene, molindone, and loxapine) may be used to treat acute positive symptoms in schizophrenia. In patients with established treatment-responsive, multi-episode schizophrenia, the daily dosage of typical antipsychotic medications should be in the range of 300 to 1000 chlorpromazine (a low-potency antipsychotic) equivalents daily. Patients with first-episode schizophrenia may respond to lower doses.[68] As noted earlier, typical antipsychotics are generally effective at doses well less than the FDA-specified maximum doses.[68]

Atypical antipsychotics are indicated for the treatment of acute psychosis in schizophrenia as well as maintenance therapy. Because they may have more long-term benefit than their typical counterparts and because there is a lower risk of permanent extrapyramidal side effects, they are used more commonly for maintenance than the typicals.[73] Clozapine and olanzapine, however, are not used as first-line agents because of their unfavorable side-effect profiles. Clozapine is more effective than other agents in the treatment of patients with refractory schizophrenia. It is used in people who experience persistent, clinically significant positive symptoms after 2 adequate trials of other antipsychotic agents, either typical or atypical.[68]

The daily dosage of atypical antipsychotics for an acute symptom episode is 10 to 30 mg of aripiprazole, 10 to 20 mg of olanzapine, 3 to 15 mg of paliperidone, 300 to 750 mg of quetiapine, 2 to 8 mg of risperidone, or 80 to 160 mg of ziprasidone. The maintenance dose is that found to be effective for reducing positive psychotic symptoms in the acute phase of treatment.[68]

Many typical (and atypical) antipsychotics are available in long-acting injectable form; there are no known substantial differences in efficacy in the treatment of schizophrenia, either among the available injectable medications or between depot and oral antipsychotics.[74,75] Depot medications may be used in patients who have had a prior response to oral antipsychotics (without major side effects) but have relapsed because of difficulty with medication adherence.

The risk for developing EPS caused by the use of antipsychotics is higher when treating schizophrenia compared with affective disorders because of the higher dosing and duration of antipsychotic medication use in this disease. This point is particularly true when using more potent, typical (first generation) antipsychotics at high doses.[68] Acute extrapyramidal effects are discussed earlier (see the section on mood stabilizers: antipsychotics). The most dreaded, and often irreversible, extrapyramidal side effect, tardive dyskinesia, is only associated with long-term antipsychotic therapy. Tardive dyskinesia is a syndrome of involuntary movements frequently involving the lips, tongue, jaw, face, trunk, and extremities. There are no pharmacologic interventions for tardive dyskinesia, and the only strategy to improve symptoms once it develops is to discontinue antipsychotics or switch to an antipsychotic with a low risk of tardive dyskinesia (such as an atypical agent).

Clozapine is not strongly associated with the development of extrapyramidal side effects (including tardive dyskinesia); but among all the antipsychotics, clozapine alone is associated with potentially fatal agranulocytosis, seen in 1% to 2% of treated patients. This risk is increased with age and decreases after the first 6 months of treatment.[76]

Atypical antipsychotics confer higher risks for metabolic side effects. There is significant variation among the antipsychotics used for schizophrenia; clinicians should remember that aripiprazole and ziprasidone have the best side-effect profile when it comes to the metabolic syndrome, quetiapine and olanzapine the worst, and risperidone and paliperidone intermediate.[66] Risperidone and its metabolite, paliperidone, have the highest risk of sexual side effects and hyperprolactinemia.[68]

See **Table 10** for more details about antipsychotic side effects and their management. See **Table 11** for details of medication interactions with antipsychotic use (**Box 6**).

Use in Mood Disorders

In addition to their dopaminergic effects, antipsychotics have serotonergic and noradrenergic activity and are efficacious in mood disorders with and without psychosis.[77] Atypical antipsychotics are an effective therapy for bipolar depression[61–64] and for augmentation of treatment-refractory nonpsychotic unipolar depression.[78–80] Both typicals and atypicals can be used for psychotic depression.[81–84] See **Table 9** for details about dosing of antipsychotic medications for affective disorders. See the antipsychotic section of "Mood stabilizer medications" for more details about the use of antipsychotics for bipolar disorder.

Many atypical and typical antipsychotics, combined with antidepressants, have been shown to be efficacious in the acute treatment of unipolar depression with

---

Box 6
Clinical pearls for the use of antipsychotics for schizophrenia

- Typical antipsychotics are generally efficacious for schizophrenia at doses far lower than the FDA-specified maxima.

- First-generation lower-potency typical antipsychotics (such as chlorpromazine, dosed in hundreds of milligrams) are less likely to cause extrapyramidal symptoms but may cause more metabolic side effects than their higher-potency counterparts.[130,131]

- Classifying antipsychotics into 2 distinct classes (typical and atypical of first generation and second generation) may be somewhat misleading in that the indications and side-effect profiles both overlap and are heterogeneous within the classes. One valid distinction, however, is that the atypical class carries less risk of extrapyramidal side effects.

- Drugs in both classes cause metabolic side effects, with the worst offenders being the atypicals olanzapine and quetiapine.

- Clozapine is least likely to cause metabolic side effects or tardive dyskinesia but carries the additional life-threatening risk of agranulocytosis.[68] For this reason, it is reserved only for treatment-refractory psychotic disease.

- There is wide cost variation among atypical antipsychotics, which are on the whole more expensive than their typical counterparts. Generic formulations are available for some, but not all, second-generation antipsychotics; clinicians should consider cost when selecting agents.

psychotic features.[81–84] There have not been head-to-head trials of different combinations, but the combination of sertraline plus olanzapine has been studied in the largest number of patients.[83] In psychotic depression, antipsychotics are not used for maintenance or suppression therapy and are typically discontinued after 4 months of sustained recovery.[85]

Atypical antipsychotics have been studied in treatment-refractory unipolar depression without psychosis.[78,79,86,87] A large meta-analysis of 16 randomized trials demonstrated overall effectiveness of aripiprazole, olanzapine, quetiapine, and risperidone when any of these agents were added to an antidepressant in nonpsychotic patients failing monotherapy. There was no appreciable difference among the antipsychotics studied, although these were not compared head to head.[80] A more recent randomized double-blind placebo-controlled trial of 225 patients with treatment-refractory depression evaluated the efficacy and tolerability of very-low-dose aripiprazole added to antidepressant monotherapy. This study demonstrated good tolerability of aripiprazole at this dose for this indication, but the efficacy was very marginal.[88]

Finally, quetiapine monotherapy has been proven effective in nonpsychotic depression; but the benefit is small, and the side-effect profile limits its use when first-line therapies are available (**Box 7**).[89–91]

Use in Geriatrics for Dementia-Related Behaviors and Symptoms

Antipsychotics are used to treat psychotic symptoms caused by a variety of organic neurologic and psychiatric disease.[92–94] In this section, the authors focus on the use of antipsychotics in elderly patients with dementia.

Both typical and atypical antipsychotics have been used for symptom management in patients with organic dementing diseases.[92,93,95–98] However, antipsychotics have been used frequently to treat psychotic and behavioral problems among elderly patients with dementia. Reasons for treatment include hallucinations, delirium and sundowning, agitation, aggression, and wandering.

Although there is some evidence that risperidone improves symptoms of aggression, agitation, and psychosis in dementia without intolerable side effects,[99,100] 2 systematic reviews concluded that neither typical nor atypical antipsychotics have an aggregate benefit in patients with dementia.[95,101] A Cochrane review concluded that haloperidol may reduce aggressive behaviors among patients with dementia but at the expense of side effects.[102] One large multicenter trial found no benefit to offset the adverse effects of atypical antipsychotic drugs.[96] Therefore, antipsychotics should be used with caution in these patients, only for debilitating symptoms or unsafe behaviors and only after other interventions have been exhausted.

In addition to the side effects described in detail elsewhere (see the antipsychotics section in "Mood stabilizer medications" and the schizophrenia section in "Antipsychotic medications"), both typical[103] and atypical[104] antipsychotics are associated with increased stroke and all-cause mortality in patients with Alzheimer disease.[105,106] Serious adverse effects, including hospitalization and death, have been attributed not

---

Box 7
Clinical pearls for the use of antipsychotic agents for mood disorders (excluding bipolar)

- When indicated, lower doses of antipsychotics can be used in elderly patients with psychotic depression.

- When used to augment therapy in treatment-refractory unipolar depression, atypical antipsychotics can be used at doses much lower than those used for other indications.

Box 8
Clinical pearls for the use of antipsychotics in dementia-related psychosis and behaviors

- Clinicians may feel comfortable with doses and side effects of antipsychotic drugs because of their proven efficacy and widespread and longstanding use in bipolar disorder and schizophrenia; however, evidence for their use in other diseases, including unipolar depression, is much less robust. The relative risk to benefit of these medications is skewed toward risk, especially when used off label for the treatment of dementia symptoms in elderly patients.

- Clinicians should inform families of the known mortality risk associated with antipsychotics in elderly patients with dementia. When used (only for severe symptoms), doses of these drugs should be kept low and treatment duration kept short.

---

only to the long-term use of antipsychotics[106] but also to their use in the short-term; in fact, the relative mortality increase may be highest in the first 30 days of use.[103]

It is worth emphasizing here that the known side effects of antipsychotic medications are more pronounced in elderly patients, who may be particularly sensitive to anticholinergic side effects and orthostatic hypotension. Antipsychotic medications are among the drugs most frequently associated with adverse effects in long-term care facilities.[107] Geriatric patients are more likely than other adults to take multiple medications,[108] so the risk of medication interactions is higher. Additionally, patients with other forms of dementia, such as frontotemporal, parkinsonian, and Lewy body dementia, seem to be more vulnerable to the neuroleptic sides of both typical and atypical antipsychotics.[109,110]

Antipsychotics are shown to increase mortality by 1.6 to 1.7 times in this population[103,104] and are not FDA approved for this indication.[14] In fact, there is a black box warning issued from the FDA for both typical and atypical antipsychotics for dementia-related psychosis.

If used, after all nonpharmacologic interventions have been exhausted, the duration of antipsychotic therapy should be kept as short as possible and the doses as low as possible. For example, olanzapine should be initiated at 2.5 mg daily and limited to 5 mg twice daily.[96,101] Risperidone should be limited to 1 mg daily, as higher doses confer an excess risk of side effects.[101] The starting and maintenance doses of other antipsychotics should be similarly reduced in geriatric patients with dementia (**Box 8**).

SUMMARY/FUTURE DIRECTIONS

It is a positive development that patients are being assessed for and diagnosed with psychiatric conditions in the primary care setting. Improving access to mental health care for all of our patients will require PCPs to step up and manage straightforward psychiatric conditions primarily (uncomplicated depression and anxiety) and more complex conditions with the help of our colleagues in psychiatry (refractory mood disorders, bipolar disease, schizophrenia). Safe and effective management of psychiatric disorders requires a solid understanding of pharmacotherapy. Savvy providers can prepare patients for what to expect in the way of efficacy onset, side effects, risks, and medication interactions. Moreover, PCPs who understand pharmacotherapy can harness their knowledge of side effects and unique medication profiles to individually tailor medication selection for their patients.

There is much room for improvement for efficacy, safety, and tolerability of psychotropic medications. Researchers have searched for a pattern in genetic polymorphisms in the hepatic metabolism of medications to improve medication selection[111]; others are exploring the possibilities of a novel target for drug design, combining medications in a way that increases the speed of the response and reduces the side-effect burden.[112] We can develop better systems of care and use our electronic medical records to identify potential medication interactions, and remind us about monitoring.

REFERENCES

1. Qaseem A, Snow V, Denberg TD, et al. Using second-generation antidepressants to treat depressive disorders: a clinical practice guideline from the American College of Physicians. Ann Intern Med 2008;149(10):725–33.
2. Huhn M, Tardy M, Spineli LM, et al. Efficacy of pharmacotherapy and psychotherapy for adult psychiatric disorders: a systematic overview of meta-analyses. JAMA Psychiatry 2014;71(6):706–15.
3. Olfson M, Blanco C, Wang S, et al. National trends in the mental health care of children, adolescents, and adults by office-based physicians. JAMA Psychiatry 2014;71(1):81–90.
4. Paterniti S, Bisserbe JC. Pharmacotherapy for bipolar disorder and concordance with treatment guidelines: survey of a general population sample referred to a tertiary care service. BMC Psychiatry 2013;13:211.
5. Salvi V, Fagiolini A, Swartz HA, et al. The use of antidepressants in bipolar disorder. J Clin Psychiatry 2008;69(8):1307–18.
6. Henriksen AL, St Dennis C, Setter SM, et al. Dementia with Lewy bodies: therapeutic opportunities and pitfalls. Consult Pharm 2006;21(7):563–75.
7. Gartlehner G, Gaynes BN, Hansen RA, et al. Comparative benefits and harms of second-generation antidepressants: background paper for the American College of Physicians. Ann Intern Med 2008;149(10):734–50.
8. Haueis P, Greil W, Huber M, et al. Evaluation of drug interactions in a large sample of psychiatric inpatients: a data interface for mass analysis with clinical decision support software. Clin Pharmacol Ther 2011;90(4):588–96.
9. Baldwin DS, Anderson IM, Nutt DJ, et al. Evidence-based pharmacological treatment of anxiety disorders, post-traumatic stress disorder and obsessive-compulsive disorder: a revision of the 2005 guidelines from the British Association for Psychopharmacology. J Psychopharmacol 2014;28(5):403–39.
10. Bandelow B, Sher L, Bunevicius R, et al. Guidelines for the pharmacological treatment of anxiety disorders, obsessive-compulsive disorder and posttraumatic stress disorder in primary care. Int J Psychiatry Clin Pract 2012;16(2):77–84.
11. Baldwin DS, Waldman S, Allgulander C. Evidence-based pharmacological treatment of generalized anxiety disorder. Int J Neuropsychopharmacol 2011;14(5):697–710.
12. Offidani E, Guidi J, Tomba E, et al. Efficacy and tolerability of benzodiazepines versus antidepressants in anxiety disorders: a systematic review and meta-analysis. Psychother Psychosom 2013;82(6):355–62.
13. Culpepper L. The role of primary care clinicians in diagnosing and treating bipolar disorder. Prim Care Companion J Clin Psychiatry 2010;12(Suppl 1):4–9.
14. Muench J, Hamer AM. Adverse effects of antipsychotic medications. Am Fam Physician 2010;81(5):617–22.
15. Declercq T, Petrovic M, Azermai M, et al. Withdrawal versus continuation of chronic antipsychotic drugs for behavioural and psychological symptoms in older people with dementia. Cochrane Database Syst Rev 2013;(3):CD007726.
16. FDA requests boxed warnings on older class of antipsychotic drugs. 2008.

17. Gartlehner G, Hansen RA, Thieda P, et al. AHRQ comparative effectiveness reviews. Comparative effectiveness of second-generation antidepressants in the pharmacologic treatment of adult depression. Rockville (MD): Agency for Healthcare Research and Quality (US); 2007.

18. Fancher TL, Kravitz RL. In the clinic. Depression. Ann Intern Med 2010;152(9). ITC51-15. [quiz: ITC55–16].

19. Hawton K, Bergen H, Simkin S, et al. Toxicity of antidepressants: rates of suicide relative to prescribing and non-fatal overdose. Br J Psychiatry 2010;196:354–8.

20. Stahl SM. Mechanism of action of serotonin selective reuptake inhibitors. Serotonin receptors and pathways mediate therapeutic effects and side effects. J Affect Disord 1998;51(3):215–35.

21. Moura C, Bernatsky S, Abrahamowicz M, et al. Antidepressant use and 10-year incident fracture risk: the population-based Canadian Multicentre Osteoporosis Study (CaMoS). Osteoporos Int 2014;25(5):1473–81.

22. Sterke CS, Ziere G, van Beeck EF, et al. Dose-response relationship between selective serotonin reuptake inhibitors and injurious falls: a study in nursing home residents with dementia. Br J Clin Pharmacol 2012;73(5):812–20.

23. Targownik LE, Bolton JM, Metge CJ, et al. Selective serotonin reuptake inhibitors are associated with a modest increase in the risk of upper gastrointestinal bleeding. Am J Gastroenterol 2009;104(6):1475–82.

24. Loke YK, Trivedi AN, Singh S. Meta-analysis: gastrointestinal bleeding due to interaction between selective serotonin uptake inhibitors and non-steroidal anti-inflammatory drugs. Aliment Pharmacol Ther 2008;27(1):31–40.

25. FDA Drug Safety Communication: Revised recommendations for Celexa (citalopram hydrobromide) related to a potential risk of abnormal heart rhythms with high doses. 2013.

26. Reid S, Barbui C. Long term treatment of depression with selective serotonin reuptake inhibitors and newer antidepressants. BMJ 2010;340:c1468.

27. Illinois BBo. Antidepressant agents step therapy criteria with medical diagnoses option. Chicago (IL): Blue Cross and Blue Shield of Illinois; 2010.

28. Stone K. Off-label applications for SSRIs. Am Fam Physician 2003;68(3): 489–504.

29. Andrade C. Selective serotonin reuptake inhibitor drug interactions in patients receiving statins. J Clin Psychiatry 2014;75(2):e95–9.

30. Catherine M, Juurlink DN, Gomes T, et al. Selective serotonin reuptake inhibitors and breast cancer mortality in women receiving tamoxifen: a population based cohort study. BMJ 2010;340:c693.

31. Edward W, Boyer MS. The serotonin syndrome. N Engl J Med 2005;352: 1112–20.

32. Rolan PE. Drug interactions with triptans: which are clinically significant? CNS Drugs 2012;26(11):949–57.

33. Kurt Kroenke MB, Damush T. Optimized antidepressant therapy and pain self-management in primary care patients with depression and musculoskeletal pain: a randomized controlled trial. JAMA 2009;301(20):2099–110.

34. Hamon M, Bourgoin S. Pharmacological profile of antidepressants: a likely basis for their efficacy and side effects? Eur Neuropsychopharmacol 2006;16:S625–32.

35. DA F. Cytochrome P450 drug interaction table 2007.

36. Bradley AJ, Lenox-Smith AJ. Does adding noradrenaline reuptake inhibition to selective serotonin reuptake inhibition improve efficacy in patients with depression? A systematic review of meta-analyses and large randomised pragmatic trials. J Psychopharmacol 2013;27(8):740–58.

37. Pentel PR, Benowitz NL. Tricyclic antidepressant poisoning. Management of arrhythmias. Med Toxicol 1986;1(2):101–21.
38. Fiedorowicz JG, Swartz KL. The role of monoamine oxidase inhibitors in current psychiatric practice. J Psychiatr Pract 2004;10(4):239–48.
39. Reinhold JA, Mandos LA, Rickels K, et al. Pharmacological treatment of generalized anxiety disorder. Expert Opin Pharmacother 2011;12(16):2457–67.
40. Baldwin DS, Aitchison K, Bateson A, et al. Benzodiazepines: risks and benefits. A reconsideration. J Psychopharmacol 2013;27(11):967–71.
41. Yatham LN, Kennedy SH, Schaffer A, et al. Canadian Network for Mood and Anxiety Treatments (CANMAT) and International Society for Bipolar Disorders (ISBD) collaborative update of CANMAT guidelines for the management of patients with bipolar disorder: update 2009, vol. 11. Denmark: Blackwell Publishing Ltd; 2009. p. 225–55.
42. Cipriani A, Pretty H, Hawton K, et al. Lithium in the prevention of suicidal behavior and all-cause mortality in patients with mood disorders: a systematic review of randomized trials. Am J Psychiatry 2005;162(10):1805–19.
43. Griswold KS, Pessar LF. Management of bipolar disorder. Am Fam Physician 2000;62(6):1343–53, 1357–8.
44. Nolen WA, Weisler RH. The association of the effect of lithium in the maintenance treatment of bipolar disorder with lithium plasma levels: a post hoc analysis of a double-blind study comparing switching to lithium or placebo in patients who responded to quetiapine (Trial 144). Bipolar Disord 2012;15(1): 100–9.
45. Freeman MP, Freeman SA. Lithium: clinical considerations in internal medicine. Am J Med 2006;119(6):478–81.
46. Wingo AP, Wingo TS, Harvey PD, et al. Effects of lithium on cognitive performance: a meta-analysis. J Clin Psychiatry 2009;70(11):1588–97.
47. McKnight RF, Adida M, Budge K, et al. Lithium toxicity profile: a systematic review and meta-analysis. Lancet 2012;379(9817):721–8.
48. Grandjean EM, Aubry JM. Lithium: updated human knowledge using an evidence-based approach: part III: clinical safety. CNS Drugs 2009;23(5): 397–418.
49. Baek JH, Kinrys G, Nierenberg AA. Lithium tremor revisited: pathophysiology and treatment. Acta Psychiatr Scand 2014;129(1):17–23.
50. Lazarus JH. Lithium and thyroid. Best Pract Res Clin Endocrinol Metab 2009; 23(6):723–33.
51. Labbate LA, Fava M, Rosenbaum JF, et al. Drugs for treatment of bipolar disorders. In: handbook of psychiatric drug therapy. Philadelphia: Lippincott Williams & Wilkins; 2012.
52. Movig KL, Baumgarten R, Leufkens HG, et al. Risk factors for the development of lithium-induced polyuria. Br J Psychiatry 2003;182:319–23.
53. Cipriani A, Barbui C, Salanti G, et al. Comparative efficacy and acceptability of antimanic drugs in acute mania: a multiple-treatments meta-analysis. Lancet 2011;378(9799):1306–15.
54. Smith LA, Cornelius V, Warnock A, et al. Effectiveness of mood stabilizers and antipsychotics in the maintenance phase of bipolar disorder: a systematic review of randomized controlled trials. Bipolar Disord 2007;9(4):394–412.
55. Messenheimer J, Mullens EL, Giorgi L, et al. Safety review of adult clinical trial experience with lamotrigine. Drug Saf 1998;18(4):281–96.
56. Bowden CL, Asnis GM, Ginsberg LD, et al. Safety and tolerability of lamotrigine for bipolar disorder. Drug Saf 2004;27(3):173–84.

57. Arana A, Wentworth CE, Ayuso-Mateos JL, et al. Suicide-related events in patients treated with antiepileptic drugs. N Engl J Med 2010;363(6):542–51.
58. Gibbons RD, Hur K, Brown CH, et al. Relationship between antiepileptic drugs and suicide attempts in patients with bipolar disorder. Arch Gen Psychiatry 2009;66(12):1354–60.
59. Yatham LN. A clinical review of aripiprazole in bipolar depression and maintenance therapy of bipolar disorder. J Affect Disord 2011;128(Suppl 1):S21–8.
60. Weisler RH, Nolen WA, Neijber A, et al. Continuation of quetiapine versus switching to placebo or lithium for maintenance treatment of bipolar I disorder (Trial 144: a randomized controlled study). J Clin Psychiatry 2011;72(11):1452–64.
61. Suppes T, Hirschfeld RM, Vieta E, et al. Quetiapine for the treatment of bipolar II depression: analysis of data from two randomized, double-blind, placebo-controlled studies. World J Biol Psychiatry 2008;9(3):198–211.
62. Young AH, McElroy SL, Bauer M, et al. A double-blind, placebo-controlled study of quetiapine and lithium monotherapy in adults in the acute phase of bipolar depression (EMBOLDEN I). J Clin Psychiatry 2010;71(02):150–62.
63. McElroy SL, Weisler RH, Chang W, et al. A double-blind, placebo-controlled study of quetiapine and paroxetine as monotherapy in adults with bipolar depression (EMBOLDEN II). J Clin Psychiatry 2010;71(2):163 74.
64. Tohen M, Vieta E, Calabrese J, et al. Efficacy of olanzapine and olanzapine-fluoxetine combination in the treatment of bipolar I depression. Arch Gen Psychiatry 2003;60(11):1079–88.
65. Lima AR, Soares-Weiser K, Bacaltchuk J, et al. Benzodiazepines for neuroleptic-induced acute akathisia. Cochrane Database Syst Rev 2002;(1):CD001950.
66. Drugs for psychotic disorders. Treat Guidel Med Lett 2010;8(96):61–4 [quiz two pages following last numbered page].
67. Leucht S, Corves C, Arbter D, et al. Second-generation versus first-generation antipsychotic drugs for schizophrenia: a meta-analysis. Lancet 2009; 373(9657):31–41.
68. Buchanan RW, Kreyenbuhl J, Kelly DL, et al. The 2009 Schizophrenia PORT psychopharmacological treatment recommendations and summary statements. Schizophr Bull 2009;36(1):71–93.
69. Bleakley SM. Identifying and reducing the risk of antipsychotic drug interactions. Prog Neurol Psychiatry 2012;20–4.
70. Christian R, Saavedra L, Gaynes BN, et al. AHRQ comparative effectiveness reviews. Future research needs for first- and second-generation antipsychotics for children and young adults. Rockville (MD): Agency for Healthcare Research and Quality (US); 2012.
71. Lexicomp online. 2013.
72. Ray WA, Chung CP, Murray KT, et al. Atypical antipsychotic drugs and the risk of sudden cardiac death. N Engl J Med 2009;360(3):225–35.
73. Green AI, Lieberman JA, Hamer RM, et al. Olanzapine and haloperidol in first episode psychosis: two-year data. Schizophr Res 2006;86(1–3):234–43.
74. Adams CE. Systematic meta-review of depot antipsychotic drugs for people with schizophrenia. Br J Psychiatry 2001;179(4):290–9.
75. Haddad PM, Taylor M, Niaz OS. First-generation antipsychotic long-acting injections v. oral antipsychotics in schizophrenia: systematic review of randomised controlled trials and observational studies. Br J Psychiatry 2009;195(52):S20–8.
76. Alvir JM, Lieberman JA, Safferman AZ, et al. Clozapine-induced agranulocytosis. Incidence and risk factors in the United States. N Engl J Med 1993; 329(3):162–7.

77. Stahl SM, Shayegan DK. The psychopharmacology of ziprasidone: receptor-binding properties and real-world psychiatric practice. J Clin Psychiatry 2003; 64(Suppl 19):6–12.
78. Berman RM, Marcus RN, Swanink R, et al. The efficacy and safety of aripiprazole as adjunctive therapy in major depressive disorder: a multicenter, randomized, double-blind, placebo-controlled study. J Clin Psychiatry 2007;68(6): 843–53.
79. Mahmoud RA, Pandina GJ, Turkoz I, et al. Risperidone for treatment-refractory major depressive disorder: a randomized trial. Ann Intern Med 2007;147(9): 593–602.
80. Nelson JC, Papakostas GI. Atypical antipsychotic augmentation in major depressive disorder: a meta-analysis of placebo-controlled randomized trials. Am J Psychiatry 2009;166(9):980–91.
81. Rothschild AJ, Williamson DJ, Tohen MF, et al. A double-blind, randomized study of olanzapine and olanzapine/fluoxetine combination for major depression with psychotic features. J Clin Psychopharmacol 2004;24(4):365–73.
82. Wijkstra J, Burger H, van den Broek WW, et al. Treatment of unipolar psychotic depression: a randomized, double-blind study comparing imipramine, venlafaxine, and venlafaxine plus quetiapine. Acta Psychiatr Scand 2010;121(3):190–200.
83. Meyers BS. A double-blind randomized controlled trial of olanzapine plus sertraline vs olanzapine plus placebo for psychotic depression. Arch Gen Psychiatry 2009;66(8):838.
84. Müller-Siecheneder F, Müller MJ, Hillert A, et al. Risperidone versus haloperidol and amitriptyline in the treatment of patients with a combined psychotic and depressive syndrome. J Clin Psychopharmacol 1998;18(2):111–20.
85. Rothschild AJ, Duval SE. How long should patients with psychotic depression stay on the antipsychotic medication? J Clin Psychiatry 2003;64(4):390–6.
86. Corya SA, Williamson D, Sanger TM, et al. A randomized, double-blind comparison of olanzapine/fluoxetine combination, olanzapine, fluoxetine, and venlafaxine in treatment-resistant depression. Depress Anxiety 2006;23(6):364–72.
87. Bauer M, Pretorius HW, Constant EL, et al. Extended-release quetiapine as adjunct to an antidepressant in patients with major depressive disorder: results of a randomized, placebo-controlled, double-blind study. J Clin Psychiatry 2009;70(4):540–9.
88. Fava M, Mischoulon D, Iosifescu D, et al. A double-blind, placebo-controlled study of aripiprazole adjunctive to antidepressant therapy among depressed outpatients with inadequate response to prior antidepressant therapy (ADAPT-A Study). Psychother Psychosom 2012;81(2):87–97.
89. Cutler AJ, Montgomery SA, Feifel D, et al. Extended release quetiapine fumarate monotherapy in major depressive disorder: a placebo- and duloxetine-controlled study. J Clin Psychiatry 2009;70(4):526–39.
90. Bortnick B, El-Khalili N, Banov M, et al. Efficacy and tolerability of extended release quetiapine fumarate (quetiapine XR) monotherapy in major depressive disorder: a placebo-controlled, randomized study. J Affect Disord 2011; 128(1–2):83–94.
91. Weisler R, Joyce M, McGill L, et al. Extended release quetiapine fumarate monotherapy for major depressive disorder: results of a double-blind, randomized, placebo-controlled study. CNS Spectr 2009;14(6):299–313.
92. Cummings JL, Street J, Masterman D, et al. Efficacy of olanzapine in the treatment of psychosis in dementia with Lewy bodies. Dement Geriatr Cogn Disord 2002;13(2):67–73.

93. Mendez MF. Frontotemporal dementia: therapeutic interventions, vol. 24. Basel (Switzerland): KARGER; 2009. p. 168–78.
94. Bonelli RM, Wenning GK. Pharmacological management of Huntington's disease: an evidence-based review. Curr Pharm Des 2006;12(21):2701–20.
95. Lee PE, Gill SS, Freedman M, et al. Atypical antipsychotic drugs in the treatment of behavioural and psychological symptoms of dementia: systematic review. BMJ 2004;329(7457):75.
96. Schneider LS, Tariot PN, Dagerman KS, et al. Effectiveness of atypical antipsychotic drugs in patients with Alzheimer's disease. N Engl J Med 2006;355(15): 1525–38.
97. McDougle CJ, Epperson CN, Pelton GH, et al. A double-blind, placebo-controlled study of risperidone addition in serotonin reuptake inhibitor-refractory obsessive-compulsive disorder. Arch Gen Psychiatry 2000;57(8):794–801.
98. Carey PD, Vythilingum B, Seedat S, et al. Quetiapine augmentation of SRIs in treatment refractory obsessive-compulsive disorder: a double-blind, randomised, placebo-controlled study [ISRCTN83050762]. BMC Psychiatry 2005; 5(1):5
99. Tune LE. Risperidone for the treatment of behavioral and psychological symptoms of dementia. J Clin Psychiatry 2001;62(Suppl 21):29–32.
100. Brodaty H, Ames D, Snowdon J, et al. A randomized placebo-controlled trial of risperidone for the treatment of aggression, agitation, and psychosis of dementia. J Clin Psychiatry 2003;64(2):134–43.
101. Sink KM, Holden KF, Yaffe K. Pharmacological treatment of neuropsychiatric symptoms of dementia. JAMA 2005;293(5):596–608.
102. Lonergan E, Luxenberg J, Colford J. Haloperidol for agitation in dementia. Cochrane Database Syst Rev 2002;(2):CD002852.
103. Wang PS, Schneeweiss S, Avorn J, et al. Risk of death in elderly users of conventional vs. atypical antipsychotic medications. N Engl J Med 2005;353(22): 2335–41.
104. Gill SS, Bronskill SE, Normand SL, et al. Antipsychotic drug use and mortality in older adults with dementia. Ann Intern Med 2007;146(11):775–86.
105. Schneider LS, Dagerman KS, Insel P. Risk of death with atypical antipsychotic drug treatment for dementia. JAMA 2005;294(15):1934.
106. Ballard C, Hanney ML, Theodoulou M, et al. The dementia antipsychotic withdrawal trial (DART-AD): long-term follow-up of a randomised placebo-controlled trial. Lancet Neurol 2009;8(2):151–7.
107. Gurwitz JH, Field TS, Judge J, et al. The incidence of adverse drug events in two large academic long-term care facilities. Am J Med 2005;118(3):251–8.
108. Qato DM, Alexander GC, Conti RM, et al. Use of prescription and over-the-counter medications and dietary supplements among older adults in the United States. JAMA 2008;300(24):2867–78.
109. Kerrsens CJ, Pijnenburg YA. Vulnerability to neuroleptic side effects in frontotemporal dementia. Eur J Neurol 2008;15(2):111–2.
110. Aarsland D, Perry R, Larsen JP, et al. Neuroleptic sensitivity in Parkinson's disease and parkinsonian dementias. J Clin Psychiatry 2005;66(5):633–7.
111. Tansey KE, Guipponi M, Perroud N, et al. Genetic predictors of response to serotonergic and noradrenergic antidepressants in major depressive disorder: a genome-wide analysis of individual-level data and a meta-analysis. PLoS Med 2012;9(10):e1001326.
112. Rosenzweig-Lipson S, Beyer CE, Hughes ZA, et al. Differentiating antidepressants of the future: efficacy and safety. Pharmacol Ther 2007;113(1):134–53.

113. Allen MH, Hirschfeld RM, Wozniak PJ, et al. Linear relationship of valproate serum concentration to response and optimal serum levels for acute mania. Am J Psychiatry 2006;163(2):272–5.
114. Haymond J, Ensom MH. Does valproic acid warrant therapeutic drug monitoring in bipolar affective disorder? Ther Drug Monit 2010;32(1):19–29.
115. Tredget J, Kirov A, Kirov G. Effects of chronic lithium treatment on renal function. J Affect Disord 2010;126(3):436–40.
116. Gitlin MJ. Lithium-induced renal insufficiency. J Clin Psychopharmacol 1993; 13(4):276–9.
117. Rzany B, Correia O, Kelly JP, et al. Risk of Stevens-Johnson syndrome and toxic epidermal necrolysis during first weeks of antiepileptic therapy: a case-control study. Study Group of the International Case Control Study on Severe Cutaneous Adverse Reactions. Lancet 1999;353(9171):2190–4.
118. Spina E, Pisani F, Perucca E. Clinically significant pharmacokinetic drug interactions with carbamazepine. An update. Clin Pharm 1996;31(3):198–214.
119. DeVane CL, Nemeroff CB. Pharmaceuticals SB. 1998 Guide to psychotropic drug interactions. 1998.
120. Herzog AG, Blum AS, Farina EL, et al. Valproate and lamotrigine level variation with menstrual cycle phase and oral contraceptive use. Neurology 2009;72(10): 911–4.
121. Cipriani A, Rendell JM, Geddes JR. Haloperidol alone or in combination for acute mania. Cochrane Database Syst Rev 2006;(3):CD004362.
122. McElroy SL, Keck PE, Stanton SP, et al. A randomized comparison of divalproex oral loading versus haloperidol in the initial treatment of acute psychotic mania. J Clin Psychiatry 1996;57(4):142–6.
123. Quiroz JA, Yatham LN, Palumbo JM, et al. Risperidone long-acting injectable monotherapy in the maintenance treatment of bipolar I disorder. Biol Psychiatry 2010;68(2):156–62.
124. Weisler RH, Calabrese JR, Thase ME, et al. Efficacy of quetiapine monotherapy for the treatment of depressive episodes in bipolar I disorder: a post hoc analysis of combined results from 2 double-blind, randomized, placebo-controlled studies. J Clin Psychiatry 2008;69(5):769–82.
125. Adler LA, Peselow E, Rosenthal M, et al. A controlled comparison of the effects of propranolol, benztropine, and placebo on akathisia: an interim analysis. Psychopharmacol Bull 1993;29(2):283–6.
126. Caroff SN, Mann SC. Neuroleptic malignant syndrome. Med Clin North Am 1993;77(1):185–202.
127. Patteet L, Morrens M, Maudens KE, et al. Therapeutic drug monitoring of common antipsychotics. Ther Drug Monit 2012;34(6):629–51.
128. Laoutidis ZG, Luckhaus C. 5-HT2A receptor antagonists for the treatment of neuroleptic-induced akathisia: a systematic review and meta-analysis. Int J Neuropsychopharmacol 2013;17:1–10.
129. Marder SR, Essock SM, Miller AL, et al. Physical health monitoring of patients with schizophrenia. Am J Psychiatry 2004;161:1334–49 American Psychiatric Association.
130. Meyer JM, Koro CE. The effects of antipsychotic therapy on serum lipids: a comprehensive review. Schizophr Res 2004;70(1):1–17.
131. Leucht C, Kitzmantel M, Chua L, et al. Haloperidol versus chlorpromazine for schizophrenia. Cochrane Database Syst Rev 2008;(1):CD004278.

Office-Based Screening of Common Psychiatric Conditions

Sirisha Narayana, MD[a], Christopher J. Wong, MD[b],*

KEYWORDS

- Screening • Depression • Anxiety • Cost-effectiveness • Outcomes

KEY POINTS

- Depression and anxiety disorders are common and significant conditions in the general population.
- Multiple well-validated screening instruments exist, which may be easily administered in an outpatient setting. These include the Patient Health Questionnaire (PHQ)-9 for depression, the Generalized Anxiety Disorder (GAD)-7 for anxiety disorders, and the Primary Care Posttraumatic Stress Disorder Screen (PC-PTSD) for PTSD.
- Despite the availability of screening tools, the overall cost effectiveness of general screening for anxiety or depression is uncertain.
- Screening for depression is recommended by some preventive health guidelines, and is most likely cost-effective in the setting of high prevalence and the availability of treatment using a collaborative care model.

INTRODUCTION

Depression and anxiety disorders are common and significantly affect health worldwide. Treatment options including psychotherapy and pharmacotherapy have expanded and in many regions are easily accessible. Yet these disorders may be undertreated. Approximately 40% of patients screening positive for anxiety disorders were not receiving treatment in one study, and patients with depression were being treated only 50% of the time in another study, with disparities among ethnic/racial groups.[1,2] Screening is therefore an important element to consider in the effort to reduce the overall burden of depression and anxiety disorders. Multiple screening modalities have been

Funding sources: None.
Conflicts of interest: None.
[a] Division of General Internal Medicine, Department of Medicine, VA Puget Sound Health Care System, University of Washington, 1660 South Columbian Way, Seattle, WA 98108, USA;
[b] Division of General Internal Medicine, Department of Medicine, University of Washington, 4245 Roosevelt Way Northeast, Box 354760, Seattle, WA 98105, USA
* Corresponding author.
E-mail address: cjwong@uw.edu

http://dx.doi.org/10.1016/j.mcna.2014.06.002
0025-7125/14/$ – see front matter © 2014 Elsevier Inc. All rights reserved.
medical.theclinics.com

developed to facilitate diagnosis and treatment of common mental health disorders in the primary care setting. With the many options available, it is important to have an understanding of the strengths and limitations of these tools, the recommendations from major guidelines regarding screening, and where unanswered questions remain.

SCREENING ASYMPTOMATIC PATIENTS FOR PSYCHIATRIC CONDITIONS—GENERAL CONSIDERATIONS

Screening requires several conditions be present to be considered effective (**Table 1**).[3] First, the illness should be significantly burdensome in the population to warrant screening. The reported prevalence of depression and anxiety disorders is high, although estimates vary by location, classification, and duration (**Table 2** shows selected studies). Prevalence estimates should be interpreted with caution. Variations exist by country,[4] and because patients with psychiatric disorders may incur more physician visits, clinic-based point prevalence estimates are generally higher than those using population-based methods (eg, generalized anxiety disorder had a 3.1% prevalence in a community sample vs 7.6% in a clinic-based sample).[1,5] Second, a highly sensitive and specific screening test that is easy to administer must exist. Third, the illness should be identified by screening at a treatable stage or a stage in which early treatment is more effective than later treatment. The concept of early treatment is more complex with psychiatric illnesses: by definition patients are symptomatic, but the natural history of common psychiatric conditions is varied; they may have potentially lifelong

Table 1 Conceptual framework for psychiatric disease screening		
Criteria	**Nonpsychiatry Examples**	**Comparison with Psychiatric Disease Screening**
Condition causes significant burden in the population	Rare but severe: phenylketonuria in newborns Common and causing morbidity: diabetes, hypertension	Similar to diabetes and hypertension, depression and anxiety disorders are common (see **Table 2**) and cause substantial morbidity
An easy-to-administer, effective screening test exists	Blood pressure Fasting glucose or A1c	Screening tools are readily available, generally consist of questionnaires
Early treatment is more effective than later treatment	Cancer screening: goal is to identify disease at an earlier stage at which treatment is more effective Diabetes: goal is to identify disease before it is symptomatic to initiate treatment and prevent complications	In contrast, by definition there is no asymptomatic stage for depression and anxiety disorders Varied natural history: waxing/waning, episodic/self-limited, lifelong
Benefits of screening tests and subsequent treatment outweigh potential harms, at acceptable cost	Mammography: Harms include radiation, follow-up imaging, biopsies, worry. Optimal target population and interval still debated	Harms of screening tools themselves generally minimal; harms and costs are associated with subsequent treatment

Table 2 Prevalence of common psychiatric disorders		
	12-mo Prevalence[5] (%)	Lifetime Prevalence[8] (%)
Any mood disorder[a]	9.5	20.8
Major depressive disorder	6.7	16.6
Any anxiety disorder[b]	18.1	28.8
Generalized anxiety disorder	3.1	5.7
PTSD	3.5	6.8
ADHD	4.1	8.1

Abbreviation: ADHD, attention-deficit and hyperactivity disorder.
[a] Includes major depressive disorder, dysthymia, and bipolar I and II disorders.
[b] Includes panic disorder, agoraphobia without panic, specific phobia, social phobia, generalized anxiety disorder, obsessive-compulsive disorder, separation anxiety disorder. Posttraumatic stress disorder subtracted from the published total because it is now classified as a trauma- and stressor-related disorder.

conditions such as generalized anxiety disorder, with waxing and waning severity, or episodic with a self-limited course as with major depressive disorder. Fourth, the screening tests and treatment must have clinically meaningful benefits that outweigh potential harms to a patient at an acceptable cost to society. For the purposes of this review, the third and fourth criteria are considered together as general effectiveness.

Case Definitions

Unless specified otherwise, this review discusses screening tools validated against structured diagnostic interviews. Most of the tools described later were tested against the Diagnostic and Statistical Manual of Mental Disorders (DSM)-III, the DSM-IV, or World Health Organization (WHO) definitions. The newer DMS-V diagnostic criteria for a major depressive episode and generalized anxiety disorder have only minor differences compared with those of DSM-IV, not expected to substantially affect the performance of these measures.[6,7]

DEPRESSION
Burden of Disease

The 12-month prevalence of major depressive disorder in the United States is estimated at 6.7%, and the lifetime prevalence of any mood disorder is approximately 20%.[5,8] Depression is estimated as the fourth leading cause of disability adjusted life years worldwide.[4]

Screening Tools

General population
Many screening tools exist for depressive disorders (**Table 3**). Selected tools are discussed below.

PHQ-9 and PHQ-2 The PHQ-9 evolved from the full Primary Care Evaluation of Mental Disorders (PRIME-MD) instrument developed in the early 1990s to diagnose depression, anxiety, somatoform disorder, and alcohol and eating disorders.[9] The PRIME-MD necessitated significant investment of physician-patient time (>11 minutes) and led to the shorter PHQ,[10] and subsequently the PHQ-9, the 9-item depression module from the full PHQ (**Box 1**). It is scored 0 to 27, with a score of 10 or more indicating a possible depressive disorder. Scores of 5, 10, 15, and 20 represented mild, moderate,

Table 3
Selected tools and considerations for depression screening

Population	Tools	Description
General population/primary care	PHQ-9 PHQ-2 Others	PHQ-9 and PHQ-2 freely available Screening recommended by USPSTF if treatment resources available
Veterans	PHQ-9 PHQ-2	The Veterans Affairs administration recommends yearly screening of veterans for depression using the PHQ-2[66] with follow-up as needed with PHQ-9 and a full assessment; and those at higher risk of developing depression (patients with hepatitis C beginning interferon treatment or patients post-MI) be given the PHQ-9 when depression is suspected Use caution in screening patients older than 75 y because instruments may not perform as well as between the ages of 65 and 75 y[67]
Medical comorbidities	Various, including PHQ-9, PHQ-2, HADS, BDI, Montgomery and Asberg Depression Rating Scale, others	Increased rates of depression in patients with central nervous system disease, cardiovascular disease, and malignancy[68-71] Up to 20% of patients with myocardial infarction meet DSM-IV criteria for major depression. The American Heart Association advocates for screening for depression after MI. Approximately half of post-MI depression resolves without treatment. Some evidence of treatment efficacy in patients poststroke, post-MI[68-75] The PHQ-9 and HADS have been studied in patients with coronary disease and are comparable in effectiveness for screening[76] The PHQ-9 has been used in multiple medical settings, including rheumatology, ophthalmology, and spinal cord injury[77]
Elderly	PHQ-9 PHQ-2 GDS	GDS score >5: sensitivity 0.92, specificity 0.81 for major depression
Addiction	PHQ-9, others	Consider screening in patients with substance use disorders
Psychiatric comorbidities	PHQ-9, others	Consider screening in patients with other psychiatric conditions, including anxiety disorders and PTSD

Abbreviations: GDS, Geriatric Depression Scale; HADS, Hospital Anxiety and Depression Scale; MI, myocardial infarction.

Box 1
Patient health questionnaire-9

Over the Last 2 wk, How Often Have You Been Bothered by Any of the Following Problems?	Not At all	Several Days	More Than Half the Days	Nearly Every Day
1. Little interest or pleasure in doing things	0	1	2	3
2. Feeling down, depressed, or hopeless	0	1	2	3
3. Trouble falling or staying asleep, or sleeping too much	0	1	2	3
4. Feeling tired or having little energy	0	1	2	3
5. Poor appetite or overeating	0	1	2	3
6. Feeling bad about yourself — or that you are a failure or have let yourself or your family down	0	1	2	3
7. Trouble concentrating on things, such as reading the newspaper or watching television	0	1	2	3
8. Moving or speaking so slowly that other people could have noticed? Or the opposite — being so fidgety or restless that you have been moving around a lot more than usual	0	1	2	3
9. Thoughts that you would be better off dead or of hurting yourself in some way	0	1	2	3
	0 +	_____ +	_____ +	_____
			=Total Score:	_____

If you checked off any problems, how difficult have these problems made it for you to do your work, take care of things at home, or get along with other people?

Not difficult at all   Somewhat difficult   Very difficult   Extremely difficult

From The Patient Health Questionnaire (PHQ) Screeners. Available at: http://www.phqscreeners.com/overview.aspx?Screener=02_PHQ-9. Accessed May 1, 2014.

---

moderately severe, and severe depression, respectively. To make the diagnosis of major depression, at least one of the first two questions must score a two or greater; this includes anhedonia and feelings of low mood/depression. The PHQ-9 module aligns closely with the DSM-IV diagnosis of depression and accordingly includes a question of whether symptoms impair functioning. At a cutoff score of 10, the PHQ-9 was found to have 0.88 sensitivity and specificity, and a likelihood ratio of 7.1, in the population studied (mean age 30–40 years, mostly white women with few medical comorbidities).[11] The validity of the PHQ-9 has been further demonstrated in a general population.[12] Subsequent meta-analyses confirmed high sensitivity of the PHQ-9, although one study did demonstrate a lower specificity of 0.77, possibly due to a lower prevalence of depression in the population studied.[13] Despite the heterogeneity of the studies in terms of settings (community, primary care, and hospital specialties), the properties of the PHQ-9 for major depression were consistent across this range.[14] The PHQ-2 consists of only the first 2 items of the PHQ-9; a PHQ-2 score of 3 or more has a sensitivity of 0.83 and a specificity of 0.92 for major depression.[15] The increased specificity of the PHQ-2 may be better for screening larger populations. However, a comparison of these 2 instruments has not yet been conducted. In addition, the PHQ-9 may also be used to monitor treatment response.

Other scales The Beck Depression Inventory for Primary Care is a 7-item scale adapted from the 21-item Beck Depression Inventory (BDI). It has a 0.97 sensitivity and 0.99 specificity for a score of 4 or more but requires a license fee for use.[16] The World Health Organization Five is a 5-item scale that was found to be slightly more sensitive but less specific than the brief PHQ in a study of 400 primary care patients.[17] There are increasing numbers of studies of its use in different populations, and it is also freely available online in all languages. The Mental Health Inventory is a 5-item mental health tool that was used as a comparison for the validity of the PHQ, but it is not specific for depression.[11] Single-question screening methods have a low sensitivity of 0.32 but a high specificity of 0.97 and thus cannot be relied on as an effective screening tool.[18]

Comparisons of the various screening instruments have been conducted. In 38 studies involving 32,000 patients in primary care settings, depression instruments were found to be comparably effective (this included PHQ-9, BDI, and the Geriatric Depression Screen, among others) with a median likelihood ratio positive of 3.3 and were quick to use (administration times ranged from <2 to 6 minutes).[19,20]

Effectiveness of screening for depression

Data are conflicting as to whether general population– or primary care–based screening leads to improved patient outcomes. A systematic review of randomized trials of screening questionnaires administered by research assistants did not show any change in physician diagnoses or interventions; these studies used the BDI, General Health Questionnaire, and the Zung Self-Rating Depression Scale.[21] A more recent review for the US Preventive Services Task Force (USPSTF) found that there was only one fair-quality randomized controlled trial that directly assessed whether screening for depression among adults in primary care reduces morbidity or mortality and showed mixed results.[22,23] Based on data from four different trials, screening was thought to be effective when ancillary staff was involved in depression care and extra efforts were made to enroll patients in specialty mental health treatment.[22] A Cochrane review in 2005 concluded that screening and case-finding instruments, when administered without any additional care structure, had little impact on the overall recognition rates of depression, management of depression (or intervention with antidepressants), and outcomes from depression.[24] No evidence was found to address the harms of screening specifically. Potential harms include stigma and psychological effects of false-positive results of diagnoses and unnecessary treatment with and exposure to side effects of antidepressant medications. Some studies, but not all, showed concern for a possible increase in upper gastrointestinal bleeding in older adults when taking selective serotonin reuptake inhibitors (SSRIs) and nonsteroidal antiinflammatory medications together.[22] There is no definitive evidence that suicidal behavior increases with second-generation SSRIs, although there is evidence that there is increased risk under the age of 25 years and decreased risk over the age of 65 years.[22]

Screening for depression was found to be cost-effective only in settings of high prevalence of depression and high treatment and remission rates. Costs were high for annual screening but were lower for screening every 5 years and only truly cost-effective for one-time screening.[25] Pearls for depression screening are listed in **Box 2**.

ANXIETY DISORDERS
Burden of Disease

Anxiety disorders have a 12-month prevalence of 18% and a lifetime prevalence as high as 29% (see **Table 2**).[5,8] Morbidity includes a high degree of interference with life activities; increased number of physician visits, especially if there are somatic symptoms; and decreased functional status.[1]

Box 2
Screening for depression: pearls

1. There is reasonable evidence to support screening general primary care populations for depression.

2. Although there are many published screening tools for depression, the PHQ-9 and the PHQ-2 are good choices because of their good operating characteristics, free availability, and ease of use for patient self-administration.

3. A cutoff score of 10 or more for the PHQ-9 (sensitivity and specificity 0.88) and 3 or more for the PHQ-2 (sensitivity 0.83, specificity 0.92) is reasonable in the general population. The PHQ-2 may be favored if time of administration or length of a questionnaire is a concern.

4. Efficacy is likely increased with access to treatment, including collaborative care models where available.

5. Consider assessment for suicidality and bipolar disorder for confirmed diagnoses.

6. Consider comorbid assessment for anxiety disorders, either after diagnosis of depression or as part of the initial screening strategy.

7. Consider screening in selected populations, include those with cardiovascular disease such as poststroke and post–myocardial infarction, central nervous system disease, chronic pain, and cancer.

Screening Tools

Beck anxiety inventory

Selected tools and considerations are listed in **Table 4**. The Beck Anxiety Inventory (BAI) is a 21-item, patient-completed questionnaire, developed to discriminate anxiety disorders from depressive disorders in an outpatient psychiatric clinic.[26] Its questions primarily report somatic symptoms. An abbreviated version, the Beck Anxiety Inventory-Primary Care (BAI-PC), has subsequently been developed, and, although

Table 4
Selected tools and considerations for screening for anxiety disorders

Population	Tools	Description
General population/ primary care	GAD-7 GAD-2	GAD-7 and GAD-2 freely available
Medical comorbidities	GAD-7, others	Consider assessment for chronic somatic symptoms such as headache syndromes, chronic pain, gastrointestinal disorders Somatic symptoms such as gastrointestinal symptoms have been found to have a high prevalence of anxiety disorders in primary care[78,79]
Addiction	GAD-7, GAD-2	Perform better as general screens for anxiety disorders than for GAD specifically[80]
Elderly	GAD-7 Geriatric Anxiety Inventory Short Form (GAI-SF)	Consider using a lower cutoff score of 5–7 if using the GAD-7 GAI-SF: sensitivity 0.75, specificity 0.84
Psychiatric comorbidities	GAD-7, others	Consider screening for those with depressive disorders, other anxiety spectrum disorders, PTSD

a follow-up study has been completed, it has not been extensively retested using diagnostic interviews as the gold standard.[27,28]

Hospital anxiety and depression scale

Hospital anxiety and depression scale (HADS) was developed to screen medical patients for psychiatric conditions. Despite its name, it has also been validated in primary care populations. The optimal cutoff score for the anxiety subscale (HADS-A) is approximately 8, with a sensitivity and specificity in the 0.70 to 0.90 range.[29]

Generalized anxiety disorder-7

GAD-7 is another patient-completed questionnaire (**Box 3**).[30] Unlike the BAI, its criteria closely mirror the DSM-IV definition of generalized anxiety disorder, with the exception that it asks for a symptom report for the prior 2 weeks rather than for 6 months. As would be expected, using higher cutoffs of the GAD-7 yields lower sensitivity but higher specificity. A follow-up study found that it also performed well in identifying PTSD, panic disorder, and social anxiety disorder, with a sensitivity of 0.80 and a specificity of 0.76 at a cutoff of 7; for GAD alone, a cutoff score of 10 maintained sensitivity while improving specificity.[1] This tool has been shortened further to the GAD-2, a 2-item questionnaire for which a score of 3 has a sensitivity of 0.86 and a specificity of 0.83 for generalized anxiety disorder.[1]

Multistage screening tools

The Symptom Driven Diagnostic System–Primary Care (SDDS-PC) was developed as a 16-item, patient-completed screening tool for multiple mental health disorders in primary care.[31] In the initial study, it had 0.85 sensitivity and 0.60 specificity for generalized anxiety disorder, with lower sensitivity and higher specificity for panic disorder.[31] Although the performance of SDDS-PC is comparable with that of GAD-7 as an initial screen, it was designed to necessitate nurse or physician follow-up using a proprietary assessment module. Similarly, the PRIME-MD tool, as discussed earlier for

---

Box 3
Generalized anxiety disorder-7

Over the Last 2 wk, How Often Have You Been Bothered by the Following Problems?	Not At All	Several Days	More Than Half the Days	Nearly Every Day
1. Feeling nervous, anxious or on edge	0	1	2	3
2. Not being able to stop or control worrying	0	1	2	3
3. Worrying too much about different things	0	1	2	3
4. Trouble relaxing	0	1	2	3
5. Being so restless that it is hard to sit still	0	1	2	3
6. Becoming easily annoyed or irritable	0	1	2	3
7. Feeling afraid as if something awful might happen	0	1	2	3
	0 +	_____ +	_____ +	_____
				=Total Score: _____

If you checked off any problems, how difficult have these problems made it for you to do your work, take care of things at home, or get along with other people?

Not difficult at all   Somewhat difficult   Very difficult   Extremely difficult

From The Patient Health Questionnaire (PHQ) Screeners. Available at: http://www. phqscreeners.com/overview.aspx?Screener=03_GAD-7.

depression, also contains a screen for anxiety disorders but was designed to be used with additional modules.[9] The PRIME-MD later evolved into the PHQ and then the shorter PHQ-9 and GAD-7. Neither SDDS-PC nor PRIME-MD is freely available for routine use, and the efficacy of using only the screening portion of such tools for anxiety disorders in a real-world setting is unknown.

Effectiveness of Screening for Anxiety

There are few cost-benefit studies available to guide implementation of screening of anxiety and depression. Small ambulatory studies showed that screening for anxiety is feasible and led to increased diagnoses even in training clinics but lacked cost-effectiveness data.[32] The collaborative care model is likely an effective intervention for both depression and anxiety,[33] with data supporting cost-effectiveness for depression,[34] equivocal results for panic disorder,[35] but lacking adequate studies for other anxiety disorders. Cost-effectiveness data are needed, as screening may identify illness of lesser severity, whereas more severe illnesses may present clinically without the need for screening. The shorter screening tests such as the PHQ-9 and GAD-7 only take minutes for the patient to complete and the provider to review, and its perceived utility is acceptable to patients.[10] Pearls for anxiety disorder screening are shown in **Box 4**.

OTHER COMMON PSYCHIATRIC CONDITIONS

Common mental health conditions encountered in the primary care office setting, including the neurodevelopmental disorder adult attention-deficit and hyperactivity disorder (ADHD) and the trauma-related disorder PTSD, are briefly discussed in the following sections. Substance use disorder (formerly substance use and dependence in DMS-IV) is not covered in this review.

ADHD
Burden of Disease

ADHD was originally thought to be primarily a pediatric disorder, whereas 40% to 60% of children with ADHD have symptoms that persist into adulthood.[36,37] ADHD is thought to have a prevalence of approximately 4% in the adult population (see **Table 2**).[5] In adulthood, symptoms of hyperactivity are less pronounced compared

---

Box 4
Screening for anxiety disorders: pearls

1. Anxiety disorders are widely prevalent, and there are freely available screening tools for use in primary care settings.

2. Despite wide prevalence and availability of proven screening tools, there is no conclusive evidence to support cost-effectiveness of screening general populations for anxiety disorders.

3. The GAD-7, using a cutoff of 10 or more, is a reasonable screen for generalized anxiety disorder (sensitivity 0.89, specificity 0.82). If a shorter screen is desired, the 2-item GAD-2 at a cutoff of 3 or more is an option (sensitivity 0.86, specificity 0.83).

4. The GAD-7 also screens for other disorders, including panic disorder and PTSD; it is critical to follow up this screening tool with an accurate clinical assessment.

5. Although not specifically screening, consider assessment for anxiety disorders in patients presenting with unexplained somatic symptoms.

6. Consider screening in patients with other psychiatric conditions, including depression and PTSD, as well as substance use disorders.

with those of inattention.[37] The DSM-V diagnosis of ADHD emphasizes pervasive symptoms of inattention, hyperactivity, and impulsivity affecting least 2 domains of daily life (eg, work and home).[6] Diagnosis is based on clinical evaluation, which should include assessment of other psychiatric illnesses and substance abuse, impact of these symptoms on daily functioning, and a developmental history.

Screening Tools

Several self-reporting measures exist for ADHD, but none are sufficient for diagnosis alone. The New York University ADHD Program advocates the use of Adult Self-Report Scale V1.1 from WHO. It consists of a total of 18 questions that correlate to DSM diagnostic criteria for ADHD, and the screener portion has 6 questions that patients can self-report. In a small study of 154 respondents, the screener questions were found to have a sensitivity of 0.69 and a specificity of 1.0, with an accuracy of 98%.[38] Subsequent validity studies showed strong concordance with clinician diagnoses.[39,40]

The Wender Utah Rating Scale (WURS) was originally found to have a sensitivity of 0.86, but subsequent studies showed a sensitivity of 0.72 and a specificity of 0.58, suggesting that it misclassifies about half of those without ADHD.[41,42] The Connors' Adult ADHD Rating Scales (CAARS) has separate scales for the patient and for completion by an observer such as a spouse, friend, or parent, so that physicians can gather corroborative data. Each scale has a screening, short, and long form. The Current Symptoms Scale asks about adult patients' behaviors in the last 6 months. It also has a separate scale for patients and for an observer. It is unclear whether any of these scales are superior.[43] In a 2011 systematic review that included 14 scales for ADHD, CAARS and WURS had the best psychometric properties. Firm conclusions were limited because of the poor quality of many of the studies identified.[44]

Effectiveness of screening for ADHD

More data are needed to clarify the value of screening for ADHD and the best tool for screening. Controversy exists about the diagnosis given that the symptoms of ADHD are challenging to differentiate from those of other psychiatric diagnoses or substance abuse. The Adult Self-Report Scale Screener shows considerable promise, and physicians should be alerted to its potential and for clinical signs of ADHD in their patients (Box 5).

POSTTRAUMATIC STRESS DISORDER
Burden of Disease

The overall lifetime prevalence of PTSD is approximately 7%,[8] higher in veterans[45] and other risk groups. PTSD is associated with functional impairment, increased mental health care utilization, and increased psychiatric comorbidities.[45]

Box 5
Screening for ADHD: pearls

1. ADHD is now considered a neurodevelopmental disorder in the DSM-V, with a prevalence of approximately 4% in adults.

2. There are several screening tools published for ADHD for patient or caregiver/observer report. The Adult Self-Report Scale V1.1 from the World Health Organization is freely available.

3. Although there are available tools for screening for ADHD, there is not sufficient evidence with regard to burden of illness or cost-effectiveness to support screening general populations.

Screening Tools

Screening tools for conditions such as generalized anxiety disorder may also be effective at screening for PTSD. For the office-based setting, if screening for anxiety disorders is performed, then use of the GAD-7 is a reasonable option. There are numerous screening tools for PTSD specifically, with validation in different populations, including at-risk groups such as veterans. The US Department of Veterans Affairs endorses several screening tools, including the BAI-PC, PC-PTSD, Short Form of the PTSD Checklist–Civilian Version (PCL-C), Short Screening Scale for Short Post-Traumatic Stress Disorder Rating Interview (PTSD), Startle, Physiological arousal, Anger, and Numbness (SPAN), Short Post-Traumatic Stress Disorder Rating Interview (SPRINT), and the Trauma Screening Questionnaire.[46] Of these, the 4-item PC-PTSD (**Box 6**) is available online through the US Department of Veterans Affairs Web site[47] and has been widely used in the veterans affairs (VA) system, whereas the other tools are either proprietary or require request from the researchers.

The PC-PTSD has been validated in the primary care setting at the VA with a sensitivity of 0.78 and specificity of 0.87 at a recommended cutoff of 3 (out of 4).[48] Alternatively, there are PTSD-specific screens that are available online that patients may complete on their own. The VA patient portal uses a version of the 17-item PCL specific for the veteran population.[49] Each question has a 5-point Likert scale ranging from not at all to extremely for possible PTSD symptoms. The recommended cutoff ranges from 30 to 50, depending on the population studied and the

---

Box 6
Primary care PTSD screen

Description

The PC-PTSD is a 4-item screen that was designed for use in primary care and other medical settings and is currently used to screen for PTSD in veterans at the VA. The screen includes an introductory sentence to cue respondents to traumatic events. The authors suggest that in most circumstances the results of the PC-PTSD should be considered "positive" if a patient answers "yes" to any 3 items. Those screening positive should then be assessed with a structured interview for PTSD. The screen does not include a list of potentially traumatic events.

Scale

Instructions:
In your life, have you ever had any experience that was so frightening, horrible, or upsetting that, in the past month, you:

1. Have had nightmares about it or thought about it when you did not want to?
   YES/NO

2. Tried hard not to think about it or went out of your way to avoid situations that reminded you of it?
   YES/NO

3. Were constantly on guard, watchful, or easily startled?
   YES/NO

4. Felt numb or detached from others, activities, or your surroundings?
   YES/NO

Current research suggests that the results of the PC-PTSD should be considered "positive" if a patient answers "yes" to any three items.

From Prins A, Ouimette P, Kimerling R, et al. The primary care PTSD screen (PC–PTSD): development and operating characteristics. Prim Care Psych 2004;9(1):9–14.

gold standard used to evaluate it, although a repeat study found that a cutoff of 60 maximized diagnostic efficiency (percentage of cases correctly diagnosed), albeit at a low sensitivity of 0.56 and a specificity of 0.92.[50] For screening purposes, if identifying the greatest percentage of cases is prioritized, a lower cutoff may be considered.

Effectiveness of screening for PTSD

Use of PTSD screens in general primary care populations outside the VA setting is less certain. Unlike the VA system, many primary care systems may not have access to specialized PTSD treatment; screening may not be desired if there is not readily available and effective treatment. These tools (PC-PTSD, PCL) may be considered if the clinical presentation includes symptoms suggestive of PTSD, although such use would not be strictly screening. Although some online Web sites use the 17-item questionnaire, the 4-item PC-PTSD may be a better initial screen for an in-office setting, especially if it would take additional time to complete in conjunction with screens for other conditions (**Box 7**).

LIMITATIONS OF EXISTING EVIDENCE

Despite the burden of disease and the availability of effective screening tools, there are still significant considerations in implementing these tools in clinical practice.

Optimal Cutoffs for Screening Tools

Most questionnaire-based screening tools use a quantitative scoring system. Operating characteristics such as the area under the curve vary depending on the population studied and the gold standard used and accordingly affect the optimal cutoff score. In addition, there is a value judgment in defining the optimal cutoff score. If one places a priority on sensitivity, assuming there is a readily available way to identify true diagnoses, then one would seek a sensitivity more than 0.9 and accept a lower specificity; the positive likelihood ratio of a positive result at such a cutoff would generally be low. Conversely, one may attempt to optimize both the sensitivity and specificity, accepting a lower sensitivity to preserve a higher specificity. Using the GAD-7 as an example, a cutoff score of 5 for screening of generalized anxiety disorder alone yields a sensitivity of 0.97 and a specificity of 0.57, whereas the suggested cutoff score of 10 still preserves reasonable sensitivity of 0.89 but improves the specificity markedly to 0.82. Thus, it is straightforward to recommend a cutoff score of 10; the small decrement in sensitivity, still at nearly 0.90, is an acceptable trade-off to improve the specificity to more than 0.80. However, if one uses the GAD-7 as a combined screen for generalized anxiety disorder, panic disorder, social anxiety disorder, and

---

Box 7
Screening for PTSD: pearls

1. PTSD has a significant burden and there are freely available screening tools.

2. Despite its prevalence, the best evidence for testing and most common strategies use a targeted screening approach.

3. Screening is likely most effective when performed where there are adequate resources for treatment of PTSD.

4. The PC-PTSD is a short, 4-item, freely available screening tool that has a sensitivity of 0.78 and specificity of 0.87 at a recommended cutoff of 3/4, best studied in veterans.

PTSD, the choice of cutoff is a bit more difficult; the cutoff score of 5 has a 0.90 sensitivity and 0.63 specificity, but increasing the cutoff score to 10 markedly diminished the sensitivity to 0.68 while increasing the specificity to 0.88. Thus, if one uses the GAD-7 as a screen for these multiple anxiety spectrum conditions, a midrange cutoff of 7 (sensitivity 0.80, specificity 0.76) might be more reasonable. The cutoff score to be used depends on the intended clinical use.

Funding Source

Many screening tool studies, including the PRIME-MD (and subsequently the PHQ), GAD-7, SDDS-PC, and PDI-4, were developed in conjunction with pharmaceutical companies or had researchers with pharmaceutical company relationships, raising the possibility of bias toward increased diagnoses that would lead to increased drug therapy.

Screening for One Diagnosis or More

There remains a question as to whether screening tools are more useful to assess for a single diagnosis or whether it is better to screen for multiple diagnoses at once. Even screens for one type of disorder have been found to be effective as screens for other diagnoses, thus rendering a decreased specificity. The BAI, for example, was designed to distinguish between depression and anxiety but in other studies tested positive for both; similarly, a depression scale, the Center for Epidemiologic Studies Depression Scale (CES-D), tested positive for patients with anxiety.[51] The GAD-7 was developed to screen for generalized anxiety disorder, but it also could be used to simultaneously screen for panic disorder, social anxiety disorder, and PTSD. In addition to the effect screening multiple diagnoses might have on operating characteristics, one must also consider the time it takes to complete the screening tools, as well as the clinical capabilities to treat all the diagnoses effectively. Broader screens such as the PDI-4, a self-completed 17-item screening tool that screens for major depressive episode, generalized anxiety disorder, ADHD, and bipolar affective disorder type 1, and the My Mood Monitor checklist, which screens for depression, bipolar spectrum disorders, and anxiety disorders, may prove useful pending further validation studies.[52,53]

THE ELDERLY

Late-life depression is often underdiagnosed and subsequently undertreated. Well-studied tools in the geriatric population include the PHQ-9 and the 15-item Geriatric Depression Scale (GDS). In a study of persons 60 years or older from primary care practices, scores of greater than 5 on the GDS had a sensitivity of 0.92 and a specificity of 0.81 for major depression.[54] In elderly primary care patients, the PHQ-9 performed comparably to the PHQ-2 and the GDS for detecting major depression. The PHQ-9 performed comparably regardless of gender or race and was somewhat better for younger elders and for those with fewer chronic illnesses.[55] The PHQ-2 was also validated in 8000 adults older than 65 years.[56] Overall, any of these scales perform well for screening for depression in the elderly (**Table 3**).

Studies of anxiety screening tools tended to have younger patients, however, and there is some evidence that geriatric populations may require different screening cutoffs or instruments. In the elderly, anxiety disorders may have overlapping symptoms of chronic medical conditions, and cognitive impairment may further complicate accurate identification. In elderly patients, for example, the GAD-7 may require a lower cutoff of 5 to improve sensitivity while maintaining specificity.[57] Alternatively, other assessment tools such as the Geriatric Anxiety Inventory (GAI) and its 5-item short-ened version (GAI-SF) have been validated against DSM-IV diagnostic interviews with a sensitivity of 0.75 and specificity of 0.84 (see **Table 4**).[58,59]

TARGETED VERSUS GENERAL SCREENING

Should these screening tools be used for the general population, for targeted high-risk groups, or both? Depression and anxiety disorders are of sufficient prevalence that general primary care screening would seem reasonable, despite concerns of uncer-tainty regarding definitive cost-benefit results. Comorbid psychiatric illness is com-mon both concurrently as well as associated with increased likelihood of another disorder arising later in life.[60,61] Thus, there is a rationale either to screen the general population for both depressive disorders and anxiety spectrum disorders simulta-neously or to screen for the other if one disorder is diagnosed.

Medical conditions have been associated with both depression and anxiety. Certain populations have demonstrated high rates of depression in association with medical comorbidities such as cardiovascular diseases or common social risk factors such as in veterans (see **Table 3**). Anxiety disorders may have higher prevalence in patients with other medical or psychiatric diagnoses, and there is evidence of efficacy of screening in these populations (see **Table 4**). For anxiety disorders especially, testing in these populations is more problematic with regard to screening, as the somatic symptoms may be one of the primary manifestations of an underlying anxiety or depression spectrum disorder rather than a comorbidity—whether to call this scre-ening may be merely semantic.

Finally, in the current Internet age, patients may complete screening tests online by their own initiative or prompted by insurance companies or employers and bring the results to the practitioner to review. In such settings, however, providers should clarify whether the patient completed the tool as a screen or because of a concern regarding symptoms.

NOVEL AND ALTERNATIVE SCREENING MODALITIES

In addition to traditional screening with fixed-length questionnaires given in an office-based setting, there has been development of newer techniques (**Table 5**), including computerized, adaptive testing using proprietary algorithms, screening outside of the clinic using screening tools on the Internet, or by telephone inter-view. Although promising, these methodologies continue to require further study and refinement.

RECOMMENDATIONS
General Recommendations

It is essential that a screening tool be recognized as just that, a screening process for which a positive test is not synonymous with a diagnosis but which requires additional evaluation by a trained clinician (**Box 8**). Although there are no precise data to clarify the optimal time to administer these screening tests, or in whom, preventative health visits provide an opportune time to administer screening in the general population, with consideration of targeted screening as other diagnoses arise. In most cases, these tests may be self-administered. Office staff may give these screening tools to patients with the intention to complete the test while in an appointment. Some of the screening tools have translations in multiple languages. These tests could be administered as part of a more comprehensive questionnaire that includes

Table 5
Newer methods for screening of common psychiatric conditions

Tool	Description	Potential Uses	Limitations
Computerized adaptive testing	Computer-based questions ask follow-up questions depending on the response. Duration may vary depending on assessed accuracy of diagnosis	Internet-based screening in the office or at home	Need for computer, language capabilities, not widely available
Telephone	Using same screening tools, but administered by phone	Outreach to patients with barriers to coming in to the office	Patients would still need to be seen to clarify diagnosis and to start treatment; uncertain utilization of recourses
Internet-based screening	Could be done by clinic, by Internet at large (eg, advocacy or nonprofit sites, but could also be from pharmaceutical companies), or by insurance companies	Patient completed, may be more efficient for patient to complete at home	Less data for real-world use and how to integrate into clinical setting

nonpsychiatric conditions, although it is uncertain whether that strategy will affect accuracy or completion rates of the psychiatric screening tool.

Depression Screening

Given inconclusive data on efficacy and cost-effectiveness, official recommendations for screening for depression differ widely. Data suggest that screening is most effective in a collaborative care model (ie, integrated care with a medical doctor, case manager, and mental health specialist).[33] Although the effectiveness of

Box 8
Screening for psychiatric conditions: general pearls

1. Published properties (sensitivity, specificity) of screening tools depend on the population studied and may be different in clinical practice.

2. Positive test results are not synonymous with a diagnosis. Positive screen results must be followed by clinical assessment for a diagnosis, as only a portion of patients testing positive have a confirmed diagnosis.

3. Increasingly, these tools are able to be self-administered by patients, either in a clinical encounter or outside the office.

4. As many of these tools are widely available on the Internet, patients may find these tools themselves and bring results to the attention of their providers.

5. The optimal time for and method of screening is unknown. Preventive health visits represent an opportunity to administer screening tests.

6. Consider targeted screening depending on the condition and the populations represented in a given clinical practice.

screening without ancillary staff support is unclear, screening with the tools currently available requires little investment on the part of the practitioner and confers minimal immediate harm to patients themselves. Therefore, it is reasonable to screen for depression in the primary care setting, although it is best when ancillary support staff and specialist referral are available. The most readily usable screening tool is likely the PHQ-9 given its free availability, brief administration time, correlation with the DSM-IV criteria, and ability to track progress. Many current electronic systems, such as that in the Veterans Administration, use the PHQ-2 as a preliminary screen/clinical reminder, which, if positive, prompts the physician or care provider to complete a PHQ-9 or conduct a more thorough clinical interview. One may consider screening in populations such as veterans, those with postmyocardial infarction, poststroke, selected other medical conditions, and those with comorbid psychiatric illness (see **Table 3**). Positive diagnoses on further assessment should be assessed for suicidality, and screening for bipolar disorder should also be considered (screening for bipolar disorder specifically is not reviewed in this article) (see **Box 2**).

Recommendations from major organizations

The USPSTF recommends routine depression screening for all average-risk patients when there is sufficient staff-assisted depression care supports in place to ensure proper diagnosis, treatment, and follow-up (**Table 6**).[62] In contrast, because of concerns for a high rate of false-positive diagnoses and harms of unnecessary treatment and absence of high-quality evidence for the effectiveness of screening for depression, the Canadian Task Force on Preventative Health Care (CTFPHC) revised its guidelines in 2013 and recommend against routine screening of average-risk and increased-risk individuals (although this is a weak recommendation based on very-low-quality evidence).[63] Neither the USPSTF nor the CTFPHC make any recommendations on which screening test to use. The United Kingdom National Institute for Health and Clinical Excellence (NICE) guidelines suggest a targeted approach, screening only those individuals at risk for depression (including those with a history of depression or a chronic physical health problem with functional impairment), using the 2 PHQ-2 questions for screening.[64]

Anxiety Screening

Although conclusive cost-effectiveness is lacking, given the prevalence of the disease, the available treatment, and the multitude of screening tools, it is reasonable to consider screening for anxiety disorders in the office-based setting. Owing to its ease of administration, good performance characteristics, and free distribution, the GAD-7 is a reasonable first screening tool for anxiety disorders in the primary care setting. In addition to considering use at preventive health visits, one may consider screening as an adjunctive tool in patients with depression, addiction, and unexplained somatic symptoms, with the caution that this strategy of use, while effective at identifying cases, is not well validated with respect to cost-effectiveness and patient outcomes. The ideal cutoff score for GAD-7 for generalized anxiety disorder is probably 10 or more, with a sensitivity of 0.89 and specificity of 0.82. If one's practice has sufficient resources to treat other anxiety spectrum disorders, it may be reasonable to use a lower cutoff point of 7 to provide more sensitivity in identifying the additional conditions of panic disorder, social anxiety disorder, and PTSD (0.80 sensitivity and 0.76 specificity). If screening a general population as part of other screening questions, the GAD-2 may be more feasible to administer in the office because of its shorter length, with a follow-up GAD-7 for positive screens.

Table 6
Recommendations from major organizations regarding screening for selected psychiatric conditions

Condition	Organization	Recommendation	Screening Tool	Strength of Recommendation
Depression	US Preventive Services Task Force (USPSTF) (2009)	Routine depression screening for all average-risk patients when there is sufficient staff-assisted depression care support in place to ensure proper diagnosis, treatment, and follow-up	Not specified	Grade B: Recommended, high certainty that the net benefit is moderate or moderate certainty that the net benefit is moderate to substantial
	Canadian Task Force on Preventative Health Care (CTFPHC) (2013)	Recommends against routine screening of average-risk and increased-risk individuals	N/A	Weak recommendation, very-low-quality evidence
	United Kingdom National Institute for Health and Clinical Excellence (NICE) (2009)	Screen those at risk for depression (ie, history of depression, diabetes or coronary heart disease, disability, or dementia)	PHQ-2	Not specified
Anxiety disorders	USPSTF	Not addressed	N/A	N/A
	CTFPHC	Not addressed	N/A	N/A
	United Kingdom National Institute for Health and Clinical Excellence (NICE) (2011)	Assess in "people presenting with anxiety or significant worry," in patients who seek care frequently who have somatic symptoms, chronic physical health problems, or "are repeatedly worrying about a wide range of different issues"[65]	None specified	Not specified

Recommendations from major organizations

The NICE guidelines from the United Kingdom recommend considering the diagnosis of GAD in "people presenting with anxiety or significant worry," and in patients who seek care frequently who have somatic symptoms, chronic physical health problems, or "are repeatedly worrying about a wide range of different issues" (see **Table 6**).[65] However, these guidelines do not advocate for a particular screening method. The USPSTF, in its recommendation for screening for depression, mentions anxiety as a comorbid psychological condition that may merit increased depression screening, but there is no separate screening guideline for anxiety disorders.[62] Guidelines will likely continue to evolve as more research into cost-effectiveness is conducted.

SUMMARY

Depression and anxiety disorders remain significant conditions in the primary care setting and in the general population. Screening tools for depression and anxiety disorders are freely available with acceptable sensitivity and specificity. Screening tools for other conditions including ADHD and PTSD also exist. Novel screening methods, including Internet-based and computerized adaptive testing, are in development and may be promising tools in the future. Despite the availability of these tools and a need to improve the mental health of patients, the utility of widespread use of screening for depression and anxiety disorders in the primary care, office-based setting is uncertain, and guidelines have reached different conclusions. The best evidence for cost-effectiveness currently is for screening of major depression as part of the collaborative care model for treatment. Targeted screening is another reasonable approach in patients with comorbid psychiatric conditions or certain medical conditions.

Despite unanswered questions, with further research, a growing literature, and increased awareness of mental health, there is every reason for optimism for the future of mental health screening.

REFERENCES

1. Kroenke K, Spitzer RL, Williams JB, et al. Anxiety disorders in primary care: prevalence, impairment, comorbidity, and detection. Ann Intern Med 2007; 146(5):317–25.
2. González HM, Vega WA, Williams DR, et al. Depression care in the United States: too little for too few. Arch Gen Psychiatry 2010;67(1):37–46.
3. Dans LF, Silvestre MA, Dans AL. Trade-off between benefit and harm is crucial in health screening recommendations. Part I: general principles. J Clin Epidemiol 2011;64(3):231–9.
4. World Health Organization. The world health report 2001: mental health: new understanding, new hope. Geneva (Switzerland): 2001. p. 23–9.
5. Kessler RC, Chiu WT, Demler O, et al. Prevalence, severity, and comorbidity of 12-month DSM-IV disorders in the National Comorbidity Survey Replication. Arch Gen Psychiatry 2005;62:617–27.
6. First M, editor. American Psychiatric Association: diagnostic and statistical manual of mental disorders. 4th edition. 2000. Available at: http://STAT!Ref. Online Electronic Medical Library.
7. American Psychiatry Association. Diagnostic and statistical manual of mental disorders. 4th Edition, Text Revision. Washington, DC, American Psychiatric Association, 2000. Available at: http://dsm.psychiatryonline.org/data/PDFS/dsm-iv_tr.pdf. Accessed June 25, 2014.

8. Kessler RC, Berglund P, Demler O, et al. Lifetime prevalence and age-of-onset distributions of DSM-IV disorders in the National Comorbidity Survey Replication. Arch Gen Psychiatry 2005;62(6):593–602.

9. Spitzer RL, Williams JB, Kroenke K, et al. Utility of a new procedure for diagnosing mental disorders in primary care. The PRIME-MD 1000 study. JAMA 1994;272(22):1749–56.

10. Spitzer RL, Kroenke K, Williams JB. Validation and utility of a self-report version of PRIME-MD: the PHQ primary care study. Primary Care Evaluation of Mental Disorders. Patient Health Questionnaire. JAMA 1999;282(18):1737–44.

11. Kroenke K, Spitzer RL, Williams JB. The PHQ-9. J Gen Intern Med 2001;16(9): 606–13.

12. Martin A, Rief W, Klaiberg A, et al. Validity of the brief patient health questionnaire mood scale (PHQ-9) in the general population. Gen Hosp Psychiatry 2006;28(1):71–7.

13. Wittkampf KA, Naeije L, Schene AH, et al. Diagnostic accuracy of the mood module of the Patient Health Questionnaire: a systematic review. Gen Hosp Psychiatry 2007;29(5):388–95.

14. Gilbody S, Richards D, Brealey S, et al. Screening for depression in medical settings with the Patient Health Questionnaire (PHQ): a diagnostic meta-analysis. J Gen Intern Med 2007;22(11):1596–602.

15. Kroenke K, Spitzer RL, Williams JB. The patient health questionnaire-2: validity of a two-item depression screener. Med Care 2003;41(11):1284–92.

16. Steer RA, Cavalieri TA, Leonard DM, et al. Use of the beck depression inventory for primary care to screen for major depression disorders. Gen Hosp Psychiatry 1999;21(2):106–11.

17. Henkel V, Mergl R, Kohnen R, et al. Identifying depression in primary care: a comparison of different methods in a prospective cohort study. BMJ 2003; 326(7382):200–1.

18. Mitchell AJ, Coyne JC. Do ultra-short screening instruments accurately detect depression in primary care? A pooled analysis and meta-analysis of 22 studies. Br J Gen Pract 2007;57(535):144–51.

19. Williams JW, Pignone M, Ramirez G, et al. Identifying depression in primary care: a literature synthesis of case-finding instruments. Gen Hosp Psychiatry 2002;24(4):225–37.

20. Williams JW, Noël PH, Cordes JA, et al. Is this patient clinically depressed? JAMA 2002;287(9):1160–70.

21. Gilbody SM, House AO, Sheldon TA. Routinely administered questionnaires for depression and anxiety: systematic review. BMJ 2001;322(7283):406–9.

22. O'Connor EA, Whitlock EP, Beil TL, et al. Screening for depression in adult patients in primary care settings: a systematic evidence review. Ann Intern Med 2009;151(11):793–803.

23. Williams JW, Mulrow CD, Kroenke K, et al. Case-finding for depression in primary care: a randomized trial. Am J Med 1999;106(1):36–43.

24. Gilbody S, House AO, Sheldon TA. Screening and case finding instruments for depression. Cochrane Database Syst Rev 2005;(4):CD002792.

25. Valenstein M, Vijan S, Zeber JE, et al. The cost-utility of screening for depression in primary care. Ann Intern Med 2001;134(5):345–60.

26. Beck AT, Epstein N, Brown G, et al. An inventory for measuring clinical anxiety: psychometric properties. J Consult Clin Psychol 1988;56(6):893–7.

27. Benjamin S, Herr NR, McDuffie J, et al. Performance characteristics of self-report instruments for diagnosing generalized anxiety and panic disorders in

primary care: a systematic review. Washington, DC: Department of Veterans Affairs (US); 2011.

28. Mori D, Lambert JF, Niles BL, et al. The BAI–PC as a screen for anxiety, depression, and PTSD in primary care - Springer. J Clin Psychol Med Settings 2003;10: 187–92.

29. Bjelland I, Dahl AA, Haug TT, et al. The validity of the Hospital Anxiety and Depression Scale. An updated literature review. J Psychosom Res 2002;52(2): 69–77.

30. Spitzer RL, Kroenke K, Williams JB, et al. A brief measure for assessing generalized anxiety disorder: the GAD-7. Arch Intern Med 2006;166(10):1092–7.

31. Broadhead WE, Leon AC, Weissman MM, et al. Development and validation of the SDDS-PC screen for multiple mental disorders in primary care. Arch Fam Med 1995;4(3):211–9.

32. Zupancic M, Yu S, Kandukuri R, et al. Practice-based learning and systems-based practice: detection and treatment monitoring of generalized anxiety and depression in primary care. J Grad Med Educ 2010;2(3):474–7.

33. Archer J, Bower P, Gilbody S, et al. Collaborative care for depression and anxiety problems. Cochrane Database Syst Rev 2012;(10):CD006525.

34. Katon WJ, Schoenbaum M, Fan MY, et al. Cost-effectiveness of improving primary care treatment of late-life depression. Arch Gen Psychiatry 2005;62(12):1313–20.

35. Katon WJ, Roy-Byrne P, Russo J, et al. Cost-effectiveness and cost offset of a collaborative care intervention for primary care patients with panic disorder. Arch Gen Psychiatry 2002;59(12):1098–104.

36. Faraone SV, Biederman J, Mick E. The age-dependent decline of attention-deficit hyperactivity disorder: a meta-analysis of follow-up studies. Psychol Med 2006;36(2):159–65.

37. Solomon CG, Volkow ND, Swanson JM. Adult attention deficit–hyperactivity disorder. N Engl J Med 2013;369(20):1935–44.

38. Kessler RC, Adler L, AMES M, et al. The World Health Organization Adult ADHD Self-Report Scale (ASRS): a short screening scale for use in the general population. Psychol Med 1999;35(2):245–56.

39. Kessler RC, Adler LA, Gruber MJ, et al. Validity of the World Health Organization Adult ADHD Self-Report Scale (ASRS) Screener in a representative sample of health plan members. Int J Methods Psychiatr Res 2007;16(2):52–65.

40. Adler LA, Spencer T, Faraone SV, et al. Validity of pilot Adult ADHD Self-Report Scale (ASRS) to rate adult ADHD symptoms. Ann Clin Psychiatry 2006;18(3): 145–8.

41. Ward MF, Wender PH, Reimherr FW. The Wender Utah Rating Scale: an aid in the retrospective diagnosis of childhood attention-deficit hyperactivity disorder. Am J Psychiatry 1993;150(6):885–90.

42. McCann BS, Scheele L, Ward N, et al. Discriminant validity of the Wender Utah Rating Scale for attention-deficit/hyperactivity disorder in adults. J Neuropsychiatry Clin Neurosci 2000;12(2):240–5.

43. Murphy KR, Adler LA. Assessing attention-deficit/hyperactivity disorder in adults: focus on rating scales. J Clin Psychiatry 2004;65(Suppl 3):12–7.

44. Taylor A, Deb S, Unwin G. Scales for the identification of adults with attention-deficit hyperactivity disorder (ADHD): a systematic review. Res Dev Disabil 2011;32:924–38.

45. Magruder KM, Frueh BC, Knapp RG, et al. Prevalence of posttraumatic stress disorder in Veterans Affairs primary care clinics. Gen Hosp Psychiatry 2005; 27(3):169–79.

46. PTSD Screening Instruments - PTSD: National Center for PTSD [Internet]. Available at: http://www.ptsd.va.gov/professional/pages/assessments/list-screening-instruments.asp. Accessed January 12, 2014.
47. PTSD: National Center for PTSD [Internet]. Available at: http://www.ptsd.va.gov/professional/pages/assessments/pc-ptsd.asp. Accessed January 12, 2014.
48. Prins A, Ouimette P, Kimerling R, et al. The primary care PTSD screen (PC–PTSD): development and operating characteristics. Prim Care Psych 2004; 9(1):9–14.
49. My HealtheVet [Internet]. Available at: https://www.myhealth.va.gov/mhv-portal-web/anonymous.portal?_nfpb=true&_pageLabel=mentalHealth&contentPage=mh_screening_tools/PTSD_SCREENING.HTML. Accessed January 12, 2014.
50. Keen SM, Kutter CJ, Niles BL, et al. Psychometric properties of PTSD Checklist in sample of male veterans. J Rehabil Res Dev 2008;45(3):465–74.
51. McQuaid JR, Stein MB, McCahill M, et al. Use of brief psychiatric screening measures in a primary care sample. Depress Anxiety 2000;12(1):21–9.
52. Houston JP, Kroenke K, Faries DE, et al. A provisional screening instrument for four common mental disorders in adult primary care patients. Psychosomatics 2011;52(1):48–55.
53. Gaynes BN, DeVeaugh-Geiss J, Weir S, et al. Feasibility and diagnostic validity of the M-3 checklist: a brief, self-rated screen for depressive, bipolar anxiety, and post-traumatic stress disorders in primary care. Ann Fam Med 2010;8(2): 160–9.
54. Lyness JM, Noel TK, Cox C, et al. Screening for depression in elderly primary care patients. A comparison of the Center for Epidemiologic Studies-Depression Scale and the Geriatric Depression Scale. Arch Intern Med 1997; 157(4):449–54.
55. Phelan E, Williams B, Meeker K, et al. A study of the diagnostic accuracy of the PHQ-9 in primary care elderly. BMC Fam Pract 2010;11(1):63.
56. Li C, Friedman B, Conwell Y, et al. Validity of the Patient Health Questionnaire 2 (PHQ-2) in Identifying Major Depression in Older People. J Am Geriatr Soc 2007;55(4):596–602.
57. Wild B, Eckl A, Herzog W, et al. Assessing generalized anxiety disorder in elderly people using the GAD-7 and GAD-2 scales: results of a validation study. Am J Geriatr Psychiatry 2013. [Epub ahead of print].
58. Pachana NA, Byrne GJ, Siddle H, et al. Development and validation of the Geriatric Anxiety Inventory. Int Psychogeriatr 2007;19(1):103–14.
59. Byrne GJ, Pachana NA. Development and validation of a short form of the Geriatric Anxiety Inventory–the GAI-SF. Int Psychogeriatr 2011;23(1):125–31.
60. Kessler RC, Berglund PA, Dewit DJ, et al. Distinguishing generalized anxiety disorder from major depression: prevalence and impairment from current pure and comorbid disorders in the US and Ontario. Int J Methods Psychiatr Res 2002;11(3):99–111.
61. Kessler RC, Gruber M, Hettema JM, et al. Co-morbid major depression and generalized anxiety disorders in the National Comorbidity Survey follow-up. Psychol Med 2008;38(3):365–74.
62. U.S. Preventive Services Task Force. Screening for depression in adults: U.S. preventive services task force recommendation statement. Ann Intern Med 2009;151(11):784–92.
63. Canadian Task Force on Preventive Health Care, Joffres M, Jaramillo A, et al. Recommendations on screening for depression in adults. CMAJ 2013;185(9): 775–82.

64. National Institute for Health and Clinical Excellence. Depression: treatment and management of depression in adults and depression in adults with a chronic physical health problem. Manchester (United Kingdom): 2009. Available at: http://www.nice.org.uk/CG90. Accessed December 26, 2013.
65. National Collaborating Centre for Mental Health (UK). Generalised anxiety disorder in adults: management in primary, secondary and community care. National clinical guideline number 113. Leicester (United Kingdom): British Psychological Society & The Royal College of Psychiatrists; 2011.
66. Whooley MA, Avins AL, Miranda J, et al. Case-finding instruments for depression. Two questions are as good as many. J Gen Intern Med 1997;12(7):439–45.
67. VA/DoD essentials for depression screening and assessment in primary care. 2010. Available at: http://www.healthquality.va.gov/mdd/. Accessed December 26, 2013.
68. Moussavi S, Chatterji S, Verdes E, et al. Depression, chronic diseases, and decrements in health: results from the World Health Surveys. Lancet 2007; 370(9590):851–8.
69. Kravitz RL, Ford DE. Introduction: chronic medical conditions and depression—the view from primary care. Am J Med 2008;121(11):S1–7.
70. Katon WJ. Clinical and health services relationships between major depression, depressive symptoms, and general medical illness. Biol Psychiatry 2003;54(3):216–26.
71. Lichtman JH, Bigger JT, Blumenthal JA, et al. Depression and coronary heart disease: recommendations for screening, referral, and treatment: a science advisory from the American Heart Association Prevention Committee of the Council on Cardiovascular Nursing, Council on Clinical Cardiology, Council on Epidemiology and Prevention, and Interdisciplinary Council on Quality of Care and Outcomes Research: Endorsed by the American Psychiatric Association. Circulation 2008;118(17):1768–75.
72. Hackett ML, Anderson CS, House A, et al. Interventions for treating depression after stroke. Cochrane Database Syst Rev 2008;(4):CD003437.
73. Glassman AH, O'Connor CM, Califf RM, et al. Sertraline treatment of major depression in patients with acute MI or unstable angina. JAMA 2002;288(6):701–9.
74. Ziegelstein RC. Depression in patients recovering from a myocardial infarction. JAMA 2001;286(13):1621–7.
75. Berkman LF, Blumenthal J, Burg M, et al. Effects of treating depression and low perceived social support on clinical events after myocardial infarction: the Enhancing Recovery in Coronary Heart Disease Patients (ENRICHD) Randomized Trial. JAMA 2003;289(23):3106–16.
76. Stafford L, Berk M, Jackson HJ. Validity of the Hospital Anxiety and Depression Scale and Patient Health Questionnaire-9 to screen for depression in patients with coronary artery disease. Gen Hosp Psychiatry 2007;29(5):417–24.
77. Kroenke K, Spitzer RL, Williams JB, et al. The patient health questionnaire somatic, anxiety, and depressive symptom scales: a systematic review. Gen Hosp Psychiatry 2010;32(4):345–59.
78. Löwe B, Spitzer RL, Williams JB, et al. Depression, anxiety and somatization in primary care: syndrome overlap and functional impairment. Gen Hosp Psychiatry 2008;30(3):191–9.
79. Mussell M, Kroenke K, Spitzer RL, et al. Gastrointestinal symptoms in primary care: prevalence and association with depression and anxiety. J Psychosom Res 2008;64(6):605–12.
80. Delgadillo J, Payne S, Gilbody S, et al. Brief case finding tools for anxiety disorders: validation of GAD-7 and GAD-2 in addictions treatment. Drug Alcohol Depend 2012;125:37–42.

Major Depression

Susan M. Bentley, DO[a],*, Genevieve L. Pagalilauan, MD[b],
Scott A. Simpson, MD, MPH[a]

KEYWORDS

- Major depression • Primary care • Diagnosis • Management • Pharmacotherapy

KEY POINTS

- MDD has a lifetime prevalence of 16% in the United States and 25% in those with chronic diseases. Though the natural history of MDD is to eventually remit, 30% or more have refractory or treatment resistant depression and even in those whose depression remits, there is a high rate of recurrence.
- The Patient Health Questionnaire 2 (PHQ2) and PHQ9 are validated and reasonably sensitive screening tools for MDD. The PHQ9 can also be used to monitor symptoms and direct adjustment of treatment.
- Medical conditions, substance abuse, grief, sleep disorders, and other psychiatric conditions can both co occur and mimic the symptoms of MDD. Providers should assess for the presence of these conditions when diagnosing MDD and consider co-morbid conditions in order to tailor management interventions.
- Of the lifestyle interventions for depression, exercise, and relaxation therapy have the best evidence.
- Psychotherapy effectively treats MDD. While no one type of psychotherapy is thought to be superior to others, there are important differences in the philosophy and approach to different types of therapy that should be considered when recommending psychotherapy for patients.
- Most antidepressants are similar in efficacy, though escitalopram and sertraline may confer a slight advantage. Clinicians should consider patient preferences, cost, side effects, and medication interactions when recommending pharmacotherapy interventions.

INTRODUCTION

Here we review the presentation and treatment of major depressive disorder (MDD) among adults in the primary care setting. To build on prior reviews of epidemiology,[1]

Conflict of Interest: G. Pagalilauan is a reviewer in Johns Hopkins Practical Reviews in Internal Medicine.
[a] Department of Psychiatry & Behavioral Sciences, Harborview Medical Center, Box 359896, 325 9th Avenue, Seattle, WA 98104, USA; [b] Department of Medicine, Division of General Internal Medicine, Roosevelt General Internal Medicine Clinic, University of Washington Medical Center, 4245 Roosevelt Way North East, Seattle, WA 98105
* Corresponding author.
E-mail address: sbentley@u.washington.edu

pharmacotherapy,[2] and other facets of MDD in primary care,[3-6] we focus on the clinical application of research evidence and treatment guidelines, the identification and differential diagnosis of major depression, and resultant treatment strategies. Other work more specifically addresses depression among children[7] and the elderly.[8,9]

THE SYNDROME OF MAJOR DEPRESSION AND ITS PRESENTATION

For research and clinical purposes, MDD is most commonly diagnosed by criteria in the Diagnostic and Statistical Manual (DSM).[10] Largely unchanged in the new DSM 5th edition (DSM-5), the criteria specify that 5 of 9 symptoms be present for a 2-week period and represent a change in functioning. **Box 1** summarizes the DSM-5 criteria for MDD. The most significant differences in DSM-5 include new emphasis on hopelessness as a feature of depression and the removal of the "bereavement exclusion," described in more detail later.[11]

Through type and severity specifiers, the DSM-5 allows for 14 categorizations of depression. Although the clinical value of this subtyping remains uncertain, it does illustrate the varying clinical symptomatology of MDD[11] and highlights diagnostic challenges. As an example, **Box 2** describes the "with anxious distress" specifier for depressive disorders in DSM- 5.

DEPRESSION SUBTYPES

Other DSM-5 depressive disorder specifiers include atypical features of mood reactivity—significant weight gain or increased appetite, hypersomnia, leaden paralysis, and longstanding patterns of interpersonal rejection sensitivity. This symptom cluster can occur in up to one-third of patients with major depression.[12,13] In clinical trials and community samples, atypical depression has been correlated with female sex,

---

Box 1
DSM-5 diagnostic criteria for major depression

A. Five (or more) of the following symptoms present during the same 2-week period and represent a change from previous functioning; at least one of the symptoms is either (1) depressed mood or (2) anhedonia

B. Symptoms cause clinically significant distress or impairment in social, occupational, or other important areas of functioning

C. Episode is not attributable to the physiologic effects of a substance or another medical condition

  1. Depressed mood most of the day (eg, feels sad, empty, hopeless)

  2. Markedly diminished interest or pleasure in almost all activities nearly every day

  3. Significant appetite changes or significant weight loss or gain

  4. Insomnia or hypersomnia nearly every day

  5. Psychomotor agitation or retardation

  6. Fatigue or loss of energy

  7. Feelings of worthlessness or excessive guilt

  8. Diminished ability to think or concentrate or indecisiveness

Adapted from Diagnostic and statistical manual of mental disorders. 5th edition. Washington, DC: American Psychiatric Association; 2013.

Box 2
DSM- 5 "with anxious distress" specifier for depressive disorders

With anxious distress: presence of at least 2 the following symptoms during most days of depressive episode

1. Feeling tense or keyed up

2. Feeling unusually restless

3. Difficulty concentrating because of worry

4. Fear that something awful might happen

5. Feeling that individual may lose control of him/herself

Note: anxious distress is a prominent feature of bipolar disorder and MDD. High levels associated w/higher suicide risk, longer duration of illness, greater likelihood of poor treatment response. Specification of severity is useful for treatment planning and monitoring.

Mild: 2 symptoms

Moderate: 3 symptoms

Moderate-Severe: 4 or 5 symptoms

Severe: 4 or 5 symptoms w/motor agitation

Adapted from Diagnostic and statistical manual of mental disorders. 5th edition. Washington, DC: American Psychiatric Association; 2013.

---

younger age of onset, family history of depression, greater anxiety including specific phobias, somatoform disorders, substance abuse, personality disorders, and suicide attempts.[12,14–18] It may be difficult for primary care providers to recognize atypical depression, as patients can often improve when circumstances are favorable and show a reactive, not depressed, affect. The epidemiology of atypical depression, along with the new DSM-5 specifier for MDD "with anxious distress," reminds clinicians that anxiety symptoms are often comorbid with MDD. Melancholic features include pronounced anhedonia, early morning awakening, and depression that is worse in the morning.[10] Psychotic symptoms often include mood congruent themes of personal inadequacy, guilt, disease, punishment, or death.[10]

DETERMINATION OF DEGREE OF IMPAIRMENT

Although culture may influence the predominant symptom presentation of depression, there is no strong underlying epidemiologic evidence to support a predictable cultural pattern.[19,20] A World Health Organization survey of primary care patients suggests a wide variation in prevalence of major depression across 14 countries (from 1.6% to 26.3%).[21] This variation likely reflects differences in the threshold of functional impairment used to make the diagnosis rather than varying symptomatology.

The presence of "clinically significant distress or impairment" is crucial for the diagnosis of depression. However, there is marked variability and subjectivity in both the individual clinician's determination and the patient's manifestations of impairment and distress. In practice, the patient's report of subjective distress is often considered sufficient for fulfilling this criterion, but there is ongoing debate and research seeking to constitute an appropriate diagnostic threshold for MDD.[22–24] Patients in studies of major depression describe impairment as less satisfaction at work, at leisure, and among family members.[25–28] Additional markers of function and impairment recognized in patients with MDD include changes in sexual drive and decline in physical function and physical health. Patients may say, "Things seem dark," "more difficult," or that they are "just not interested." Patients describe their distress or impairment as cognitive dysfunction causing difficulty keeping track of things or focusing on work. However, distress and functional impairment, although sensitive for MDD, are not specific and do not differentiate depression from other diagnoses.

EPIDEMIOLOGY AND COURSE OF MDD

Depression is a common and complicated illness. The lifetime prevalence of MDD in the United States is about 16%[29] in a given year; about 7% of the population will experience an episode of MDD, half of which are moderate in severity.[30,31] A Finnish study of primary care patients endorsing at least 2 current symptoms of depression found that current MDD was present in 66% of cases. The annual prevalence rate is up to 25% in patients with chronic medical illness.[32] Risk factors are multifactorial and include genetic, medical, social, and environmental factors.

The course of MDD reflects this complexity: initial presentation can include a variety of physical symptoms including pain (headache, musculoskeletal, abdominal/pelvic), neurovegetative mood symptoms (see **Box 1**), and cognitive changes. The course of MDD is variable with some patients rarely experiencing a remission (>2 months with no or only a few mild symptoms) and others with having many years with few or no symptoms between discrete depressive episodes. Distinguishing patients who present during an exacerbation of chronic depressive symptoms from those with recent onset of symptoms is important in anticipating illness trajectory. Recent onset of symptoms is a strong determinant of near-term recovery. Many patients who have only been depressed for a few months may be expected to recover spontaneously. Chronicity of symptoms decreases the likelihood that full remission will follow treatment. Lower recovery rates are also associated with psychotic features, symptom severity, prominent anxiety, and personality disorders.

Most patients with symptoms of MDD do eventually improve. Recovery typically begins within 3 months of symptoms onset for about 40% of patients with MDD and within 1 year for approximate 80%. A prospective, observational study of 174 outpatients with MDD found that more than 70% achieved remission: 43% remitted by 6 months and maintained remission over 3 years, 40% fluctuated between periods of depression and remission, and a significant minority (17%) remained depressed without periods of improvement.[33] These data are similar in proportion to the 33% of subjects who did not to respond after 4 treatment steps in the Sequenced Treatment Alternatives to Relieve Depression (STAR*D) trial but lower than seen in the Finnish cohort.[34,35] Residual depressive symptoms—fatigue, cognitive impairment, and insomnia—may persist even after successful treatment.[36–38] Persistence of symptoms after treatment heightens the risk for recurrence of a major depressive episode.

Unfortunately, depression is highly recurrent. In a prospective study of greater than 300 patients who had recovered from an episode of MDD, 64% experienced at least 1 additional episode of MDD with the greatest risk of recurrence in the first months after recovery. The probability of recurrence decreased as the period of remission progressed. A history of recurrent depressive episodes is the most predictive risk factor for additional episodes of MDD, and each recurrence increases the risk of experiencing another episode by 16%.[39]

SCREENING

Depression is common and frequently goes undetected in primary care settings without screening. The US Preventive Services Task Force and other agencies recommend the use of standardized screening instruments for the diagnosis of MDD in outpatient practice, screening all patients at routine visits.[40,41] The Department of Veterans Affairs recommends screening for MDD annually.[42] Factors in the choice of screening instruments include the diagnostic accuracy for the target population and pragmatic constraints such as the ease of administration/interpretation, such as number of questions and reading level requirements. Short screens that can be completed by patients while waiting for their visits or administered by staff during check-in for vital signs are practical and efficient.

The use of the Patient Health Questionnaire-2 (PHQ-2), a 2-item screener, is frequently suggested. It can be administered either written or verbally with yes/no or scaled responses. The PHQ-2 is based on the stem, "Over the last 2 weeks, how often have you been bothered by any of the following problems... (1) Little interest or pleasure in doing things...and (2) Feeling down, depressed, or hopeless."[43] Patients answer from 0 (not at all) to 3 (nearly every day) to for both questions, and a score of 3 or greater (out of 0) has a sensitivity of more than 00% for MDD. A yes on either portion also indicates possible depression. A positive screening result should be followed up with further evaluation to diagnose depression. **Box 3** summarizes risk factors for MDD. Patients with multiple risk factors on by history may be a higher prevalence population worthy of attention when targeting depression screening efforts.

The longer PHQ-9 (**Table 1**) is slightly more sensitive and allows clinicians to track depressive symptoms over time. It can also be used to educate patients as to the various symptoms of depression.[44,45] Depression severity is scored 0, 1, 2, and 3, to the response categories of not at all, several days, more than half the days, and nearly every day, respectively, with total scores in a range of 0 to 27. Scores of 10 or higher indicate a possible depressive disorder. The question of whether depressive symptoms are impairing function is important in establishing a DSM-based diagnosis. However, like other screening tools, the PHQ-9 is not sufficiently accurate to establish a definitive diagnosis for depression. Scores indicating a positive screening result should prompt a thoughtful assessment of treatment considerations.

Box 3
Selected risk factors for depression

Prior depressive episode

Family history

Gender (female)

Age (younger)

Race (white)

Childbirth (ie, postpartum depression)

Childhood trauma/adversity

Stressful life events

Poor social support

Serious medical illness

Cognitive impairment/dementia

Substance use (illicit, prescription)

Adapted from Kendler KS, Gardner CO, Prescott CA. Toward a comprehensive developmental model for major depression in men. Am J Psychiatry 2006;163(1):115.

Table 1
Use of PHQ9 in Initial Depression Management

Name:			Date:	
Over the last 2 wk, how often have you been bothered by any of the following problems?	Not at all	Several days	More than half the days	Nearly every day
Little interest or pleasure in doing things	0	1	2	3
Feeling down, depressed, or hopeless	0	1	2	3
Trouble falling or staying asleep, or sleeping too much	0	1	2	3
Feeling tired or having little energy	0	1	2	3
Poor appetite or overeating	0	1	2	3
Feeling bad about yourself, or that you are a failure, or have let yourself or your family down	0	1	2	3
Trouble concentrating on things, such as reading the newspaper or watching television	0	1	2	3
Moving or speaking so slowly that other people could have noticed? Or the opposite, being so fidgety or restless that you have been moving around a lot more than usual	0	1	2	3
Thoughts that you would be better off dead or of hurting yourself in some way	0	1	2	3
Total ___ =	—	+ ___	+ ___	+ ___

PHQ-9 Score ≥10: Likely major depression.
Depression score ranges:
5 to 9: mild
10 to 14: moderate
15 to 19: moderately severe
≥20: severe

If you checked off any problems, how difficult have these problems made it for you to do your work, take care of things at home, or get along with other people?	Not difficult at all ___	Somewhat difficult ___	Very difficult ___	Extremely difficult ___

PHQ-9 Score	PHQ-9 Interpretation Depression Severity	Initial Treatment Considerations
0–4	None-minimal	None
5–9	Mild	Monitor/repeat PHQ-9 at follow up
10–14	Moderate	Consider counseling, +/− pharmacotherapy, follow-up 4–6 wk
15–19	Moderately Severe	Active treatment with pharmacotherapy +/− psychotherapy, close follow-up 2–4 wk
20–27	Severe	Address acute safety concerns. Immediate initiation of pharmacotherapy, follow-up 1 wk or sooner. Consider expedited referral to a mental health specialist for psychotherapy and/or collaborative management

From The Patient Health Questionnaire (PHQ) Screeners. Available at: http://www.phqscreeners.com/overview.aspx?Screener=02_PHQ-9. Accessed July 17, 2014.

Attention to screening is variably supported in the literature. Screening is recommended by the US Preventive Services Task Force for patients if there is adequate availability of appropriate treatment and staff assistance, such as having a nurse highlight a patient's depression screener to the provider.[40,46] The psychometric properties of available screening tools are detailed elsewhere.[47]

PATHOPHYSIOLOGY

Although the diagnosis is made through clinical examination, major depression correlates with numerous biological measures signifying the MDD's complex pathophysiology. The classic monoamine hypothesis of depression posits a relative deficiency of monoamine neurotransmitter activity, particularly serotonin, in the synaptic cleft. Several excellent reviews describe emerging, more complex neurobiological models involving multiple neurotransmitter systems.[48–50] Depression correlates with hypersensitization of α adrenergic receptors (with resulting decrease in serotonin), and antidepressant treatment results in β adrenergic receptor downregulation along with desensitization of inhibitory serotonin receptors.[48–50] These changes affect longer-term adaptive neuronal changes that correlate with the therapeutic response time for antidepressants; reduced brain-derived neurotropic factor activity may account for morphologic changes and impaired neuroplasticity in depressed patients. The hypothalamic-pituitary-adrenal axis has also been implicated; depressed patients have elevated cortisone levels, fail to respond to dexamethasone suppression tests, and have enlarged pituitary and adrenal glands. Depressed patients have less rapid eye movement, stage 3, and stage 4 sleep perhaps resulting from the observed increase in proinflammatory cytokines (interleukin-1, interleukin-6, and tumor necrosis factor). Family and twin studies suggest some genetic contribution to major depression—the effect appears stronger for recurrent or early-occurring depression—but the mechanism of this effect remains unclear, and genetic effects are not likely stronger than environmental stressors.[51 53] This increasingly sophisticated biological understanding may soon—but not yet—guide depression treatment selection and predict response.[54]

IDENTIFICATION, COMORBIDITY, AND DIFFERENTIAL DIAGNOSIS

Many symptoms of major depression are shared by other medical and psychiatric illnesses, complicating diagnosis.[32] Alternative diagnostic schemes have been proposed that substitute or ignore the somatic symptoms of depression in the presence of medical illness.[55,56] But, the more traditional criteria remain widely used even under such circumstances. It is better to err on the side of sensitivity given the implications of missing major depression, and major depression often manifests as multiple somatic complaints in the primary care setting.

Substance Use Disorder

Anyone in whom depression is suspected must be screened for substance dependence including marijuana, prescription drug diversion, and especially alcohol. Substance dependence is common among patients with depression, may induce or exacerbate depressed mood and associated symptoms, and is an additional risk factor for suicide.[57–59] In a telephone survey of the general population comparing short screeners for alcohol use disorders, the Rapid Alcohol Problems Screen 4 was the most sensitive (0.86 for alcohol dependence) and had high specificity (0.95 for dependence).[60] The Rapid Alcohol Problems Screen 4 is positive if the patient answers yes to 1 of 4 questions: Have you felt guilt or remorse after drinking? Has a friend or family member ever told you about things you said or did while drinking that you did not remember? Have you failed to do what was normally expected of you because of drinking? Do you sometimes take a drink when you first get up in the morning?

General Medical Conditions

Many medical conditions cause depressive symptoms like fatigue, changes in eating and sleeping pattern, and even hyper/hypoactivity, but these medical illnesses are less likely to induce cognitive distortions typical of major depression (low mood, anhedonia, feelings of guilt). Hence, these medical conditions can mimic symptoms of depression, but with careful history taking and use of screening tools like the PHQ9, as well as appropriate medical work-up, these conditions should be distinguished as independent from MDD. Complicating matters, is the strong co-morbid association between depression and some medical conditions such as COPD, acute MI, and chronic kidney disease.[61] Delirium can induce depressive episodes, and a thorough medical investigation is warranted for patients with disorientation, difficulty maintaining consciousness or wakefulness, abnormal vital signs or physical examination, or a new psychiatric diagnosis after age 40.[62,63] Initial testing for depression might include a complete blood count (testing for anemia and infection), basic metabolic panel (hyponatremia, renal failure, dehydration), liver function tests (hepatic encephalopathy), thyroid-stimulating hormone (hypothyroidism), and a pregnancy test (as changes related to pregnancy maybe misattributed to somatic manifestations of MDD, ie, fatigue, weight gain, changes in appetite, and sleep).

Prescription Medications

Medications associated with MDD include steroids, anticonvulsants, benzodiazepines, nonsteroidal anti-inflammatory drugs, dopamine, and clonidine.[42] Polypharmacy can also contribute to depressive spectrum symptoms.

Adjustment Disorders and Demoralization

Adjustment disorders occur when patients experience significant distress in the presence of an identifiable life stressor but do not exhibit the range of symptoms necessary for the diagnosis of depression. Similarly, a syndrome of demoralization has been recognized among medically ill patients struggling with feelings of hopelessness, helplessness, and incompetence.[64–66] As opposed to those with depression, demoralized patients are not usually anhedonic and quickly recover with abatement of the stressor. Patients who initially have an adjustment or demoralization disorder may progress to depression; patients who fulfill criteria for MDD merit the formal diagnosis and appropriate treatment.

Sleep Disorders

Insomnia or hypersomnia are cardinal symptoms of major depression; however, primary sleep disorders may mimic depression. Patients with obstructive sleep apnea describe difficulty with concentration, mood, and energy but are able to enjoy activities and lack the negative cognitive distortions of depression. Insomnia and parasomnia may underlie many symptoms of depression, and brief therapeutic interventions for insomnia may augment the efficacy of depression treatment.[67]

Posttraumatic Stress Disorder

Patients with posttraumatic stress disorder (PTSD) complain of difficulty forming close relationships, envisioning a plan for their futures, poor sleep, and anhedonia. Focusing on these symptoms could lead a primary care physician (PCP) to diagnose MDD.

However, patients with PTSD will also report re-experiencing and hypervigilance symptoms (eg, startling easily). Appropriate treatment of PTSD requires different pharmacotherapeutic and psychotherapeutic approaches than for MDD.

Grief and Bereavement

Grief is "the mainly emotional response to bereavement," "an almost universal life event."[68,69] In response to the loss of a loved one, it is natural for patients to experience sadness, guilt, and thoughts of joining the deceased. Psychotic experiences such as temporarily experiencing hallucinations in which the deceased is perceived as present (eg, seeing the deceased sitting in a favorite chair) may also occur. These symptoms can be associated with complicated grief particularly if out of proportion or inconsistent with religious, cultural, or age-appropriate norms. Clinicians should suspect pathologic major depression when feelings of sadness worsen rather than improve, or there is significant impairment in functioning, psychotic experiences unrelated to the deceased, or prominent feelings of worthlessness and anhedonia. Whereas the previous DSM-IV test revision specified that bereavement should not last longer than 2 months, DSM-5 does not specify a time period by which grief is expected to normally resolve and recognizes that "the exercise of clinical judgment" is necessary to distinguish normal grief from a major depressive disorder. Bereaved patients are at higher risk of new depression, substance use, suicide, and mortality.[68,70]

Minor and Persistent Depression

Patients may describe long-standing depressive symptoms that do not fulfill criteria for MDD because of insufficient symptom duration, intensity, or impairment. With some variation in quality or duration, these states have been described as minor or subsyndromal depression, dysthymic disorder, and, now in DSM-5, persistent depressive disorder.[71,72] Chronic dysthymia can be associated with significant impairment,[73,74] and 4 in 5 patients also experience a major depressive episode.[75] Moreover, these syndromes may be less amenable to traditional treatments.[76,77] MDD merits treatment if present, and chronically depressed patients should be referred for psychotherapy.[78]

Personality

Many patients report a depressive pattern in response to life circumstances but lack anhedonia or blunted affect. Asking these patients "When was the last time you felt good?" often evokes a response of "years." The duration of depressive symptoms may be quite long, even lifelong, without a clear temporal course. These clues should raise suspicion for personality characteristics underlying the depressive symptoms. A combination of negative affect, somatization, and social inhibition has been described as Type D personality and subsequently associated with poor psychosocial and health outcomes.[79–81] Type D personality can be a helpful psychological construct for clinicians to consider, although not a pathologic diagnosis in DSM-5.

Astute clinicians will appreciate that many of the above diagnoses can be comorbid with MDD—more than half of patients with MDD have another psychiatric diagnosis, most commonly an anxiety or personality disorder.[30,34] Regardless of comorbidity, MDD should be treated. Comorbidity can impact treatment resistance and functional impairment and may manifest as new psychiatric symptoms in a patient whose depressed mood is otherwise improving. When multiple diagnoses are present, there is no evidence to guide which diagnosis should be treated first.

SUICIDE, DEPRESSION, AND ASSESSMENT

Depression is strongly associated with completed suicide, and suicide assessment is intrinsic to any evaluation of the depressed patient.[82,83] In a prospective 5-year study of patients with major depressive disorder, nearly 15% of subjects attempted suicide at least once.[84] This risk increased 21 times during periods of active depression compared with periods in remission. The lifetime risk of death by suicide among patients with major depression, cited to be as high as 6%, is comparable to the risk of those with schizophrenia or alcoholism.[85,86] Primary care providers must be familiar with suicide risk assessment, as 23% to 45% of patients completing suicide are last seen by a nonpsychiatric provider.[87,88]

Because completed suicide is a very rare event, predicting suicide completion is not possible. Rather, assessment centers on risk stratification, which begins with asking the patient about suicidal thoughts or ideation. In one analysis of data from a managed care system, outpatients who reported thoughts of death or self-harm nearly every day on the PHQ-9 screener were 10 times more likely to attempt suicide in the following year.[89] The excellent review by McDowell and colleagues[87] of suicide risk assessment in the primary care setting endorses a model based on low-, medium-, and high-risk stratification.[90] Low-risk patients have no prior suicide attempts or suicidal ideation or have suicidal ideation without a plan or intent; these patients require outpatient follow-up. Medium-risk patients endorse suicidal ideation and a plan but not rehearsals or intent. These patients should be referred to psychiatry, at least, or perhaps the emergency room if other pressing risk factors are present (eg, a lack of close social supports,[82] impulsivity, philosophic reasons for dying,[91] or active alcohol use disorder[91]). High-risk patients have a suicide plan and the intent to complete suicide concurrent with agitation, psychosis, or recent suicide attempt. High-risk patients require constant observation in clinic while transportation to emergency treatment is arranged. Clinicians should document the reasoning underlying their risk assessment and interventions taken.[87]

TREATMENT AND MANAGEMENT

Several modalities have evidence for efficacy in the treatment of MDD. These include behavioral interventions/self-care strategies, psychotherapy in its many forms, and psychopharmacologic interventions.

The quantification of severity in MDD can help guide management strategies (**Table 1**) not only for initial therapy but also for ongoing management once the diagnosis has been made.

Behavioral Interventions and Self-Care

Many patients are opposed to treating depressive symptoms with psychotherapy or medications. Some patients have had adverse reactions to medications, and others may not have access to resources or the time necessary for traditional interventions. These patients seek to start with interventions they can initiate on their own or with alternative support.

Although the increase in the diagnosis of depression over the last several decades discussed above may be owing to improved screening and awareness by patients and providers, it may also reflect a true increase in the incidence and prevalence of MDD in society. Hidaka[92] makes a case that compared with 40 to 50 years ago, Western societies eat more calorie-dense nutrition-poor foods and exercise less. The article evidenced the association between depression and a modern lifestyle to also include isolation from a family unit, less meaningful social interactions in a community, sleep-wake disruption, inadequate exposure to sunlight, and high stress levels. In short, depression may be increasing because more people today are undernourished yet obese, isolated, lonely, stressed, and sedentary. It follows that attempts to reverse these possible drivers of depression may treat or prevent the condition.

Diet

An excellent review by Sarris and colleagues[93] in 2014 summarizes the evidence for lifestyle medicine for depression. Cross-sectional and longitudinal studies conducted in multiple international sites evidence the association between the Western diet and the likelihood for depression development; unfortunately, insufficient studies assess if changing diet will treat depression. A randomized, controlled study is currently looking at this question, and those results are expected in 2015.

Exercise

Unlike dietary intervention, exercise has been studied more extensively as an intervention for MDD but yielded mixed outcomes.[93] Fortunately, a 2013 Cochrane review looks at exercise interventions for the treatment of depression.[94] For the purposes of the review, exercise is defined as "planned, structured repetitive bodily movement done to improve or maintain one or more components of physical fitness." Pooled outcomes of 35 trials comparing exercise with no intervention show that exercise provides a moderate positive effect, but methodologic problems are noted for several trials. Looking only at the 6 high-quality trials in the review, the effect of exercise diminishes, and although positive, is no longer statistically significant. Interestingly, exercise was noninferior to both psychotherapy (7 trials) and pharmacotherapy (4 trials) for MDD. Notably, the National Institute for Health and Clinical Excellence 2009 guidelines recommend a structured group-based physical activity program as low intensity intervention for mild-to-moderate MDD.[95] Yoga, which combines exercise and mindfulness practices is also moderately effective.[93] In practical terms, exercise is a low-cost, relatively low-risk intervention to recommend to patients, although clinicians should be mindful about the exercise capacity of those who suffer from other medical comorbidities.

Sleep

The relationship between MDD and sleep is complicated as illustrated by the manifestations of insomnia and hypersomnia in MDD. There is strong correlation with sleep disruption and mood disorders, and insomnia in one review predicts a 2-fold increased risk for MDD.[93] The review by Sarris and colleagues[93] notes that most studies on intervention for sleep disturbance in MDD are focused on sleep hygiene, cognitive behavioral therapy and pharmacotherapy interventions. A small randomized, controlled trial (RCT) shows cognitive behavioral therapy added to antidepressant therapy to address sleep disturbance increases remission rates from 33% in the control arm to 61% in the intervention arm.[96] A small but interesting surgical study found that 75% of depressed patients receiving corrective surgical intervention for obstructive sleep apnea experienced remission of their MDD.[97] So, although it is well evidenced that disruptions in sleep contribute to and are manifestations of MDD and other psychiatric disorders, the evidence remains sparse that treating sleep derangements primarily will effectively treat MDD. Currently, clinicians should consider treatment of sleep abnormalities an adjunctive approach to treating MDD and not a first- or even second-line measure.

Alcohol and tobacco use

Alcohol use disorder and MDD appear to have a reciprocal relationship—the presence of one doubles the risk of the other.[93] The same review shows abstinence from alcohol rapidly alleviates depressive symptoms. A 2014 systematic review and meta-analysis of 26 studies found that maintaining smoking cessation for greater than 6 weeks statistically reduces (measured in standard mean difference) depression (−0.25), anxiety (−0.37), and mixed anxiety and depression states (−0.31) and improves psychological quality of life (+0.22).[98]

Other lifestyle interventions

A systematic review (15 studies) and meta-analysis of 11 RCTs on relaxation techniques, including progressive muscle relaxation, relaxation imagery, and autogenic training, found relaxation therapy moderately reduces self-reported depression ratings and trends toward a benefit in clinician-reported depression ratings (2 studies).[99] Meditation,[93] music therapy,[100] and animal-assisted therapy[101] have some evidence for benefit in the treatment of MDD. However, lifestyle interventions require more robust RCTs before most clinicians will recommend them with confidence.

Psychotherapy for MDD

Psychotherapy is a well-studied intervention for MDD. Many forms of psychotherapy including cognitive behavioral therapy, behavioral activation therapy, interpersonal psychotherapy, problem-solving therapy, nondirective counseling, and psychodynamic therapy show effectiveness in the treatment of MDD.[102] No one type of psychotherapy is thought to be superior to another for MDD.

The efficacy of psychotherapy in the setting of high placebo response rates seen in studies calls into question the true clinical benefit of the intervention. Two recent meta-analyses attempted to determine if psychotherapy has meaningful effectiveness compared with placebo. Huhn and colleagues[103] found acute phase psychotherapy had a moderate effect size (standard mean difference, 0.58) compared with placebo or no treatment. A 2014 meta-analysis looked at the absolute number of patients that no longer met the diagnosis of depression, response, and remission rates based on the Beck Depression Rating Scale and the Hamilton Depression Rating Scale (highly validated scales for depression severity and diagnosis). After psychotherapy interventions, 62% of study patients no longer met criteria for MDD compared with 43% of controls and 48% of patients receiving care as usual. The authors reported that psychotherapy added a 14% additional benefit for resolving depression over usual care.

PCPs can offer more direction to patients than a referral to psychotherapy. There are practical considerations and important differences among the forms of psychotherapy that should be considered before referral. First, patients should understand their insurance benefits. Some insurers will cover mental health benefits including psychotherapy but may preferentially cover a particular type of psychotherapy or therapist (preferred providers). Secondly, there are differences in the premise and approach of different types of psychotherapy (**Table 2**) that may confer certain advantages and disadvantages depending on the patient's philosophy, level of insight, willingness to participate, and preferences.[104] Lastly, other practical considerations like proximity to work and home, therapist reputation, and a patient's prior experiences with psychotherapy may drive the selection of the type of therapy and the therapist.

Pharmacotherapy

Nonpsychiatrists are responsible for 64% of psychotropic medication prescriptions to adults in the United States.[105] PCPs are increasingly responsible for both diagnosing and pharmacologically managing conditions like depression with or without the help of mental health specialists.[106] However, specific training during residency and

Table 2
Psychotherapy types: advantages and disadvantages

Type of Psychotherapy	Description	Advantages	Disadvantages
Cognitive behavioral therapy	Based on a premise that thoughts and behaviors are modifiable. Patients learn "rational" thoughts and "adaptive" behaviors. Homework is assigned 8–16 sessions	• Well validated and studied • Insurers are more likely to pay for it because of measurable goals • Short-term and interactive	• Patients struggling with motivation or resistance may struggle with the expectation of active participation • Does not address psychic conflict • Requires a skilled therapist
Interpersonal therapy	Based on the premise that current interpersonal conflicts drive psychiatric symptoms. The focus is on short-term, present-focused interpersonal skills, communication, and coping. Key areas are: • Grief • Role transition • Interpersonal conflicts • Interpersonal deficits	• Short-term • Behaviorally specific treatment plans • Measurable goals • Patients learn strategies for effective living • More likely to be covered by insurers	• Patients must actively participate • Patients must implement change in behaviors • Does not address intrapsychic conflict
Psychodynamic therapy	Freudian theory that difficulties are caused by internal and unconscious conflicts, often rooted in childhood experiences, repeating in the present and during the therapy relationship. Coming to terms with loss/grief is a major focus.	• Helpful in patients with unconscious or internal conflict • Time-limited sessions are available	• Less helpful in people without unconscious conflict • May not be helpful in severe psychopathology, psychotic symptoms, severe personality disorders
Client-centered therapy	Insight-oriented approach that focuses on the present not past. The therapist approach is nondirective, with empathetic active listening, rephrasing, and reflecting the patient's emotions and statements.	• Accepted by patients because they feel unconditional acceptance • Models healthy relationships	• Less scientifically based • Unclear treatment endpoints • May not be helpful in severe depression • Does not address intrapsychic conflict

Data from Bea SM, Tesar GE. A primer on referring patients for psychotherapy. Cleve Clin J Med 2002;69(2):113–27.

continuing medical education on the topic of psychopharmacology is highly variable among providers.

General approach
In general, first- and second-generation antidepressants have equal efficacy with 60% to 70% of patients responding (symptoms >50% improved) to therapy.[107] Second-generation medications like selective serotonin reuptake inhibitors (SSRIs), serotonin–norepinephrine reuptake inhibitors (SNRIs), bupropion, and mirtazapine are preferred over first-generation medications (tricyclic antidepressants [TCAs] and monoamine oxidase inhibitors [MAOIs]) because of their less problematic side effects and reduced risk for fatality in overdose situations.[108,109] Antidepressants are best evidenced for more severe depression[77] and have been used as monotherapy or in combination with psychotherapy and other modalities of care (see **Table 1**).

After a systematic review found minimal differences in efficacy among the second-generation antidepressants,[110] the American College of Physicians 2008 Guidelines recommended that providers consider side effects (to avoid or to harness for the benefit of the patient), cost, and patient preference in selecting a first-line antidepressant.[111] This advice remains sound in general, but the specific pharmacodynamics of medications within and among classes help to explain both the effectiveness and tolerability of antidepressants. Understanding these differences can help guide providers to tailor medication management to the specific needs of patients.

Once an antidepressant has been initiated, the PHQ-9 should be tracked at follow-up and can be used to guide adjustments in dosages and changes to the overall regimen. Four to 6 weeks after medication initiation, if the PHQ-9 score decreases by 5 or more the current treatment should be continued. For score reduction between 2 and 4 increasing the dose of the medication should be considered, and for score reductions of less than 2, switching or augmenting the medication should be considered. A common pitfall for PCPs is not pushing antidepressant medication dosages to therapeutic levels before considering them a failure. Up to one-third of patients require 10 weeks at a therapeutic antidepressant level to experience a response.[112]

As providers have many options of electronically based medication references specific medication dosing is not covered in this review. These tools should be employed to confirm starting doses, usual treatment doses, and maximum doses of antidepressants. Dose adjustments based on liver and kidney function, and safety in the setting of pregnancy or lactation should also be reviewed prior to selection of a medication.

The goal of treatment is for full remission of major depression. PCPs should familiarize themselves with terms commonly used in psychiatry, including partial response, response, remission, and recovery (**Table 3**).

Table 3
Grading response to treatment

Grade	Definition
No response	<25% reduction[a]
Partial response	20%–50% reduction[a]
Response	>50% reduction
Remission	Asymptomatic for 2 wk
Recovery	Asymptomatic for 6 mo

[a] Reduction in the initial score from a validated instrument – Examples include PHQ9, Hamilton Depression Rating Scale, Beck Depression Inventory.

Mechanism of action, efficacy and tolerability

In 2009 a systematic review of 117 RCTs found that mirtazapine (highest efficacy), escitalopram, venlafaxine, and sertraline, were most efficacious statistically versus 12 antidepressants assessed (although not specifically based on head-to-head trials). The same review found escitalopram, sertraline, citalopram, and bupropion were the best tolerated medications based on having the lowest dropout rates in studies (in order with the lowest dropout rate first). The superiority of escitalopram and sertraline over comparator antidepressants was further substantiated in a pair of Cochrane Review articles, although the lead author was the same for all 3 reviews.[113,114] Hence, all other considerations being equal, PCPs can consider escitalopram and sertraline statistically superior to other choices for first-line therapy based on a combination of high efficacy and tolerability in studies. However, as with many studies, the impact of these statistical differences in real life clinical differences for patients is unclear.

Escitalopram may be easier to tolerate because it binds in a highly selective way to 5-hydroxytryptamine (5-HT) serotonin reuptake receptors, whereas most SSRIs bind with varying degrees to both 5-HT and the noradrenaline (NA) receptor that modulates norepinephrine reuptake inhibition.[115] In general, the more neurotransmitter effects an antidepressant causes, the more side effects it causes as well. For example, MAOIs, some of the most difficult to tolerate antidepressants, not only modulate serotonin and norepinephrine, they are also anticholinergic like TCAs, antihistaminic, and affect tyramine levels. Sertraline and escitalopram may be more efficacious than some because, except for paroxetine and duloxetine, they are the most potent in their binding to 5-HT.[115] Interestingly, sertraline is also a significant dopamine reuptake inhibitor.

Table 4 summarizes the mechanisms of action of antidepressants and the implications for common side effects related to those mechanisms. Table 5 highlights common side effects and the antidepressants most likely to cause them. Notably, the primary reason for discontinuation of antidepressants cited in studies is nausea and vomiting.[110] Fortunately, nausea and vomiting resolve within 2 weeks of initiation or a dose increase and can be mitigated with lower initial doses and taking medication with food.[116] As the preliminary nausea resolves, many antidepressants including SSRIs, TCAs, MAOIs, and mirtazapine cause weight gain; the least likely to do so are bupropion and SNRIs.

If PCPs understand antidepressant side effects well they can counsel patients on the specific risks and benefits of classes and specific medications. Identification of deal-breaker side effects, like sexual dysfunction for some patients, can help to eliminate some choices. It is helpful to counsel patients that SSRI side effects like nausea, vomiting, diarrhea, and headache tend to resolve over time, but fatigue, weight gain, and sexual dysfunction can be more chronic.[116] It is important to adequately prepare patients for nearly immediate experience of side effects and the delay in the experience of improved mood.

Serious side effects

Common side effects listed above are problematic for quality of life but rarely have significant clinical long-term harm. However, antidepressants are not innocuous, and there are several serious side effects worth highlighting.

SSRIs have been found in observational studies to cause upper gastrointestinal bleeding especially in combination with NSAIDs.[117] This risk increases with the concurrent use of other substances that accelerate ulcer formation, such as alcohol and corticosteroids, and is reduced with acid suppression medications including proton pump inhibitors and H2 blockers.[118]

Table 4
Antidepressant side effects related to affected neuroamine

Serotonin (5-HT reuptake inhibition) • SSRIs, SNRIs, TCAs (clomipramine), MAOIs, mirtazapine	• Abdominal upset, diarrhea • Sexual dysfunction • Short-term anxiety • Sleep disturbances
Norepinephrine (Na reuptake inhibition) • Most SSRIs, SNRIs, TCAs (desipramine, maprotiline), unique mechanism, MAOI	• Elevated blood pressure • Dry mouth • Constipation
Dopamine (DA reuptake inhibition) • Sertraline, bupropion, mirtazapine, MAOIs, venlafaxine (at high doses)	• Hyperprolactinemia • Extrapyramidal symptoms • Sexual dysfunction • Cognitive dysfunction • Galactorrhea, gynecomastia
Acetylcholine (Muscarinic receptor blockade) • TCAs, paroxetine	Head, Eyes, Ears, Nose and Throat (HEENT): dry eyes, blurred vision, dry mouth, acute narrow angle glaucoma Cardiovascular: sinus tachycardia Gastrointestinal: constipation Genitourinary: urinary retention Neuro: memory dysfunction
Histamine (H1 receptor blockade) • TCAs	• Sedation • Weight gain
Alpha-1 adrenergic receptor (antagonism) • TCAs, nefazodone	• Orthostatic hypotension • Dizziness • Reflex tachycardia

Data from Refs.[115,128–130]

Table 5
Antidepressants and common side effects

Side Effect	Medications	Clinical Pearl
Nausea and vomiting	Venlafaxine highest. Common in multiple antidepressants.	• Use extended release formulation of venlafaxine to reduce nausea • Start at lower doses • Take with food
Diarrhea	Sertraline > paroxetine	Consider using in patients with constipation
Weight gain	TCAs/MAOIs, mirtazapine > paroxetine	Consider using in patients with anorexia or unintentional weight loss
Somnolence	Trazodone > mirtazapine	Use in patients with concurrent insomnia. Dose at night.
Dizziness	Venlafaxine > sertraline, duloxetine	Consider bedtime dosing
Headache	Venlafaxine > bupropion, paroxetine, sertraline, escitalopram	
Sexual dysfunction	Sertraline > venlafaxine > citalopram > paroxetine Bupropion and mirtazapine do not have this effect	May require dose reduction or medication switch
Insomnia	Bupropion > sertraline, fluoxetine, paroxetine, venlafaxine	Take in the morning

Data from Refs.[110,116]

Hyponatremia is most apt to occur around 2 weeks after initiation of an SSRI.[110] The highest risk populations for hyponatremia are women older than 65, especially those taking diuretics or medications that interact with the liver metabolism of antidepressants. In US Food and Drug Administration case reports, fluoxetine was most frequently reported (70%). Clinicians should consider checking a chemistry panel 2 weeks after initiation in high-risk populations or any patient manifesting typical signs and symptoms of hyponatremia.

Falls and fractures have been reported with SSRI use. A 2014 Canadian prospective cohort study of 6600 postmenopausal women found that use of SSRIs or SNRIs increased the risk for fragility fractures (hazard ratio, 1.88) even after controlling for history of falls and bone mineral density in the spine and hip (hazard ratio, 1.68).[119] Given the prevalence of antidepressant medication use and the morbidity and mortality associated with osteoporotic fractures (especially of the hip), clinicians should consider the risk/benefit ratio of antidepressant therapy in at risk populations for osteoporosis.

Serotonin syndrome is a rare but potentially fatal condition that arises from the use of multiple serotonergic medications. A seminal New England Journal of Medicine review in 2005 describes a clinical triad of mental status changes, autonomic hyperactivity, and neuromuscular abnormalities that characterize the syndrome.[120] The review describes neuromuscular changes that start with symptoms of akathisia then progress to tremor, clonus, and finally rigidity; autonomic changes that include tachycardia, hypertension, diaphoresis and hyperthermia; and mental status changes that progress from agitation and hypervigilance to overt delirium. Recognizing the correlation between these symptoms and signs and interacting medications or recreational substance use is imperative, because the treatment only is supportive with the immediate discontinuation of the offending agents. Culprit medications include all antidepressants but also triptans, lithium, buspirone, antiemetics, drugs of abuse including ecstasy, and opiates (eg, methadone, fentanyl, meperidine).[121] A good resource for determining the safety of medications use, including antidepressants, during lactation is the National Institute of Health sponsored site - LacMed- http://toxnet.nlm.nih.gov/newtoxnet/lactmed.htm. The nuances of antidepressant safety during pregnancy are beyond the scope of this review. Clinicians need to weigh the risks of birth defects that have been reported in case-reports or cohort studies such as persistent pulmonary hypertension, and cardiac defects with the risks of untreated depression on the health of the mother and unborn fetus.

Medication interactions

Many antidepressants are metabolized through the hepatic cytochrome P450 system (TCAs, fluoxetine, paroxetine, venlafaxine) and are susceptible to medication interactions. Complicating matters, some antidepressants are cytochrome P450 inhibitors (fluoxetine, paroxetine, bupropion, duloxetine).[122,123] Given the risks of these interactions, PCPs should check for medication interactions whenever initiating an antidepressant or adding a different medication to a medication regimen that already includes an antidepressant.

Treatment-resistant depression

Unfortunately, approximately 30% to 40% of patients will not respond to first-line antidepressant interventions. Treatment-resistant depression (TRD) by strict definition is the failure to respond to adequate doses and duration of therapy of 2 different antidepressants from 2 different classes.[124] More liberal definitions have been used in studies and in practice. Taking a complete psychiatric history with detailed information on number of prior episodes of major depression; comorbid psychiatric, medical, and substance use disorders; and history of antidepressant use including highest dose achieved, duration of therapy, and experience with efficacy and side effects is helpful for the ongoing treatment of patients with refractory depression. Many patients report a history of not responding to an antidepressant but never used the medication long enough or never achieved a therapeutic dose to determine efficacy.

The 2006 STAR*D trial is the best study on the medication management of TRD and suggests a reasonable approach. After failure to respond to citalopram, 25% of subjects experienced remission with switching medications to another SSRI or to a different class of medications (venlafaxine, bupropion).[125] Alternatively, 30% of subjects experienced remission with augmentation of the SSRI with bupropion or buspirone (although buspirone had higher dropout rates).[126] After failing to improve with the switch of medications, or augmentation, an additional 25% had remission of symptoms with augmentation with liothyronine (triiodothyronine) versus 16% with lithium.[127] Switching antidepressants instead of augmenting at this stage had lower efficacy with 13% remission with mirtazapine and 20% with nortriptyline.[35] By the fourth attempt at a medication change in the study, adding or changing medications to this highly refractory group had low remissions rates of 7% to 14%.[112]

The take-home points for PCPs are to consider switching medications or using an augmenting agent if patients do not reach remission. However, if patients have refractory symptoms after 2 to 3 medication changes, they should be seen by a psychiatrist for assistance in the management of TRD.

A dose-equivalent, immediate medication switch can occur if medications are changed to one in the same class (eg, sertraline 150 mg to escitalopram 20 mg). If the new medication is of a different class, a cross-tapering strategy can be used (eg, sertraline 200 mg to venlafaxine XR 150 mg). During the first week, half the dose of the first antidepressant can be used at the same time as half the therapeutic equivalent dose of the second antidepressant (eg, sertraline 100 mg and venlafaxine XR 75 mg). After this crossover week, the first antidepressant is discontinued and the second antidepressant is increased to the full therapeutic equivalent dose (eg, discontinue sertraline, increase venlafaxine XR to 150 mg). If providers are unfamiliar with use of augmenting agents, they should seek the advice of a psychiatrist to discuss dose initiation, titration, and monitoring of medications like triiodothyronine and lithium.

SUMMARY

Depression is a common and morbid condition seen frequently in primary care settings. PCPs are increasingly responsible for the diagnosis and management of this condition. Well-validated and time-effective screening modalities exist and should be used in the ambulatory setting as long as adequate access to support and interventions is available. Although MDD is usually episodic, it confers significant harm, and the specific symptoms and degree of functional impairment experienced by patients is variable. Characterizing the severity of symptoms helps with determining an optimal management plan.

Lifestyle, psychotherapy, and pharmacotherapy interventions are effective for the treatment of MDD. Options should be discussed with patients so that an appropriate and acceptable strategy can be mutually determined. Adherence to psychotherapy and pharmacotherapy can be improved by engaging patients in the risks, benefits, timing, and practical implications of each approach. Side effects are the most common reason for discontinuation of medication therapy, but providers can tailor the choice of medications to best fit the individual needs of patients. The goals of therapy are to reach remission, but approximately one-third of patients experience refractory symptoms. PCPs should be familiar with strategies to address TRD depression but also acknowledge when MDD symptoms are either too severe or refractory for primary management by a generalist.

There are many opportunities to improve the care of depressed patients in the primary care setting. Education and understanding by providers about the identification and management of MDD is just one step. Cultural and societal stigmas continue to hamper the care of many patients; ongoing public health campaigns and parity of access and coverage for mental health is necessary to meet the needs of patients. Improvements in drug design can address the delay in efficacy and the problematic side-effect profile of antidepressants to improve efficacy and tolerability of pharmacologic approaches to care.

REFERENCES

1. Craven MA, Bland R. Depression in primary care: current and future challenges. Can J Psychiatry 2013;58:442–8.
2. Bostwick JM. A generalist's guide to treating patients with depression with an emphasis on using side effects to tailor antidepressant therapy. Mayo Clin Proc 2010;85:538–50.
3. Fancher TL, Kravitz RL. In the clinic. Depression. Ann Intern Med 2010;152: ITC51-15 [quiz: ITC5–6].
4. Weihs K, Wert JM. A primary care focus on the treatment of patients with major depressive disorder. Am J Med Sci 2011;342:324–30.
5. Salazar WH. Management of depression in the outpatient office. Med Clin North Am 1996;80:431–55.
6. Hermanns N, Caputo S, Dzida G, et al. Screening, evaluation and management of depression in people with diabetes in primary care. Prim Care Diabetes 2013; 7:1–10.
7. Lima NN, do Nascimento VB, de Carvalho SM, et al. Childhood depression: a systematic review. Neuropsychiatr Dis Treat 2013;9:1417–25.
8. Park M, Unutzer J. Geriatric depression in primary care. Psychiatr Clin North Am 2011;34:469–87, ix–x.
9. Unutzer J, Park M. Older adults with severe, treatment-resistant depression. JAMA 2012;308:909–18.
10. American Psychiatric Association. Diagnostic and statistical manual of mental disorder. 5th edition. Arlington (VA): American Psychiatric Association; 2013.
11. Uher R, Payne JL, Pavlova B, et al. Major depressive disorder in dsm-5: implications for clinical practice and research of changes from DSM-IV. Depress Anxiety 2014;31(6):459–71.
12. Novick JS, Stewart JW, Wisniewski SR, et al. Clinical and demographic features of atypical depression in outpatients with major depressive disorder: preliminary findings from STAR*D. J Clin Psychiatry 2005;66:1002–11.
13. Pae CU, Tharwani H, Marks DM, et al. Atypical depression: a comprehensive review. CNS Drugs 2009;23:1023–37.
14. Blanco C, Vesga-Lopez O, Stewart JW, et al. Epidemiology of major depression with atypical features: results from the National Epidemiologic Survey on Alcohol and Related Conditions (NESARC). J Clin Psychiatry 2012;73:224–32.

15. The ICD-10 classification of mental and behavioural disorders. World Health Organization. 2010. Available at: http://www.who.int/classifications/icd/en/. Accessed January 12, 2014.

16. Barlow DH. Clinical handbook of psychological disorders: a step-by-step treatment manual. 4th edition. New York: Guilford Press; 2008.

17. Hollon SD. What is cognitive behavioural therapy and does it work? Curr Opin Neurobiol 1998;8:289–92.

18. Haaga DA, Beck AT. Perspectives on depressive realism: implications for cognitive theory of depression. Behav Res Ther 1995;33:41–8.

19. Das AK, Olfson M, McCurtis HL, et al. Depression in African Americans: breaking barriers to detection and treatment. J Fam Pract 2006;55:30–9.

20. Lewis-Fernandez R, Das AK, Alfonso C, et al. Depression in US Hispanics: diagnostic and management considerations in family practice. J Am Board Fam Pract 2005;18:282–96.

21. Simon GE, Goldberg DP, Von Korff M, et al. Understanding cross-national differences in depression prevalence. Psychol Med 2002;32:585–94.

22. Wakefield JC, Schmitz MF. When does depression become a disorder? Using recurrence rates to evaluate the validity of proposed changes in major depression diagnostic thresholds. World Psychiatry 2013;12:44–52.

23. Maj M. When does depression become a mental disorder? Br J Psychiatry 2011; 199:85–6.

24. Parker G. Classifying clinical depression: an operational proposal. Acta Psychiatr Scand 2011;123:314–6.

25. Kennedy SH, Dickens SE, Eisfeld BS, et al. Sexual dysfunction before antidepressant therapy in major depression. J Affect Disord 1999;56:201–8.

26. Zilcha-Mano S, Dinger U, McCarthy KS, et al. Changes in well-being and quality of life in a randomized trial comparing dynamic psychotherapy and pharmacotherapy for major depressive disorder. J Affect Disord 2014;152–154:538–42.

27. IsHak WW, Greenberg JM, Balayan K, et al. Quality of life: the ultimate outcome measure of interventions in major depressive disorder. Harv Rev Psychiatry 2011;19:229–39.

28. Clarke DM, Currie KC. Depression, anxiety and their relationship with chronic diseases: a review of the epidemiology, risk and treatment evidence. Med J Aust 2009;190:S54–60.

29. Kessler RC, Berglund P, Demler O, et al. The epidemiology of major depressive disorder: results from the National Comorbidity Survey Replication (NCS-R). JAMA 2003;289:3095–105.

30. Kessler RC, Chiu WT, Demler O, et al. Prevalence, severity, and comorbidity of 12-month DSM-IV disorders in the National Comorbidity Survey Replication. Arch Gen Psychiatry 2005;62:617–27.

31. Vuorilehto M, Melartin T, Isometsa E. Depressive disorders in primary care: recurrent, chronic, and co-morbid. Psychol Med 2005;35:673–82.

32. Meader N, Mitchell AJ, Chew-Graham C, et al. Case identification of depression in patients with chronic physical health problems: a diagnostic accuracy meta-analysis of 113 studies. Br J Gen Pract 2011;61(593):e808–20.

33. Stegenga BT, Kamphuis MH, King M, et al. The natural course and outcome of major depressive disorder in primary care: the PREDICT-NL study. Soc Psychiatry Psychiatr Epidemiol 2012;47:87–95.

34. Vuorilehto MS, Melartin TK, Isometsa ET. Course and outcome of depressive disorders in primary care: a prospective 18-month study. Psychol Med 2009; 39:1697–707.

35. Rush AJ, Trivedi MH, Wisniewski SR, et al. Acute and longer-term outcomes in depressed outpatients requiring one or several treatment steps: a STAR*D report. Am J Psychiatry 2006;163(11):1905–17.
36. Zajecka J, Kornstein SG, Blier P. Residual symptoms in major depressive disorder: prevalence, effects, and management. J Clin Psychiatry 2013;74:407–14.
37. Gilman SE, Dupuy JM, Perlis RH. Risks for the transition from major depressive disorder to bipolar disorder in the National Epidemiologic Survey on Alcohol and Related Conditions. J Clin Psychiatry 2012;73:829–36.
38. Salvatore P, Baldessarini RJ, Khalsa HM, et al. Predicting diagnostic change among patients diagnosed with first-episode DSM-IV-TR major depressive disorder with psychotic features. J Clin Psychiatry 2013;74:723–31.
39. Solomon DA, Keller MB, Leon AC, et al. Multiple recurrences of major depressive disorder. Am J Psychiatry 2000;157(2):229.
40. U.S. Preventive Services Task Force. Screening for depression in adults: U.S. preventive services task force recommendation statement. Ann Intern Med 2009;151:784–92.
41. MacMillan HL, Patterson CJ, Wathen CN, et al. Screening for depression in primary care: recommendation statement from the Canadian Task Force on Preventive Health Care. CMAJ 2005;172:33–5.
42. Group MoMW. VA/DoD clinical practice guideline for management of major depressive disorder (MDD). Department of Veterans Affairs, Department of Defense; 2009.
43. Kroenke K, Spitzer RL, Williams JB. The Patient Health Questionnaire-2: validity of a two-item depression screener. Med Care 2003;41:1284–92.
44. Unutzer J, Park M. Strategies to improve the management of depression in primary care. Prim Care 2012;39:415–31.
45. Kroenke K, Spitzer RL, Williams JB. The PHQ-9: validity of a brief depression severity measure. J Gen Intern Med 2001;16:606–13.
46. Jarjoura D, Polen A, Baum E, et al. Effectiveness of screening and treatment for depression in ambulatory indigent patients. J Gen Intern Med 2004;19:78–84.
47. Maurer DM. Screening for depression. Am Fam Physician 2012;85:139 44.
48. Chopra K, Kumar B, Kuhad A. Pathobiological targets of depression. Expert Opin Ther Targets 2011;15:379–400.
49. Soskin DP, Cassiello C, Isacoff O, et al. The inflammatory hypothesis of depression. FOCUS: The Journal of Lifelong Learning in Psychiatry 2012;10:413–21.
50. Prins J, Olivier B, Korte SM. Triple reuptake inhibitors for treating subtypes of major depressive disorder: the monoamine hypothesis revisited. Expert Opin Investig Drugs 2011;20:1107–30.
51. Shyn SI, Hamilton SP. The genetics of major depression: moving beyond the monoamine hypothesis. Psychiatr Clin North Am 2010;33:125–40.
52. Sullivan PF, Neale MC, Kendler KS. Genetic epidemiology of major depression: review and meta-analysis. Am J Psychiatry 2000;157:1552–62.
53. Kendler KS, Kessler RC, Walters EE, et al. Stressful life events, genetic liability, and onset of an episode of major depression in women. Am J Psychiatry 1995;152:833–42.
54. El-Hage W, Leman S, Camus V, et al. Mechanisms of antidepressant resistance. Front Pharmacol 2013;4:146.
55. Endicott J. Measurement of depression in patients with cancer. Cancer 1984;53:2243–9.
56. Bjelland I, Dahl AA, Haug TT, et al. The validity of the Hospital Anxiety and Depression Scale. An updated literature review. J Psychosom Res 2002;52:69–77.

57. Blanco C, Alegria AA, Liu SM, et al. Differences among major depressive disorder with and without co-occurring substance use disorders and substance-induced depressive disorder: results from the National Epidemiologic Survey on Alcohol and Related Conditions. J Clin Psychiatry 2012;73:865–73.

58. Magidson JF, Wang S, Lejuez CW, et al. Prospective study of substance-induced and independent major depressive disorder among individuals with substance use disorders in a nationally representative sample. Depress Anxiety 2013;30:538–45.

59. Bolton JM, Belik SL, Enns MW, et al. Exploring the correlates of suicide attempts among individuals with major depressive disorder: findings from the national epidemiologic survey on alcohol and related conditions. J Clin Psychiatry 2008;69:1139–49.

60. Cherpitel CJ. Screening for alcohol problems in the U.S. general population: comparison of the CAGE, RAPS4, and RAPS4-QF by gender, ethnicity, and service utilization. Rapid Alcohol Problems Screen. Alcohol Clin Exp Res 2002;26:1686–91.

61. Gleason OC, Pierce AM, Walker AE, et al. The two-way relationship between medical illness and late-life depression. Psychiatr Clin North Am 2013;36(4): 533–44.

62. Gregory RJ, Nihalani ND, Rodriguez E. Medical screening in the emergency department for psychiatric admissions: a procedural analysis. Gen Hosp Psychiatry 2004;26:405–10.

63. Olshaker JS, Browne B, Jerrard DA, et al. Medical clearance and screening of psychiatric patients in the emergency department. Acad Emerg Med 1997;4: 124–8.

64. Griffith JL, Gaby L. Brief psychotherapy at the bedside: countering demoralization from medical illness. Psychosomatics 2005;46:109–16.

65. Sansone RA, Sansone LA. Demoralization in patients with medical illness. Psychiatry (Edgmont) 2010;7:42–5.

66. O'Keeffe N, Ranjith G. Depression, demoralisation or adjustment disorder? Understanding emotional distress in the severely medically ill. Clin Med 2007;7: 478–81.

67. Wagley JN, Rybarczyk B, Nay WT, et al. Effectiveness of abbreviated CBT for insomnia in psychiatric outpatients: sleep and depression outcomes. J Clin Psychol 2013;69:1043–55.

68. Stroebe M, Schut H, Stroebe W. Health outcomes of bereavement. Lancet 2007; 370:1960–73.

69. Nagraj S, Barclay S. Bereavement care in primary care: a systematic literature review and narrative synthesis. Br J Gen Pract 2011;61:e42–8.

70. Sung SC, Dryman MT, Marks E, et al. Complicated grief among individuals with major depression: prevalence, comorbidity, and associated features. J Affect Disord 2011;134:453–8.

71. Howland RH, Schettler PJ, Rapaport MH, et al. Clinical features and functioning of patients with minor depression. Psychother Psychosom 2008;77:384–9.

72. Rodriguez MR, Nuevo R, Chatterji S, et al. Definitions and factors associated with subthreshold depressive conditions: a systematic review. BMC Psychiatry 2012;12:181.

73. Hellerstein DJ, Agosti V, Bosi M, et al. Impairment in psychosocial functioning associated with dysthymic disorder in the NESARC study. J Affect Disord 2010;127:84–8.

74. Backenstrass M, Frank A, Joest K, et al. A comparative study of nonspecific depressive symptoms and minor depression regarding functional impairment

and associated characteristics in primary care. Compr Psychiatry 2006;47: 35–41.

75. Klein DN, Shankman SA, Rose S. Ten-year prospective follow-up study of the naturalistic course of dysthymic disorder and double depression. Am J Psychiatry 2006;163:872–80.

76. Ackermann RT, Williams JW Jr. Rational treatment choices for non-major depressions in primary care: an evidence-based review. J Gen Intern Med 2002;17: 293–301.

77. Fournier JC, DeRubeis RJ, Hollon SD, et al. Antidepressant drug effects and depression severity: a patient-level meta-analysis. JAMA 2010;303(1):47–53.

78. Cuijpers P, Sijbrandij M, Koole SI, et al. The efficacy of psychotherapy and pharmacotherapy in treating depressive and anxiety disorders: a meta-analysis of direct comparisons. World Psychiatry 2013;12:137–48.

79. Denollet J. Type D personality. A potential risk factor refined. J Psychosom Res 2000;49:255–66.

80. Mols F, Denollet J. Type D personality in the general population: a systematic review of health status, mechanisms of disease, and work-related problems. Health Qual Life Outcomes 2010;8:9.

81. Denollet J, Sys SU, Stroobant N, et al. Personality as independent predictor of long-term mortality in patients with coronary heart disease. Lancet 1996;347: 417–21.

82. Li Z, Page A, Martin G, et al. Attributable risk of psychiatric and socio-economic factors for suicide from individual-level, population-based studies: a systematic review. Soc Sci Med 2011;72:608–16.

83. Hawton K, van Heeringen K. Suicide. Lancet 2009;373:1372–81.

84. Holma KM, Melartin TK, Haukka J, et al. Incidence and predictors of suicide attempts in DSM-IV major depressive disorder: a five-year prospective study. Am J Psychiatry 2010;167:801–8.

85. Harris EC, Barraclough B. Suicide as an outcome for mental disorders. A meta-analysis. Br J Psychiatry 1997;170:205–28.

86. Inskip HM, Harris EC, Barraclough B. Lifetime risk of suicide for affective disorder, alcoholism and schizophrenia. Br J Psychiatry 1998;172:35–7.

87. McDowell AK, Lineberry TW, Bostwick JM. Practical suicide risk management for the busy primary care physician. Mayo Clin Proc 2011;86(8):792–800.

88. Smith EG, Kim HM, Ganoczy D, et al. Suicide risk assessment received prior to suicide death by Veterans health administration patients with a history of depression. J Clin Psychiatry 2013;74:226–32.

89. Simon GE, Rutter CM, Peterson D, et al. Does response on the PHQ-9 depression questionnaire predict subsequent suicide attempt or suicide death? Psychiatr Serv 2013;64:1195–202.

90. Suicide assessment five-step evaluation and triage (SAFE-T). Substance Abuse and Mental Health Services Administration U.S. Department of Health and Human Services; 2009. p. 2.

91. Beck AT, Steer RA. Clinical predictors of eventual suicide: a 5- to 10-year prospective study of suicide attempters. J Affect Disord 1989;17:203–9.

92. Hidaka BH. Depression as a disease of modernity: explanations for increasing prevalence. J Affect Disord 2012;140(3):205–14.

93. Sarris J, O'Neil A, Coulson CE, et al. Lifestyle medicine for depression. BMC Psychiatry 2014;14:107.

94. Cooney GM, Dwan K, Greig CA, et al. Exercise for depression. Cochrane Database Syst Rev 2013;(9):CD004366.

95. Pilling S, Anderson I, Goldberg D, et al. Depression in adults, including those with a chronic physical health problem: summary of NICE guidance. BMJ 2009;339:b4108.

96. Manber R, Edinger JD, Gress JL, et al. Cognitive behavioral therapy for insomnia enhances depression outcome in patients with comorbid major depressive disorder and insomnia. Sleep 2008;31(4):489–95.

97. Ishman SL, Benke JR, Cohen AP, et al. Does surgery for obstructive sleep apnea improve depression and sleepiness? Laryngoscope 2014. [Epub ahead of print].

98. Taylor G, McNeill A, Girling A, et al. Change in mental health after smoking cessation: systematic review and meta-analysis. BMJ 2014;348:g1151.

99. Jorm AF, Morgan AJ, Hetrick SE. Relaxation for depression. Cochrane Database Syst Rev 2008;(4):CD007142.

100. Kamioka H, Tsutani K, Yamada M, et al. Effectiveness of music therapy: a summary of systematic reviews based on randomized controlled trials of music interventions. Patient Prefer Adherence 2014;8:727–54.

101. Kamioka H, Okada S, Tsutani K, et al. Effectiveness of animal-assisted therapy: a systematic review of randomized controlled trials. Complement Ther Med 2014;22(2):371–90.

102. Cuijpers P, van Straten A, Andersson G, et al. Psychotherapy for depression in adults: a meta-analysis of comparative outcome studies. J Consult Clin Psychol 2008;76(6):909–22.

103. Huhn M, Tardy M, Spineli LM, et al. Efficacy of Pharmacotherapy and Psychotherapy for Adult Psychiatric Disorders: A Systematic Overview of Meta-analyses. JAMA psychiatry 2014.

104. Bea SM, Tesar GE. A primer on referring patients for psychotherapy. Cleve Clin J Med 2002;69(2):113–4, 117–8, 120–2, 125–7.

105. Olfson M, Blanco C, Wang S, et al. National trends in the mental health care of children, adolescents, and adults by office-based physicians. JAMA Psychiatry 2014;71(1):81–90.

106. Mojtabai R, Olfson M. National trends in long-term use of antidepressant medications: results from the U.S. National Health and Nutrition Examination Survey. J Clin Psychiatry 2014;75(2):169–77.

107. Gartlehner G, Hansen RA, Thieda P, et al. AHRQ Comparative Effectiveness Reviews. Comparative effectiveness of second-generation antidepressants in the pharmacologic treatment of adult depression. Rockville (MD): Agency for Healthcare Research and Quality (US); 2007.

108. Hawton K, Bergen H, Simkin S, et al. Toxicity of antidepressants: rates of suicide relative to prescribing and non-fatal overdose. Br J Psychiatry 2010;196:354–8.

109. Stahl SM. Mechanism of action of serotonin selective reuptake inhibitors. Serotonin receptors and pathways mediate therapeutic effects and side effects. J Affect Disord 1998;51(3):215–35.

110. Gartlehner G, Gaynes BN, Hansen RA, et al. Comparative benefits and harms of second-generation antidepressants: background paper for the American College of Physicians. Ann Intern Med 2008;149(10):734–50.

111. Qaseem A, Snow V, Denberg TD, et al. Using second-generation antidepressants to treat depressive disorders: a clinical practice guideline from the American College of Physicians. Ann Intern Med 2008;149(10):725–33.

112. Rush AJ. STAR*D: what have we learned? Am J Psychiatry 2007;164(2):201–4.

113. Cipriani A, Santilli C, Furukawa TA, et al. Escitalopram versus other antidepressive agents for depression. Cochrane Database Syst Rev 2009;(2):CD006532.

114. Cipriani A, La Ferla T, Furukawa TA, et al. Sertraline versus other antidepressive agents for depression. Cochrane Database Syst Rev 2009;(2):CD006117.
115. Hamon M, Bourgoin S. Pharmacological profile of antidepressants: a likely basis for their efficacy and side effects? Eur Neuropsychopharmacol 2006;16:S625–32.
116. Gharbia SAP. Common side effects of antidepressants. Available at: http://www.pdrhealth.com/antidepressants/common-side-effects-of-antidepressants.
117. Loke YK, Trivedi AN, Singh S. Meta-analysis: gastrointestinal bleeding due to interaction between selective serotonin uptake inhibitors and non-steroidal anti-inflammatory drugs. Aliment Pharmacol Ther 2008;27(1):31–40.
118. Targownik LE, Bolton JM, Metge CJ, et al. Selective serotonin reuptake inhibitors are associated with a modest increase in the risk of upper gastrointestinal bleeding. Am J Gastroenterol 2009;104(6):1475–82.
119. Moura C, Bernatsky S, Abrahamowicz M, et al. Antidepressant use and 10-year incident fracture risk: the population-based Canadian Multicentre Osteoporosis Study (CaMoS). Osteoporos Int 2014;25(5):1473–81.
120. Edward W, Boyer MS. The Serotonin syndrome. N Engl J Med 2005;352: 1112–20.
121. Rolan PE. Drug interactions with triptans: which are clinically significant? CNS Drugs 2012;26(11):949–57.
122. Andrade C. Selective serotonin reuptake inhibitor drug interactions in patients receiving statins. J Clin Psychiatry 2014;75(2):e95–9.
123. DA F. Cytochrome P450 drug interaction table. 2007. Accessed at: http://medicine.iupui.edu/clinpharm/ddis/main-table/.
124. Souery D, Papakostas GI, Trivedi MH. Treatment-resistant depression. J Clin Psychiatry 2006;67(Suppl 6):16–22.
125. Rush AJ, Trivedi MH, Wisniewski SR, et al. Bupropion-SR, sertraline, or venlafaxine-XR after failure of SSRIs for depression. N Engl J Med 2006; 354(12):1231–42.
126. Trivedi MH, Fava M, Wisniewski SR, et al. Medication augmentation after the failure of SSRIs for depression. N Engl J Med 2006;354(12):1243–52.
127. Nierenberg AA, Fava M, Trivedi MH, et al. A comparison of lithium and T(3) augmentation following two failed medication treatments for depression: a STAR*D report. Am J Psychiatry 2006;163(9):1519–30 [quiz: 1665].
128. Bijlsma EY, Chan JS, Olivier B, et al. Sexual side effects of serotonergic antidepressants: mediated by inhibition of serotonin on central dopamine release? Pharmacol Biochem Behav 2014;121c:88–101.
129. Yildiz A, Gonül AS, Tamam L. Mechanism of actions of antidepressants: beyond the receptors. Bull Clin Psychopharmacol 2002;12:194–200.
130. Damsa C, Bumb A, Bianchi-Demicheli F, et al. "Dopamine-dependent" side effects of selective serotonin reuptake inhibitors: a clinical review. J Clin Psychiatry 2004;65(8):1064–8.

Anxiety Disorders in Primary Care

Heidi Combs, MD, MS*, Jesse Markman, MD, MBA

KEYWORDS

- Anxiety disorders • Primary care • Generalized anxiety disorder • Panic disorder
- Social anxiety disorder • Posttraumatic stress disorder
- Obsessive-compulsive disorder

KEY POINTS

- Anxiety disorders are the most common psychiatric condition presenting to primary care practitioners.
- Patients with anxiety disorders present significant costs in terms of healthcare use, loss of workforce productivity, disability, and quality of life.
- Detection of anxiety disorders in primary care is poor and can be improved with use of available screening tools.
- Effective management for each of the anxiety disorders is available, but currently underused, leaving patients in a less-than-optimally treated state.

INTRODUCTION

Anxiety disorders, the most common psychiatric diagnosis in the United States, have an estimated prevalence of 13.3%.[1] Even though potentially and significantly debilitating, these conditions often command less attention than higher-profile affective and psychotic illnesses. Supporting the serious nature of these conditions is the study by Kroenke and coworkers[2] of 965 randomly selected patients in primary care clinics. The study found 19.5% had at least one anxiety disorder. As the number of anxiety diagnoses rose, accompanying impairment correspondingly increased. These conditions are also associated with elevated divorce rates, greater unemployment, a diminished sense of well-being, and increased reliance on public assistance.[3] Significantly, suicide risk elevates with acute and chronic anxiety disorders.[4]

Patients with anxiety disorders often seek treatment from primary care providers (PCP).[5] They may present with medically unexplained symptoms, making identification of the correct diagnosis a challenge. The patient may be oblivious to recognizing

Department of Psychiatry and Behavioral Sciences, Harborview Medical Center, University of Washington, 325 9th Avenue Box 359911, Seattle, WA 98103, USA
* Corresponding author.
E-mail address: hcombs@uw.edu

Med Clin N Am 98 (2014) 1007–1023
http://dx.doi.org/10.1016/j.mcna.2014.06.003
medical.theclinics.com

their symptom as anxiety and the correct diagnosis becomes easier to miss. Given that 25% to 50% of primary care clinic patients present with medically unexplained symptoms, it is important for the PCP to screen for psychiatric illnesses, including anxiety disorders.[6]

Adequate treatment is necessary. Effective management for each of the anxiety disorders is available, but currently underused, leaving patients in a less-than-optimally treated state. For example, in Kroenke's sample of 965 patients, 41% with anxiety disorders went untreated.[2]

This article reviews epidemiology, screening tools, impact on patients, costs, and treatment of each of the major anxiety disorders.

METHODS

A PubMed literature search was conducted in September and October of 2013 using the following terms: "Anxiety Disorders and Primary Care," "Generalized Anxiety Disorder and Primary Care," "Social Anxiety Disorder and Primary Care," "Post Traumatic Stress Disorder and Primary Care," and "Obsessive-Compulsive Disorder and Primary Care." Abstracts from articles on adults, written in English and published within the past 5 years, were reviewed for relevance. Additional articles and texts were identified from references found in the bibliographies of appropriate manuscripts.

DIAGNOSTIC CHALLENGES

PCPs often miss the accurate diagnosis of anxiety disorders. In a study of 840 primary care patients, rates of misdiagnosis were 85.8% for panic disorder (PD), 71% for generalized anxiety disorder (GAD), and 97.8% for social anxiety disorder (SAD).[7] The first step in making an accurate diagnosis is to understand the disorder. **Table 1** contains a brief description of the key features of the major anxiety disorders. Unfortunately, patient descriptions of their symptoms can mislead even the most astute physician. Patients may report physical or psychological distress, including somatic complaints, pain, sleep disturbance, and depression,[8] but are unaware that they are actually experiencing anxiety. Wittchen and colleagues[9] noted that only 13.3% of patients with GAD presented with anxiety symptoms as a chief complaint, whereas somatic concerns were described 47.8% of the time. **Table 2** contains a case illustrating a common presentation for a person with GAD. Screening for key symptoms associated with the disorder can help identify the diagnosis. Patients with anxiety disorders also have high rates of coexisting additional mental illnesses, further complicating the diagnostic process.

CO-OCCURRING MENTAL DISORDERS

Co-occurring mental conditions are commonly found in patients with anxiety disorders. These can be disorders of mood, substance use, psychosis, or another anxiety disorder. It is estimated that up to 90% of persons with GAD experience one or more comorbid psychiatric diagnoses.[11] Stein and coworkers[12] found that in patients with posttraumatic stress disorder (PTSD), major depression is seen in 61% of patients, GAD in 39%, social phobia in 17%, PD in 6%, and substance use disorders in 22% of patients. Additionally, the presence of comorbid psychiatric conditions worsens prognosis. Patients with multiple psychiatric diagnoses experience lower remission rates, increased rate of suicide, and higher use of health care.[8,11]

Table 1
Key diagnostic features of various anxiety disorders

Diagnosis	Key Features Including Signs/Symptoms[10]
Generalized anxiety disorder	Excessive, uncontrolled anxiety/worry about several things that interfere with ability to function. In addition, worry accompanied by other symptoms, such as fatigue, muscle tension, irritability, restlessness, and sleep disturbance.
Social anxiety disorder	Marked anxiety or fear in social settings where there is risk of scrutiny or judgment. Results in avoidance of situation or enduring situation with marked distress.
Panic disorder	Recurrent panic attacks described as unexpected waves of anxiety associated with multiple physical and cognitive symptoms. Common symptoms include elevated heart rate, shortness of breath, trembling, abdominal distress, dizziness, and fear of death or losing control.
Posttraumatic stress disorder	After trauma exposure person experiences symptoms that can include intrusive thoughts of trauma, negative mood, dissociation, avoiding thinking about the trauma or external reminders of it, and hyperarousal.
Obsessive-compulsive disorder	Presence of unwanted recurrent intrusive thoughts or images and/or repetitive behaviors or mental acts, such as counting or checking performed to reduce anxiety. These thoughts/acts impair function or are significantly time-consuming.

Data from American Psychiatric Association, DSM-5 Task Force. Diagnostic and statistical manual of mental disorders: DSM-5. Arlington (VA): American Psychiatric Association; 2013.

Table 2
Case and key diagnostic features

Case	Key Diagnostic Features
A 36-year-old woman comes in with a chief complaint of insomnia. She feels constantly on edge and finds it hard to fall asleep because of concern about her parents. She also experiences muscle stiffness and shoulder and back pain. On questioning, she describes unremitting worry that something terrible will happen to her elderly parents. The patient lives in a state distant from her parents. There is a family history of cardiovascular disease and she worries they will die of heart attacks. The patient calls her parents multiple times a day to check in with them and feels extremely anxious if she cannot reach them. She also worries about how her kids are doing in school even though they are getting good grades, and about her finances even though she is in good standing financially. She has been experiencing the worry for 5 y. She has missed multiple days of work because of her incapacitating worry.	She experiences multiple symptoms associated with the worry including feeling on edge, sleep disturbance, muscle stiffness, shoulder pain The worry is uncontrolled The worry is about multiple things 5-y history indicating chronic problem It is impairing function as evidenced by missing multiple days of work

HUMAN AND FINANCIAL COST

Patients with anxiety disorders present significant costs in terms of health care use, loss of workforce productivity, disability, and quality of life. The estimated direct and indirect cost of PD per 1 million persons in 2005 was between $241.7 and $287.6 billion US dollars.[13] The estimated health costs for persons with GAD are 64% higher than those without GAD, and patients with obsessive-compulsive disorder (OCD) are estimated to lose 3 years of wages because of their illness over their lifetime.[14,15] Moitra and colleagues[16] found patients with SAD had significantly impaired workplace function compared with individuals with other anxiety disorders and unemployment was twice as likely. Those who suffer from anxiety also experience disability outside of work resulting in poor quality of life and diminished life satisfaction.

IMPACT OF SUBTHRESHOLD SYMPTOMS

Multiple studies describe that persons suffering from anxiety symptoms that are subdiagnostic threshold have significantly more impairment than those who report no symptoms.[17–20] Problems these patients encounter include poor perceived health, psychological distress, and increased use of medical services.[17–20] Predictably, data indicate that there are far more patients with subthreshold anxiety symptoms than there are patients with diagnosed, threshold disorders; yet it is questionable if this group is identified or treated.[17,19,20] Data do not yet exist for criteria for treatment in subthreshold cases.

INCREASED RISK OF SUICIDE

Practitioners associate increased risk of suicide with depression; however, many do not realize anxiety disorders also increase risk. Suicidal ideation, rates of self-injury, and suicide attempts are elevated in persons with anxiety disorders.[21–23] Bomyea and colleagues[24] found approximately 26% of patients with anxiety disorders endorsed passive suicidal ideation and 16% endorsed suicidal thoughts in the previous month. Both current and lifetime anxiety disorders confer increased suicide risk. Kahn and colleagues[4] found suicide risk among patients with anxiety disorders was increased by a factor of 10 or more compared with the general population, regardless of the type of anxiety disorder. The association between suicide and anxiety disorders underscores the importance of detection and treatment.

SCREENING TOOLS

Effective screening tools are available to detect anxiety disorders (**Table 3**). Finding time to use these adjuncts can be challenging in a busy primary care practice. Screening tools designed to address the full spectrum of co-occurring affective and anxiety disorders are especially useful. The Hospital Anxiety and Depression Scale distinguishes between depression and anxiety if both are present.[25] Other broad-based instruments, such as the PRIME-MD-PHQ, can identify anxiety and mood disorders.[26] For the case shown in **Table 2**, either of the screening tools for GAD listed in **Table 3** are appropriate.

CHANGES FROM DIAGNOSTIC AND STATISTICAL MANUAL OF PSYCHIATRIC DISORDERS-IV TO DIAGNOSTIC AND STATISTICAL MANUAL OF PSYCHIATRIC DISORDERS-V

The newest version of the Diagnostic and Statistical Manual of Psychiatric Disorders (DSM), the DSM-V, is now available.[10] Some highlights are relevant. Agoraphobia is

Table 3
Screening tools

Diagnosis	Screening Tools	Screening Question
GAD	GAD-7[27] GAD-2[28]	Do you consider yourself a worrier?
SAD	SPIN[29] Mini-SPIN[30]	When you are in a situation where people can observe you, do you feel nervous and worry that they will judge you?
PD	PHQ panic disorder scale[31]	Do you have waves of nervousness that come out of the blue and you notice things in your body like your heart goes fast or it is hard to breathe?
PTSD	PC-PTSD[32] PCL-C[33] M-3[34]	Have you experienced a trauma that still haunts you?
OCD	MINI[35] Y-BOC[35] PRIME-MD[35]	Do you have thoughts that occur over and over that really bother you? Are there things you have to do over and over, such as washing your hands, checking, or counting?

now in a category of its own rather than a qualifier for PD. The diagnosis of PTSD is no longer found in the anxiety disorder section but is now described in the section on, "Trauma and Stress-Related Disorders." In addition, the trauma can have occurred to a close family member or friend, or the trauma could be first-hand repeated or extreme exposures to details, such as those experienced by police officers. The later criteria mean that such persons as first responders could develop PTSD. OCD is now found under the classification, "Obsessive-Compulsive and Related Disorders." Although PTSD and OCD are no longer officially classified in the category of "anxiety disorders" in the DSM-V, they share the same issues of underdiagnosis and approaches to treatment so they are therefore included in this review.

EPIDEMIOLOGY, COURSE OF ILLNESS, AND PROGNOSIS
GAD

The prevalence rates for GAD in primary care settings range from 3.7% to 14.8%.[17,36] GAD accounts for 50% of anxiety disorders seen in this setting.[37] Only depression is a more commonly identified psychiatric diagnosis. GAD tends to be a chronic illness with fluctuating symptom severity. A 12-year longitudinal study found 60% of patients recovered; however, approximately half of these patients relapsed during that time.[38] Disability caused by GAD is comparable with that of major depressive disorder.[39]

SAD

The 1-month prevalence of SAD in primary care is 7%.[40] This condition is a chronic illness marked by long duration and has a rate of recovery of only 38%.[41,42] One study described the probability of recovery from SAD in 12-year follow-up as 37%; this number was lower than for GAD and PD.[38] SAD is associated with marked impairment in work productivity and decreased income.[43]

PD

The median prevalence of PD in primary care is 4% to 6%, whereas the median prevalence in the general population is 2.7%.[1,44] The course of PD is similar to other anxiety disorders in that it is chronic and relapsing. In the Harvard/Brown Anxiety Research Study, nearly one-third of patients with PD were likely to experience a recurrence within a year after recovery and another study by Simon and coworkers found that nearly half had recurrence in 2 years.[38,45,46]

PTSD

The prevalence for PTSD in primary care settings is estimated to be 11.8%.[12] This is higher than the 1-year prevalence rate of 3.5% to 6% for the general US population.[47] In Stein's study of 368 patients in a primary care clinic, 65% reported a history of exposure to a severe, potentially traumatic event. Similar to other anxiety disorders, patients with PTSD are more likely to reach out to their primary care physicians than to a mental health specialist. PTSD is a chronic condition with only one-third recovering at 1 year and one-third still experiencing symptoms 10 years after trauma exposure.[48]

OCD

OCD has an estimated lifetime prevalence of 1.6%.[1] The onset of the condition can be in adolescence; however, patients may be sufficiently embarrassed or ashamed preventing them from revealing their symptoms. Consequently, the average time to diagnosis is 11 years.[49] An estimated 70% of patients with OCD experience a chronic course, whereas only 23% experience a waxing and waning course.[49] Data vary for remission rates with treatment. In the largest trial of 213 patients, 22.1% had partial remission, 16.9% had full remission, and 59% of patients who remitted subsequently relapsed.[50]

TREATMENT

Treatment of anxiety disorders can be difficult and intimidating for the PCP. There are specific recommendations for interventions that can be accomplished without the support of psychiatrist or psychotherapist. Many options address multiple anxiety disorders. **Table 4** provides an overview of treatment options for each anxiety disorder.

PHARMACOTHERAPY

Pharmacotherapy for anxiety disorders is separated into two categories of medications each having a different purpose. The first consists of agents that aim to prevent future anxiety, whereas the second treat acute anxiety, but do not decrease future occurrences.

First-line pharmacologic treatment of anxiety disorders aims to prevent future symptoms. This is best accomplished with single-agent treatment with a selective serotonin reuptake inhibitor (SSRI) or serotonin noradrenergic reuptake inhibitor (SNRI).[51–54] These medications have been shown to be effective in reducing anxiety symptoms in multiple placebo-controlled trials, but no single agent has proved consistently more effective than others.[51–55] The choice of SSRIs and SNRIs over tricyclic antidepressants (TCAs) as first-line therapy is due largely to their lack of anticholinergic side effects and toxicity in overdose.[51] Increased tolerability does not translate to increased efficacy, however, and some experienced PCPs may be more comfortable with use of TCAs because they have been in use for more than 40 years. The antidepressant mirtazapine is an effective agent either as single agent or combined with SSRIs for augmentation.[55] Unfortunately, these medicines can require 4 to 8 weeks to show efficacy. Treatment of anxiety disorders typically requires higher doses and longer duration than indicated for unipolar depression.[56] Brief medication trials can give the false perception of failure and treatment resistance. The ability to wait for response is therefore required on the part of provider and patient.

Table 4
Treatment options

	GAD	PD	OCD	SAD	PTSD
Medication-based treatment recommendations	Daily SSRI/SNRI Anxiolytics may be needed as a bridge for severe symptoms until antidepressants provide relief	Daily SSRI/SNRI Use long-acting anxiolytics because short-acting agents are unlikely to actually abort panic attacks	Daily SSRI/SNRI Anxiolytics may be needed as a bridge for severe symptoms until antidepressants provide relief	Daily SSRI/SNRI Propranolol is useful for public speaking	Daily SSRI/SNRI Use prazosin for nightmares Anxiolytics may be needed as a bridge for severe symptoms until antidepressants provide relief Benzodiazepines are generally not recommended
Psychotherapy recommendations	Cognitive behavioral therapy	Cognitive behavioral therapy	Exposure and response prevention	Cognitive behavioral therapy	Prolonged exposure Cognitive processing therapy

Anxiolytic medications compose the second set of pharmacologic agents for treatment of acute anxiety. These medicines abort current symptoms of anxiety and do little to prevent symptom recurrence. Anxiolytics can be divided into benzodiazepines and nonbenzodiazepines.

Benzodiazepines are frequently thought of as the classic anxiolytic. This class of medication provides a wide range of choices in terms of onset of action, half-life, and the presence of an active metabolite.[57] There are no specific recommendations in terms of use of one benzodiazepine over another in the treatment of anxiety disorders. In general terms, benzodiazepines with shorter half-lives and more rapid onset of action are more likely to lead to rebound anxiety when effects of the medication wane, leading to a need to take more of the medication.[58] If possible, longer-acting benzodiazepines (ie, clonazepam) should be used in conjunction with antidepressants, when the provider needs to decrease anxiety acutely, to allow for treatment engagement, and/or treat symptoms that are threatening patient safety. If possible, treatment should be limited in duration and stopped once antidepressants lower overall anxiety levels and patients are able to engage in other forms of treatment. Although benzodiazepines are effective, physiologic dependence develops in all users so misuse poses potential problems. Tapering benzodiazepines must be gradual and can be dangerous if completed too abruptly. The withdrawal syndrome that accompanies benzodiazepine cessation closely parallels that of alcohol withdrawal. The mildest form is rebound anxiety that can be seen with reducing or missing doses and is most common with short-acting benzodiazepines (ie, alprazolam).[58] In rare cases, severe withdrawal symptoms can be seen, which can lead to seizure, coma, and death. Although exact rates of risk are unknown, severe withdrawal is rare and more likely in patients taking higher doses, for prolonged periods, and for whom the medication is discontinued abruptly.[58] Co-occurring substance use disorder is common and in such situations treatment with benzodiazepines is contraindicated.

When anxiety needs to be controlled acutely, but benzodiazepines are not indicated, there are other alternatives. The anticholinergic agent hydroxyzine, β-blocker propranolol, and gabapentin are effective alternatives as anxiolytics without abuse potential.

PSYCHOTHERAPY

Several psychotherapy modalities are effective in the treatment of anxiety disorders. The modality that has the most robust data is cognitive behavioral therapy (CBT).[59] CBT is designed to identify the maladaptive automatic thoughts and behaviors, and then restructure them through therapeutic exercises. CBT has been shown sufficiently effective for several anxiety disorders, with very limited side effects, so it is often considered first-line treatment. Disorder-specific and general protocols are created to address all major anxiety disorders.[59] Major drawbacks to therapy include difficulty in engaging the patient (a significant barrier with anxiety disorders) and limited or variable availability of well-trained therapists. With the advent of manualized therapy and computer-based therapy, treatment can now be delivered without therapists. This provides an exciting resource for rural areas or for isolated primary care physicians with limited support. Social workers, nurses, and medical assistants can be trained to provide therapy and primary care physicians can guide the patient through the protocol in a few office visits.

COMBINATION TREATMENT

Although psychotherapy and pharmacotherapy have been shown to be individually effective, studies consistently demonstrate that combination treatment gives superior results compared with either treatment alone.[51,59,60]

ADJUNCTIVE TREATMENTS

Although recognized as components of behavioral therapies, breathing exercises, muscle relaxation, and mindfulness-based meditation techniques are effective alone or in conjunction with other therapies.[61] Exercise as adjunctive therapy produces mixed results. Randomized controlled trials of exercise as treatment of anxiety disorders compared with waitlist control do show a benefit for exercise therapy. Trials that compare exercise therapy with pharmacotherapy or CBT, however, show no benefit for exercise over these traditional treatments. Although it may seem, then, that exercise may be better than no intervention, yet not superior to pharmacotherapy or psychotherapy, one cannot yet draw that conclusion. There is significant variability between the discussed studies in terms of type of exercise intervention, population, and control groups, making it difficult to draw any firm conclusions when looking at the collection of studies as a whole.[62]

COMPLEMENTARY AND ALTERNATIVE MEDICINE

A robust review of the use of complementary and alternative medicine (CAM) is outside the scope of this article, although CAM is commonly used in patients with anxiety disorders. The Coordinated Anxiety Learning and Management study reports 43% of patients relied on CAM when they believed that their symptoms were inadequately treated.[63] CAM includes such remedies as St. John's wort and kava, substances with potential negative side effects so their use should be identified by the practitioner. St. John's wort frequently interacts with medications through the P-450 system. Additionally, providers often do not recognize that combining St. John's wort with other serotonergic agents can precipitate serotonin syndrome. Kava is potentially hepato toxic.[63] PCPs should identify patients using alternative agents so they can monitor for side effects and drug-drug interactions.

USE OF RATING SCALES IN TREATMENT

Rating scales are very useful in terms of diagnosis and following treatment response, but providers should not mistake changes in rating scales as a replacement for the subjective experience of the patient. Treatment choices (ie, dose changes, medication initiation, or discontinuation) should be driven by patient choice and subjective experience of improvement or lack thereof.

SPECIFIC TREATMENTS AND RECOMMENDATIONS
GAD

The generalized nature of symptoms in GAD requires the use of pharmacotherapy oriented toward prevention. SSRIs and SNRIs are considered the mainstay of therapy.[51] Anxiolytics, although effective for a short time, have limited overall utility given that they need frequent repeat dosing as a result of accompanying rebound anxiety. Longer-acting benzodiazepines, such as clonazepam, offer some benefit, but still fail to inhibit future anxiety once the medication has worn off.[57] Severe cases of GAD may require that serotonergic medications be pushed to maximum dosage and response to medication may not appear until 12 weeks or more have elapsed.[55] Augmentation with agents, such as mirtazapine, buspirone, and even atypical antipsychotics, has been effective but this strategy is best done with psychiatric consultation.[51,55]

Psychotherapy for GAD is very effective. CBT for GAD focuses on psychoeducation and identifying and restructuring common automatic thoughts, such as catastrophizing. Several different manualized protocols have been developed and can be used in a primary care setting.[59] For patients who are particularly emotionally sophisticated and motivated, some of these protocols can be completed with very limited practitioner support or even without supervision.[64,65] Although many protocols exist, we recommend "Mastery of your anxiety and worry" as part of the "Treatments That Work" series, published by Oxford University Press, because this manual is practical, effective, and well validated. Although treatment manuals for providers are not free of charge, a single therapist's guide can be reused for hundreds of patients. A sample case of combination treatment is presented in **Table 5**.

Table 5
Generalized anxiety disorder case and treatments

Case: Treatment Generalized Anxiety Disorder	

A 36-year-old woman comes in with a chief complaint of insomnia. She feels constantly on edge and finds it hard to fall asleep because of concern about her parents. She also experiences muscle stiffness and shoulder and back pain. On questioning, she describes unremitting worry that something terrible will happen to her elderly parents. The patient lives in a state distant from her parents. There is a family history of cardiovascular disease and she worries they will die of heart attacks. The patient calls her parents multiple times a day to check in with them and feels extremely anxious if she cannot reach them. She also worries about how her kids are doing in school even though they are getting good grades, and about her finances even though she is in good standing financially. She has been experiencing the worry for 5 y. She has missed multiple days of work because of her incapacitating worry.	Initial Treatment:
	• Start SSRI or SNRI medication
	  ○ Sertraline, 25 mg PO Q day × 7 d, then increase to 50 mg PO Q day
	• Refer patient to therapist for CBT
	  ○ Therapy focused on psychoeducation and understanding safety behaviors (calling parents). Therapy also challenges automatic, catastrophic thoughts (ie, "my parents will die")

Return visit in 6 wk: Patient has mild symptom improvement, but still feels anxious	Continued treatment: • Increase sertraline to 100 mg PO Q day because symptoms have improved somewhat, but further improvement may be seen with a higher dose • May need future dose increase to 200 mg • Continued CBT protocol
Return in 12 wk: Patient completed CBT; feels appreciably improved. Worry decreased, she makes fewer calls to her parents, and chronic pain has significantly subsided. Sleep is improved and she no longer misses work. Patient would like to continue her current medication regimen as it is.	Continued treatment • Maintain sertraline at 100 mg per day for now because the patient is pleased with her improvements and would like to continue her current treatment • Return in 6 mo to assess progress

PD

Treatment of PD centers on the prevention of panic attacks and reducing anxiety about impending attacks. Treatment with SSRIs and SNRIs is effective in preventing attacks and reducing overall anxiety.[53] These agents do nothing to treat an acute attack, however, and reducing symptoms typically takes 4 to 8 weeks or longer. Severe cases of PD may require high dosing of SSRIs and prolonged treatment, but improvement can be tracked by frequency of attacks.

Providers may find that patients benefit from an agent to abort an impending attack at its onset. Benzodiazepines are the agent of choice[66]; however, these medications must be prescribed with caution. If a patient has attacks that last less than 20 minutes, limited efficacy is seen from a short-acting benzodiazepine because the agent's onset occurs after the attack has resolved. There is also evidence that use of benzodiazepines worsens the response or outcome of psychotherapy, an important treatment modality in PD.[59] Some providers find that using longer-acting benzodiazepines, such as clonazepam, may reduce overall anxiety that can contribute to or trigger attacks, but use of these agents should be reserved for cases when patients are unable to function without them or cannot otherwise tolerate the use of serotonergic medications.

Psychotherapy for PD is at least as effective a treatment as pharmacotherapy and at times superior to medication.[59] CBT for PD is the most studied and validated.[59] Although more experienced therapists have been shown to provide better outcomes for their patients, novice therapists can also be effective.[59] Online and manualized CBT protocols for PD are well-validated and can be used with limited supervision or, with certain versions, by the patient alone.[64,65] "Mastery of your anxiety and panic" is another manualized favorite from the "Treatments That Work" series, published by Oxford University Press.[67]

SAD

Medication for true SAD requires serotonergic agents. SSRIs and SNRIs are first-line choices. Positive results may not be evident for up to 8 weeks.[52] There is limited use for anxiolytic agents except for specific anxiety-provoking events (ie, public speaking) that acutely worsen symptoms. In these cases, propranolol can be used at low doses and side effects are minimal. There have been no studies, however, that demonstrate efficacy for β-blockers for the treatment of overall symptoms of SAD.[52] Benzodiazepines can be tried, but used with caution, as previously described.[52]

CBT for social phobia centers on exposure to anxiety-provoking situations to demonstrate that resulting anxiety is tolerable and not dangerous. Over time, repeated exposure leads to an overall symptom reduction and patients are able to tolerate what they could not before. This modality can be combined with cognitive restructuring techniques that examine and challenge assumptions that patients make about themselves (ie, "I will embarrass myself"). A combination of exposure and cognitive restructuring may be the most effective psychotherapy available.[59] Although effective, patients are frequently unable to engage in it on their own or with only limited provider guidance. Therapists require more extensive treatment experience than merely familiarizing themselves with a treatment manual; therefore, we recommend patient referral to a trained therapist.[59]

OCD

Pharmacologic treatment of OCD also centers on the use of serotonergic agents. SSRIs and SNRIs are first choice and treatment of adults often requires prescribing maximum dosage. Time to efficacy can be as long as 12 weeks at this dose.[55] Treatment-resistant cases of OCD may respond to higher-potency serotonergic medications, such as clomipramine, a TCA with significant serotonergic activity, or to the addition of augmentation agents, such as atypical antipsychotics.[55] These strategies should be managed by a psychiatrist. Little benefit is seen from short-acting anxiolytic medication other than in extreme cases when they are needed to reduce anxiety sufficiently severe so as the patient is inhibited from travel to a provider's office.

Exposure and response prevention therapy is the gold standard of treatment of patients with OCD.[59] This therapy consists of exposing the patient to an anxiety-provoking stimulus (ie, germs from a dirty sink) and then preventing typical response behavior (ie, hand washing). Through experience of anxiety, the patient learns that it is tolerable and response behaviors are unnecessary. Taking a patient through this type of therapy requires a highly trained therapist and a committed patient. PCPs should refer patients with OCD, willing to engage in psychotherapy, to experienced therapists whenever possible.

PTSD

Pharmacotherapy for PTSD spans several different agents because there are often multiple symptom domains that require treatment. Overall mood and anxiety symptoms associated with PTSD are well-treated by SSRIs and SNRIs.[54] These agents can also help reduce the acute hypervigilance and explosive anger outbursts that manifest with this disorder. Efficacy after starting medication is usually evident in 4 to 8 weeks.[56] Patients may require acute anxiolytics for management of immediate symptoms while serotonergic agents take effect. Benzodiazepines can be used, but have no long-term effect on PTSD and might possibly be harmful by prolonging recovery time.[54] Many patients with PTSD experience trauma-related nightmares. Treatment with prazosin is considered the first-line agent of choice, but providers should counsel patients about the risk of dizziness and orthostatic hypotension with use.[54] Treatment-resistant or complex cases of PTSD (those with severe symptoms, extreme mood variability, and psychosis) can be treated with the addition of antipsychotic agents and/or mood stabilizers, and should also be referred to a psychiatrist.

The standard of care for PTSD uses psychotherapy and medication management.[54] Multiple therapies have been developed. Two forms of therapy shown to have the best efficacy are prolonged exposure and cognitive processing therapy.[54] Prolonged exposure focuses on exposing the patient (in a real or imaginative way) to the trauma they experienced and progressively habituating the patient to the resultant anxiety. Cognitive processing therapy seeks to restructure assumptions and thoughts raised by exposure to trauma. Both therapeutic modalities require trained, experienced therapists for successful treatment.

DISCUSSION AND CONCLUSION

Anxiety disorders are prevalent and debilitating. They are often underdiagnosed and undertreated in the primary care setting. Because of their propensity to cause generalized and poorly differentiated symptoms, detection can prove difficult. Multiple, effective screening tools exist to aid the PCP in this challenge. Once identified, however, treatments are predictably effective. Protocols for managing GAD, PD, SAD, OCD, and PTSD have much in common. Even if delineation of the specific disorder is unclear, the PCP will rarely go wrong by providing a prescription for a serotonergic antidepressant and referral for psychotherapy. Psychotherapy is important for adequate treatment and many online and manualized treatments have greatly increased patients' access to care.

Although this article serves as an overview, individual cases can vary in presentation and course. Of all challenging cases, those determined to be treatment-resistant cases can be the most problematic.

In conclusion, PCPs can effectively diagnose and manage patients with a variety of anxiety disorders. Many patients would benefit from psychotherapy and/or psychopharmacology. More complex or severe anxiety disorders are best managed with consultation and collaboration with colleagues in psychiatry and psychology.

REFERENCES

1. Kessler RC, Chiu WT, Demler O, et al. Prevalence, severity, and comorbidity of 12-month DSM-IV disorders in the National Comorbidity Survey Replication. Arch Gen Psychiatry 2005;62(6):617–27. http://dx.doi.org/10.1001/archpsyc. 62.6.617.
2. Kroenke K, Spitzer RL, Williams JB, et al. Anxiety disorders in primary care: prevalence, impairment, comorbidity, and detection. Ann Intern Med 2007; 146(5):317–25.
3. Olatunji BO, Cisler JM, Tolin DF. Quality of life in the anxiety disorders: a meta-analytic review. Clin Psychol Rev 2007;27(5):572–81. http://dx.doi.org/10.1016/j. cpr.2007.01.015.
4. Khan A, Leventhal RM, Khan S, et al. Suicide risk in patients with anxiety disorders: a meta analysis of the FDA database. J Affect Disord 2002;68(2–3):183–90.
5. Harman JS, Rollman BL, Hanusa BH, et al. Physician office visits of adults for anxiety disorders in the United States, 1985-1998. J Gen Intern Med 2002;17(3):165–72.
6. Edwards TM, Stern A, Clarke DD, et al. The treatment of patients with medically unexplained symptoms in primary care: a review of the literature. Ment Health Fam Med 2010;7(4):209–21.
7. Vermani M, Marcus M, Katzman MA. Rates of detection of mood and anxiety disorders in primary care: a descriptive, cross-sectional study. Prim Care Companion CNS Disord 2011;13(2). http://dx.doi.org/10.4088/PCC.10m01013.
8. Nutt D, Argyropoulos S, Hood S, et al. Generalized anxiety disorder: a comorbid disease. Eur Neuropsychopharmacol 2006;16(Suppl 2):S109–18. http://dx.doi. org/10.1016/j.euroneuro.2006.04.003.
9. Wittchen H-U, Kessler RC, Beesdo K, et al. Generalized anxiety and depression in primary care: prevalence, recognition, and management. J Clin Psychiatry 2002;63(Suppl 8):24–34.
10. American Psychiatric Association, DSM-5 Task Force. Diagnostic and statistical manual of mental disorders: DSM-5. Arlington (VA): American Psychiatric Association; 2013.
11. Wittchen HU, Zhao S, Kessler RC, et al. DSM-III-R generalized anxiety disorder in the National Comorbidity Survey. Arch Gen Psychiatry 1994;51(5):355–64.
12. Stein MB, McQuaid JR, Pedrelli P, et al. Posttraumatic stress disorder in the primary care medical setting. Gen Hosp Psychiatry 2000;22(4):261–9.
13. Konnopka A, Leichsenring F, Leibing E, et al. Cost-of-illness studies and cost-effectiveness analyses in anxiety disorders: a systematic review. J Affect Disord 2009;114(1–3):14–31. http://dx.doi.org/10.1016/j.jad.2008.07.014.
14. Olfson M, Gameroff MJ. Generalized anxiety disorder, somatic pain and health care costs. Gen Hosp Psychiatry 2007;29(4):310–6. http://dx.doi.org/10.1016/j. genhosppsych.2007.04.004.

15. Huppert JD, Simpson HB, Nissenson KJ, et al. Quality of life and functional impairment in obsessive-compulsive disorder: a comparison of patients with and without comorbidity, patients in remission, and healthy controls. Depress Anxiety 2009;26(1):39–45. http://dx.doi.org/10.1002/da.20506.
16. Moitra E, Beard C, Weisberg RB, et al. Occupational impairment and social anxiety disorder in a sample of primary care patients. J Affect Disord 2011; 130(1–2):209–12. http://dx.doi.org/10.1016/j.jad.2010.09.024.
17. Kertz SJ, Woodruff-Borden J. Human and economic burden of GAD, subthreshold GAD, and worry in a primary care sample. J Clin Psychol Med Settings 2011; 18(3):281–90. http://dx.doi.org/10.1007/s10880-011-9248-1.
18. Olfson M, Broadhead WE, Weissman MM, et al. Subthreshold psychiatric symptoms in a primary care group practice. Arch Gen Psychiatry 1996; 53(10):880–6.
19. Pini S, Perkonnig A, Tansella M, et al. Prevalence and 12-month outcome of threshold and subthreshold mental disorders in primary care. J Affect Disord 1999;56(1):37–48.
20. Rucci P, Gherardi S, Tansella M, et al. Subthreshold psychiatric disorders in primary care: prevalence and associated characteristics. J Affect Disord 2003; 76(1–3):171–81.
21. Sareen J, Cox BJ, Afifi TO, et al. Anxiety disorders and risk for suicidal ideation and suicide attempts: a population-based longitudinal study of adults. Arch Gen Psychiatry 2005;62(11):1249–57. http://dx.doi.org/10.1001/archpsyc.62. 11.1249.
22. Chartrand H, Sareen J, Toews M, et al. Suicide attempts versus nonsuicidal self-injury among individuals with anxiety disorders in a nationally representative sample. Depress Anxiety 2012;29(3):172–9. http://dx.doi.org/10.1002/da.20882.
23. Bolton JM, Cox BJ, Afifi TO, et al. Anxiety disorders and risk for suicide attempts: findings from the Baltimore Epidemiologic Catchment area follow-up study. Depress Anxiety 2008;25(6):477–81. http://dx.doi.org/10.1002/da.20314.
24. Bomyea J, Lang AJ, Craske MG, et al. Suicidal ideation and risk factors in primary care patients with anxiety disorders. Psychiatry Res 2013;209(1):60–5. http://dx.doi.org/10.1016/j.psychres.2013.03.017.
25. Bjelland I, Dahl AA, Haug TT, et al. The validity of the Hospital Anxiety and Depression Scale. An updated literature review. J Psychosom Res 2002;52(2): 69–77.
26. Spitzer RL, Kroenke K, Williams JB. Validation and utility of a self-report version of PRIME-MD: the PHQ primary care study. Primary Care Evaluation of Mental Disorders. Patient Health Questionnaire. JAMA 1999;282(18):1737–44.
27. Spitzer RL, Kroenke K, Williams JB, et al. A brief measure for assessing generalized anxiety disorder: the GAD-7. Arch Intern Med 2006;166(10):1092–7. http://dx.doi.org/10.1001/archinte.166.10.1092.
28. Kroenke K, Spitzer RL, Williams JBW, et al. The Patient Health Questionnaire Somatic, Anxiety, and Depressive Symptom Scales: a systematic review. Gen Hosp Psychiatry 2010;32(4):345–59. http://dx.doi.org/10.1016/j.genhosppsych.2010. 03.006.
29. Connor KM, Davidson JR, Churchill LE, et al. Psychometric properties of the Social Phobia Inventory (SPIN). New self-rating scale. Br J Psychiatry 2000; 176:379–86.
30. Seeley-Wait E, Abbott MJ, Rapee RM. Psychometric properties of the mini-social phobia inventory. Prim Care Companion J Clin Psychiatry 2009;11(5): 231–6. http://dx.doi.org/10.4088/PCC.07m00576.

31. Löwe B, Gräfe K, Zipfel S, et al. Detecting panic disorder in medical and psychosomatic outpatients: comparative validation of the Hospital Anxiety and Depression Scale, the Patient Health Questionnaire, a screening question, and physicians' diagnosis. J Psychosom Res 2003;55(6):515–9.

32. Ouimette P, Wade M, Prins A, et al. Identifying PTSD in primary care: comparison of the Primary Care-PTSD screen (PC-PTSD) and the General Health Questionnaire-12 (GHQ). J Anxiety Disord 2008;22(2):337–43. http://dx.doi.org/10.1016/j.janxdis.2007.02.010.

33. Elhai JD, Gray MJ, Kashdan TB, et al. Which instruments are most commonly used to assess traumatic event exposure and posttraumatic effects?: a survey of traumatic stress professionals. J Trauma Stress 2005;18(5):541–5. http://dx.doi.org/10.1002/jts.20062.

34. Gaynes BN, DeVeaugh-Geiss J, Weir S, et al. Feasibility and diagnostic validity of the M-3 checklist: a brief, self-rated screen for depressive, bipolar, anxiety, and post-traumatic stress disorders in primary care. Ann Fam Med 2010;8(2):160–9. http://dx.doi.org/10.1370/afm.1092.

35. Fineberg NA, Krishnaiah RB, Moberg J, et al. Clinical screening for obsessive-compulsive and related disorders. Isr J Psychiatry Relat Sci 2008;45(3):151–63.

36. Olfson M. Impairment in generalized anxiety disorder. Am J Psychiatry 2000;157(12).2060–1.

37. Wittchen HU, Hoyer J. Generalized anxiety disorder: nature and course. J Clin Psychiatry 2001;62(Suppl 11):15–9 [discussion: 20–1].

38. Bruce SE, Yonkers KA, Otto MW, et al. Influence of psychiatric comorbidity on recovery and recurrence in generalized anxiety disorder, social phobia, and panic disorder: a 12-year prospective study. Am J Psychiatry 2005;162(6):1179–87. http://dx.doi.org/10.1176/appi.ajp.162.6.1179.

39. Kessler RC, DuPont RL, Berglund P, et al. Impairment in pure and comorbid generalized anxiety disorder and major depression at 12 months in two national surveys. Am J Psychiatry 1999;156(12):1915–23.

40. Stein MB, McQuaid JR, Laffaye C, et al. Social phobia in the primary care medical setting. J Fam Pract 1999;48(7):514–9.

41. Beard C, Moitra E, Weisberg RB, et al. Characteristics and predictors of social phobia course in a longitudinal study of primary-care patients. Depress Anxiety 2010;27(9):839–45. http://dx.doi.org/10.1002/da.20676.

42. Chartier MJ, Hazen AL, Stein MB. Lifetime patterns of social phobia: a retrospective study of the course of social phobia in a nonclinical population. Depress Anxiety 1998;7(3):113–21.

43. Katzelnick DJ, Greist JH. Social anxiety disorder: an unrecognized problem in primary care. J Clin Psychiatry 2001;62(Suppl 1):11–5 [discussion: 15–6].

44. Roy-Byrne PP, Stein MB, Russo J, et al. Panic disorder in the primary care setting: comorbidity, disability, service utilization, and treatment. J Clin Psychiatry 1999;60(7):492–9 [quiz: 500].

45. Keller MB, Yonkers KA, Warshaw MG, et al. Remission and relapse in subjects with panic disorder and panic with agoraphobia: a prospective short-interval naturalistic follow-up. J Nerv Ment Dis 1994;182(5):290–6.

46. Simon NM, Safren SA, Otto MW, et al. Longitudinal outcome with pharmacotherapy in a naturalistic study of panic disorder. J Affect Disord 2002;69(1–3):201–8.

47. Kessler RC, McGonagle KA, Zhao S, et al. Lifetime and 12-month prevalence of DSM-III-R psychiatric disorders in the United States. Results from the National Comorbidity Survey. Arch Gen Psychiatry 1994;51(1):8–19.

48. Kessler RC, Sonnega A, Bromet E, et al. Posttraumatic stress disorder in the National Comorbidity Survey. Arch Gen Psychiatry 1995;52(12): 1048–60.

49. Pinto A, Mancebo MC, Eisen JL, et al. The Brown Longitudinal Obsessive Compulsive Study: clinical features and symptoms of the sample at intake. J Clin Psychiatry 2006;67(5):703–11.

50. Eisen JL, Sibrava NJ, Boisseau CL, et al. Five-year course of obsessive-compulsive disorder: predictors of remission and relapse. J Clin Psychiatry 2013;74(3):233–9. http://dx.doi.org/10.4088/JCP.12m07657.

51. Reinhold JA, Mandos LA, Rickels K, et al. Pharmacological treatment of generalized anxiety disorder. Expert Opin Pharmacother 2011;12(16):2457–67. http://dx.doi.org/10.1517/14656566.2011.618496.

52. Blanco C, Bragdon LB, Schneier FR, et al. The evidence-based pharmacotherapy of social anxiety disorder. Int J Neuropsychopharmacol 2013;16(1): 235–49. http://dx.doi.org/10.1017/S1461145712000119.

53. Perna G, Guerriero G, Caldirola D. Emerging drugs for panic disorder. Expert Opin Emerg Drugs 2011;16(4):631–45. http://dx.doi.org/10.1517/14728214.2011.628313.

54. VA/DoD. Clinical practice guideline for the management of post-traumatic stress. 2010.

55. Nemeroff CB. Management of treatment-resistant major psychiatric disorders. New York: Oxford University Press; 2012.

56. Stahl S. Stahl's essential psychopharmacology: the prescriber's guide. New York: Cambridge University Press; 2011.

57. Dell'osso B, Lader M. Do benzodiazepines still deserve a major role in the treatment of psychiatric disorders? A critical reappraisal. Eur Psychiatry 2013;28(1): 7–20. http://dx.doi.org/10.1016/j.eurpsy.2011.11.003.

58. Lader M. Benzodiazapines revisited: will we ever learn? Addiction 2011;106(12): 2086–109. http://dx.doi.org/10.1111/j.1360-0443.2011.03563.x.

59. Barlow D, Barlow D. Clinical handbook of psychological disorders. New York: Guilford Press; 2008.

60. Roy-Byrne P, Craske MG, Sullivan G, et al. Delivery of evidence-based treatment for multiple anxiety disorders in primary care: a randomized controlled trial. JAMA J Am Med Assoc 2010;303(19):1921–8. http://dx.doi.org/10.1001/jama.2010.608.

61. Marchand WR. Mindfulness-based stress reduction, mindfulness-based cognitive therapy, and Zen meditation for depression, anxiety, pain, and psychological distress. J Psychiatr Pract 2012;18(4):233–52. http://dx.doi.org/10.1097/01.pra.0000416014.53215.86.

62. Bartley CA, Hay M, Bloch MH. Meta-analysis: aerobic exercise for the treatment of anxiety disorders. Prog Neuropsychopharmacol Biol Psychiatry 2013;45: 34–9. http://dx.doi.org/10.1016/j.pnpbp.2013.04.016.

63. Bystritsky A, Hovav S, Sherbourne C, et al. Use of complementary and alternative medicine in a large sample of anxiety patients. Psychosomatics 2012;53(3): 266–72. http://dx.doi.org/10.1016/j.psym.2011.11.009.

64. Lewis C, Pearce J, Bisson JI. Efficacy, cost-effectiveness and acceptability of self-help interventions for anxiety disorders: systematic review. Br J Psychiatry 2012;200(1):15–21. http://dx.doi.org/10.1192/bjp.bp.110.084756.

65. Ruwaard J, Lange A, Schrieken B, et al. The effectiveness of online cognitive behavioral treatment in routine clinical practice. PLoS One 2012;7(7):e40089. http://dx.doi.org/10.1371/journal.pone.0040089.

66. Moylan S, Giorlando F, Nordfjærn T, et al. The role of alprazolam for the treatment of panic disorder in Australia. Aust N Z J Psychiatry 2012;46(3):212–24. http://dx.doi.org/10.1177/0004867411432074.
67. Barlow D, Craske MG. Mastery of your anxiety and panic. New York: Oxford University Press; 2007.

Diagnosis and Management of Bipolar Disorder in Primary Care
A DSM-5 Update

Carolyn J. Brenner, MD*, Stanley I. Shyn, MD, PhD

KEYWORDS

- Bipolar disorder • Mood stabilizers • Mood diagnosis and screening
- Collaborative care

KEY POINTS

- Depression is the most common presentation in bipolar disorder.
- Despite a more modest prevalence in the general population, there is a substantial over-representation of bipolar disorder among primary care patients presenting for depression, making the correct identification of these patients a high priority for general providers.
- Mood stabilizer selection depends on whether a patient requires treatment for bipolar depression, mania, or mood maintenance.
- Antidepressants (ie, reuptake blockers) are not generally appropriate in bipolar depression.

INTRODUCTION

Bipolar disorder (BD) is a chronic mental illness with multiple medical and psychiatric comorbidities, significant functional impairment, high cost to the patient and to the health care system, and high rates of suicide. Bipolar and related disorders include bipolar I disorder (BD1), bipolar II disorder (BD2), and cyclothymic disorder. Primary care providers may encounter emerging symptoms of BD in undiagnosed patients or may provide ongoing treatment with mood-stabilizing medication and manage common medication-related side effects and comorbidities. Timely identification of BD, particularly in the depressive phase, can be challenging. Selection of an appropriate medication regimen and thoughtful implementation of psychoeducation and

Funding Sources: None.
Conflicts of Interest: None.
Department of Psychiatry and Behavioral Sciences, Harborview Medical Center, University of Washington, 325 Ninth Avenue, Seattle, WA 98104, USA
* Corresponding author.
E-mail address: brennerc@uw.edu

Med Clin N Am 98 (2014) 1025–1048
http://dx.doi.org/10.1016/j.mcna.2014.06.004
0025-7125/14/$ – see front matter © 2014 Elsevier Inc. All rights reserved.

medical.theclinics.com

psychotherapy can substantially improve a patient's course. Finally, we discuss the advantages of collaborative care models and when circumstances might dictate referral to a community mental health center or higher level of care.

EPIDEMIOLOGY

BD affects men and women about equally with a lifetime prevalence estimated at between 1% and 3% in the general population,[1,2] with onset typically between age 18 and the mid-20s.[3] There is a marked skew in these numbers in the clinical setting, with one study finding 9.8% of all patients waiting to be seen in an urban primary care waiting room screening positive on the Mood Disorders Questionnaire (MDQ), a screening instrument for BD.[4] A separate investigation[5] found that 26% of the patients in a cohort of consecutive patients from a family practice clinic presenting for anxiety or depression had bipolar spectrum illness diagnosed on a semistructured diagnostic interview.

Despite this disproportionate representation, BD is an often missed diagnosis given that most of its natural history, during symptomatic periods, is depressive (and frequently subsyndromal, meaning that full-episode criteria are not always maintained). Long-term longitudinal studies show that the number of weeks spent with depressive symptoms outnumber weeks spent with manic symptoms by about 3:1 in BD1[6] and outnumber weeks spent with hypomanic symptoms by about 39:1 in BD2.[7]

GENETICS

The lifetime risk of BD increases to about 8% if there is a parent or other first-degree relative with BD, and this is multiplied several-fold if there is a more extensive family history (eg, both parents). When only a single second-degree relative is affected (eg, an aunt or a grandparent), this risk recedes to close to that of general population levels.[8] Despite earlier frustrations in pedigree analyses to find markers linked to BD,[9] subsequent efforts using genomewide association (including meta-analyses of these studies) have yielded more robust genetic associations, including in genes such as *ANK3*, *CACNA1C*, *SYNE1*, and *ODZ4*.[10] The cumulative genetic contribution accounted for by these genetic polymorphisms remains small, and the underlying biology connecting these disparate loci and their corresponding gene products still remains an active area of investigation. More recent efforts examining cross-diagnostic categories have determined that there appears to be a higher genetic correlation between BD and schizophrenia than between BD and major depression.[11]

IMPACT OF BD

It has long been recognized that BD is characterized by a substantial increase in risk of suicide attempts and completions. Lifetime prevalence of at least one suicide attempt is comparable between BD1 and BD2 at about 35%.[3] Although older studies suggest that as many as 15% of bipolar patients complete suicide,[12] revised estimates place the rate of suicide completion in BD, today, closer to 7% to 8% overall (less if a patient has never been hospitalized),[13] with the risk likely higher in the BD2 subpopulation.[14] Suicide risk is believed to be highest during depressive and mixed presentations in BD[15] and further increased with concurrent substance use and anxiety disorders.[16]

Beyond suicide, BD increases the risk of multiple medical comorbidities and premature mortality. Patients with BD die, on average, 8 to 20 years earlier than their counterparts in the general population.[17,18] Aside from the contribution by higher suicide rates, this statistic is attributable to riskier behaviors and lifestyle choices and greater medication side effect burden leading to more severe medical problems and a higher rate of accidents and injuries. Bipolar patients have demonstrably higher rates of smoking, substance use, and obesity and frequently have more severe cardiovascular disease, diabetes, and chronic obstructive pulmonary disease.[18] Further complicating this picture is the observation that bipolar patients are less likely to see their primary care providers on a regular basis.[19]

DIAGNOSIS

Changes to the diagnostic criteria for bipolar spectrum illnesses in the May 2013 release of Diagnostic and Statistical Manual of Mental Disorders, Fifth Edition (DSM-5)[3] were modest, but merit special mention. Foremost among these is that manic episodes now have an additional requirement in Criterion A for "persistently increased goal-directed activity or energy" on top of expansive or irritable mood. If mood is expansive, 3 additional symptoms are required from Criterion B, which is a list that includes grandiosity, decreased sleep requirement, pressured speech, flight of ideas, distractibility, psychomotor agitation or increased goal-directed activity (interestingly, repeating the new Criterion A insertion), and excessive pleasure seeking with a "high potential for painful consequences." Four Criterion B symptoms are required if mood is irritable rather than expansive, and symptom counts are identical between manic and hypomanic episodes. One week of symptoms is required for a manic episode (unless the patient requires hospitalization, in which case this is waived), whereas a minimum of 4 days are required for a hypomanic episode. Exclusions for substances or other medical conditions are made as they were in DSM-IV.

Whereas a single manic or mixed episode was sufficient in DSM-IV for BD1,[20] a history of at least 1 manic episode is now firmly required, because the mixed episode construct no longer exists in DSM-5. Mixed episodes, instead, are now captured as a manic, hypomanic, or depressive episode "with mixed features" when 3 symptoms from the opposite pole are simultaneously present during the "majority of the days" of the called episode. Of note, elevated, but not irritable, mood can count as one of these symptoms in "depressive episode, with mixed features," but distractibility cannot—perhaps because of overlap with the impaired concentration of depression. Likewise, depressed mood can count toward mixed features in a manic or hypomanic episode, but appetite and sleep symptoms cannot, because, by definition, these can already be disrupted with the increased activation and distractibility in an upswing. Lastly, when full criteria are met for both a manic and depressive episode, by default, DSM-5 dictates that the episode is a manic episode, with mixed features.

Medication-induced mania or hypomania (eg, with an antidepressant medication), colloquially referred to as manic switch, and previously captured as "substance-induced mood disorder" in DSM-IV can now be labeled as a manic or hypomanic episode in DSM-5, as long as the requisite number of diagnostic criteria are met and the disturbance remains "at a fully syndromal level" past the expected window for persistence of the offending treatment. Short of this, an alternative diagnosis of "substance/medication-induced bipolar and related disorder" would be applied.

Bipolar II disorder requires a history of at least 1 hypomanic episode and 1 major depressive episode. Of note, an item that has not changed between the different DSM iterations is that hypomanic episodes (in contrast to manic and major depressive episodes), by definition, are not functionally impairing (the presence of psychotic features or the need for hospitalization automatically escalates a mood upswing to a manic episode). Additionally, because BD2 is functionally impairing, the source of this impairment lies in the burden caused by major depressive episodes.

Cyclothymic disorder refers to a subsyndromal variation of BD which, in DSM-IV, consisted of hypomanic episodes alternating with periods of dysthymia. In DSM-5, this has been significantly altered so that if a full hypomanic episode has occurred, cyclothymia is now excluded. A DSM-5–defined cyclothymic disorder, therefore, refers to patients whose hypomania and dysthymia are both subsyndromal and have never met full episode criteria for hypomania or major depression. Cases characterized by hypomanic episodes with or without dysthymia would, instead, be captured by a diagnosis of "other specified bipolar and related disorder" or "unspecified bipolar and related disorder" (where the former label requires an explanation of why criteria are not met for BD1 or BD2 and the latter simply highlights this fact without an accompanying reason).

Table 1 lists the nomenclature for the new DSM-5 bipolar and related disorders, along with their most closely corresponding predecessors from DSM-IV.

SCREENING

Screening for BD is often missed in primary care despite being recommended in US Food and Drug Administration (FDA) guidelines.[21] There is a strong imperative to improve detection of BD because we know that most depression is seen in primary care rather than in psychiatry; up to 10% of all visits to primary care are depression related and estimates are that as many as 64% of all clinical encounters for depression occur in this setting rather than in specialty care.[22] And, as mentioned above, most presentations of BD are for depressive symptoms. **Table 2** highlights several items that can improve detection of BD.

Table 1 DSM-5 nomenclature of bipolar and related disorders and their nearest DSM-IV equivalents	
DSM-IV	**DSM-5**
Bipolar I disorder	Bipolar I disorder
Bipolar II disorder	Bipolar II disorder
Cyclothymic disorder	Cyclothymic disorder –or– Other specified bipolar and related disorder –or– Unspecified bipolar and related disorder
BD, not otherwise specified	Other specified bipolar and related disorder –or– Unspecified bipolar and related disorder
Substance-induced mood disorder	Substance/medication-induced bipolar and related disorder
BD due to a general medical condition	Bipolar and related disorder due to another medical condition
Mood disorder, not otherwise specified	Now forced to choose among: Other specified depressive disorder –or– Unspecified depressive disorder –or– Other specified bipolar and related disorder –or– Unspecified bipolar and related disorder

In the case of "other specified" versus "unspecified," the former is used when a provider chooses to state a specific reason why criteria for a more definitive diagnosis is not met (eg, insufficient duration), whereas the latter is used when a provider elects to not detail this reason.

Data from Diagnostic and statistical manual of mental disorders. 5th edition. Washington, DC: American Psychiatric Association; 2013; and American Psychiatric Association, Task Force on DSM-IV. Diagnostic and statistical manual of mental disorders DSM-IV-TR. 4th edition, text revision. Washington, DC: American Psychiatric Association; 2000.

Table 2
Considerations that can improve the detection of BD

History	Clinical Features	Other Sources
Family history of BD, psychosis, substance issues, suicide	More recurrent episodes of depression	Collateral information (particularly about longitudinal history) from family, friends
Frequent changes of occupation	Atypical features (eg, reverse vegetative symptoms, leaden paralysis)	
Marital or relationship instability	Psychotic symptoms (including postpartum psychosis in young female patients)	
Frequent relocations		
Preponderance of financial or legal setbacks		

Clues to BD can be uncovered with the benefit of additional historians, increased frequency of depressive episodes, or unusual psychosocial morbidity, particularly with regard to unstable employment or relationships.

Data from Manning JS. Tools to improve differential diagnosis of BD in primary care. Prim Care Companion J Clin Psychiatry 2010;12(Suppl 1):17–22. http://dx.doi.org/10.4088/PCC.9064su1c.03; and Cerimele JM, Chwastiak LA, Chan YF, et al. The presentation, recognition and management of bipolar depression in primary care. J Gen Intern Med 2013;28(12):1648–56. http://dx.doi.org/10.100//s11606-013-2545-7.

Regular use of a standardized screening instrument such as the MDQ[23] or Bipolar Spectrum Diagnostic Scale (BSDS)[24] can also improve detection of BD, and, despite sometimes tenuous numbers reported for sensitivity (0.58–0.73 for the MDQ, 0.73 for the BSDS) and specificity (0.67–0.90 for the MDQ, 0.90 for the BSDS), when the pretest probability of BD is in the range of 10% to 20% (a typical probability for BD in patients presenting to primary care for a chief complaint of depression), the negative predictive value can still be quite excellent (0.92–0.97 for the MDQ, 0.97 for the BSDS).[25] This last reference highlights that the 2 instruments are very effective at ruling out BD but can be expected to overcall BD by a factor of about 2 to 3, making interpretation of a positive screening result more problematic—and requiring a more detailed interview (by a psychiatrist if the general provider is not comfortable) to formalize a bipolar diagnosis.

Even with best practices, the detection of BD remains challenging given the preponderance of depressive and subsyndromal presentations, which can precede a first manic or hypomanic episode by as many as 10 years.[26] Accurate differentiation of bipolar from unipolar illness is critical to ensure safe and proper treatment of mood symptoms, because the use of standard antidepressants is frequently insufficient and potentially dangerous in BD. Conversely, overdiagnosis can be problematic because the use of bipolar medication regimens in unipolar illness can introduce unnecessary complexity and burden.

Finally, whether the concern is for major depressive disorder (MDD) or BD, regular screening for suicidality is very important. **Table 3** provides a brief overview of risk assessment considerations.

MEDICAL WORKUP

Before diagnosing BD and starting medication, it is important to rule out any possible medical condition, substance, or medication that may induce manic symptoms.

Table 3
Risk assessment

	Factors to Consider	Potential Actions
DTS	• A particular concern on depressive and mixed/agitated presentations • Risk is elevated with past suicide attempts, current suicidal ideation, suicide rehearsal and intent, self-injurious behaviors (even when suicidal intent is not definitive), command hallucinations, and concurrent substance problems • Level of financial and psychosocial support can be exacerbating (if poor or absent) or mitigating (if abundant)	• Direct but sensitive questioning about possible thoughts of death or suicide should be conducted regularly; when present, further questioning about possible plan and intent to act are indicated • Make efforts to obtain collateral from friends/family or other providers (as permitted by the patient) • Consider increasing medication or clinical surveillance • Consider elevating level of care (eg, emergency referral or inpatient) • Chart whether the patient seems to be a low/medium/high acute risk, factors considered, and thresholds for changing the treatment plan
DTO	• Risk is incrementally increased with each successive past act of violence • Comorbid psychosis or substance use can increase DTO risk • Active suicidal ideation is a risk factor (not mitigating factor) for DTO risk	• All of the above actions for DTS are applicable here as well • Motivation and timing of a plan to harm others should be carefully explored • The provider should carefully consider if the proposed plan sounds lethal or dangerous • Depending on jurisdiction, statutes or case law may necessitate, permit, or (in rarer instances) impede a duty to warn—which can be to the intended victim, law enforcement, or both
GD	• Commonly defined as the inability to attend to food, clothing, shelter (or, sometimes, medical needs) as a result of psychiatric decompensation • Civil commitment does not necessarily empower providers to force a needed medical treatment	• As above, under DTS, efforts to obtain collateral, tailor level of clinical attention to the patient's situation, and specification of anticipated level of risk and thresholds for changing level of care • Careful exploration with the patient of intentions and plans to acquire necessities of community living

Danger to self, danger to others, and grave disability are the most frequent concerns in assessing whether a patient is at-risk because of psychiatric decompensation.

Abbreviations: DTO, danger to others; DTS, danger to self; GD, grave disability.

A comprehensive medical history and complete physical including neurologic examination is indicated, as are an accurate history of recent medications and substances (corroborated by friends or family when possible) and a urine toxicology screening. In the case of substances, intoxication and withdrawal are possible etiologies for mood symptoms, and timelines are critical in distinguishing exogenous from endogenous presentations. It is best to inquire about the presence or absence of mood symptoms during windows of extended sobriety (ideally, at least 6 months), although often such windows may either not exist or be well remembered. It should also be noted that there are high rates of comorbid substance use disorders in BD, so the 2 conditions do not preclude each other.[27] In a medically ill or geriatric patient, a hyperactive delirium should be considered if manic-like symptoms are present with no history of mania. **Table 4** summarizes potential medical and substance/medication mimics for manic presentations, and **Table 5** reviews helpful laboratory tests and their rationale in the workup of mood disorder patients.

PSYCHIATRIC COMORBIDITIES AND DIFFERENTIAL DIAGNOSIS

Psychiatric comorbidities are common with BD (particularly substance use disorders, anxiety disorders, attention deficit/hyperactivity disorder [ADHD], and impulse control disorder), are associated with worse prognosis,[28] and merit additional clinical attention and treatment. A number of psychiatric conditions are also very similar to BD, and distinguishing features are summarized in **Table 6**.

Table 4
Summary of possible bipolar mania phenocopies

Medical Conditions That Can Cause Manic Symptoms	Medications That Can Cause Manic Symptoms	Drugs of Abuse That Can Cause Manic Symptoms
Cerebrovascular disease	Antidepressants	Alcohol
Cushing's disease	Baclofen	Amphetamines
Dementia	Bromocriptine	Bath salts
Herpes encephalitis	Captopril	Cocaine
Human immunodeficiency virus (HIV) encephalitis	Cimetidine	Hallucinogens (including phencyclidine)
Hyperthyroidism	Disulfiram	Opioids
Hypothyroidism	Hydralazine	
Migraine headaches	Interferon	
Multiple sclerosis	Isoniazid	
Neoplasm	Psychostimulants	
Neurosyphilis	Steroids	
Nutritional deficiencies (B12, folate, niacin)		
Seizure disorder		
Systemic lupus erythematosus		
Traumatic brain injury		
Wilson's disease		

Examples of general medical conditions, prescription drugs, and illicit substances are provided, though the list is not exhaustive.

Table 5	
Laboratory workup and rationale for patients with a possible diagnosis of BD	
Basic metabolic panel	Helpful to have a baseline creatinine, particularly when initiating lithium, which can impact renal function; baseline fasting glucose is helpful for monitoring later metabolic effects of atypical antipsychotics
Complete blood cell count	To rule out anemia and to monitor for potential changes with medications (eg, blood dyscrasias secondary to carbamazepine, valproate)
Electrocardiogram	For baseline comparison, especially if atypical antipsychotics (which can increase QTc interval) are used
Lipids, fasting	For baseline comparison with later atypical antipsychotic use; together with fasting glucose above, may be helpful in detecting Cushing's syndrome
Liver function tests	For baseline comparison, because some agents (eg, valproate) can trigger transaminitis
Pregnancy test	To avoid teratogenic complications of pharmacotherapy
Thyroid-stimulating hormone	For baseline comparison (especially before starting lithium) but also to rule out mood dysregulation secondary to thyroid disorder
Toxicology screening	To rule out substance-induced presentations; helpful to also have a blood alcohol level with urine testing
Urinalysis	Helpful for ruling out infections, particularly in geriatric patients

PHARMACOLOGIC MANAGEMENT

Pharmacologic therapies for BD are more complex than for unipolar depression, in part because of the different faces of BD (eg, manic, depressed, mixed variants) but also because combination therapy is frequently indicated, and the medications involved carry more morbidity and risk than antidepressants. Despite requiring medications very distinct from those used in MDD, a 2007 survey of a prescription database found that for 7760 patients who received a recent diagnosis of BD and started on a single-agent, antidepressant monotherapy (49.8%) was the most common strategy, with mood stabilizer monotherapy (24.6%) a distant second.[29] Such findings highlight the need for wider implementation of evidence-based strategies, particularly in light of the general lack of appreciable benefit with standard antidepressants in the treatment of BD.[30]

Mania can be addressed with a wide array of pharmacologic options, among which are lithium, valproate, carbamazepine, and 8 of the antipsychotic agents listed in **Table 7**. Although all are more effective than placebo, monotherapy with any of these choices is frequently insufficient to reduce manic symptoms even after 3 weeks; hence, combination treatment is frequently used, particularly in more severe presentations.[31] **Table 8** provides details about dosing, monitoring, and additional clinical considerations in the choice of a mood stabilizer. Of note, all of the antipsychotics listed in **Tables 7** and **8** (with the exception of lurasidone) are vetted treatment options for acute mania, although the risk of extrapyramidal side effects (including tardive dyskinesia) and, in the case of the atypical antipsychotics, metabolic syndrome, should be weighed against the potential benefits.[32]

Longitudinal tracking of manic symptoms is not as facile as it is for depressive symptoms, but one option is to use the Young Mania Rating Scale, which the clinician completes after a 15- to 30-minute interview.[33] The MDQ and BSDS are not longitudinal instruments but, as discussed above, are for initial screening only.

Table 6
Psychiatric conditions in the differential diagnosis of BD

	Similarities	Differences
MDD	Major depressive episodes can be identical with those of BD. Decreased sleep and poor concentration (distractibility) can count toward a major depressive episode and toward a hypomanic or manic episode.	MDD does not come with a history of prior manic or hypomanic episodes, which is why it is important to inquire about these. More accurate history can come from secondary sources such as family and friends.
Anxiety disorders	Can also manifest with rapid speech/thoughts, difficulty sleeping, and psychomotor agitation.	There can be a distinction in the quality of the sleep disturbance (eg, decreased need in BD vs difficulty getting needed sleep in anxiety). Thoughts can be more ruminative in anxiety vs more capricious in mania.
ADHD	Poor concentration, racing thoughts, rapid speech, decreased sleep can be present in both ADHD and BD.	The key distinction may lie in whether these symptoms are episodic (as in BD) vs baseline/chronic (as in ADHD).
Schizophrenia	Both schizophrenia and BD can have prominent psychotic symptoms, and, even in the former, there can be fluctuations in severity. Schizophrenia can also have comorbid depression.	There is a more episodic nature to the psychotic symptoms of BD, and a clearer correlation to acute mood disturbance in BD than in schizophrenia. The depression that sometimes accompanies schizophrenia is not typically present for the majority of the illness.
Schizoaffective disorder	Mood and psychosis generally track together for most of the illness.	The key distinguishing feature (by definition) is that in schizoaffective disorder there is at least a 2-wk window in which psychotic symptoms are present without an ongoing mood disturbance.
Borderline personality disorder	Mood swings, lability, irritability, frequent suicidal ideation.	Typically, this is more situational, and flares are more short-lived in borderline personality—though it is a baseline tendency. In BD, decompensations, although more episodic, are on the order of at least 1–2 wk at a time.

Several instances (including anxiety disorders, ADHD, and borderline personality) are not necessarily mutually exclusive of a BD diagnosis.

Depression in BD is a distinct entity from depression in MDD, and its management follows an equally distinct treatment algorithm. The most critical points to emphasize are (1) there is a relative dearth in bipolar depression (compared with mania) of randomized controlled trial (RCT)-supported pharmacologic options (see **Table 7**) and (2) antidepressants (ie, reuptake blockers) are largely inappropriate and ineffective agents for this indication. The Systematic Treatment Enhancement Program for Bipolar Disorder (STEP-BD) study included a groundbreaking publication by Sachs

Table 7
Mood stabilizers and FDA-approved indications in BD

Medication	AED	Antipsychotic	Maintenance	Mania	Depression
Aripiprazole (ABILIFY)		X	X	X	
Asenapine (SAPHRIS)		X		X	
Carbamazepine extended-release (Tegretol XR)	X			X	
Haloperidol (Haldol)		X		X	
Lamotrigine (Lamictal)	X		X		
Lithium			X	X	
Lurasidone (LATUDA)		X			X
Olanzapine (Zyprexa)		X	X	X	
Olanzapine-fluoxetine (Symbyax)		X			X
Paliperidone (INVEGA)		X		X	
Quetiapine (SEROQUEL)		X	Adjunctive	X	X
Risperidone (RISPERDAL)		X		X	
Valproate (Depakote)	X			X	
Ziprasidone (GEODON)		X		X	

Abbreviations: AED, antiepileptic drug; XR, extended release.

and colleagues[30] that enrolled actively depressed BD1 and BD2 patients and randomly assigned them to either mood stabilizer plus antidepressant (in which the antidepressant was either bupropion or paroxetine) or a mood stabilizer plus placebo treatment arm. On the primary outcome measure of durable recovery (8 consecutive weeks of euthymia), there was no separation between the 2 groups. Equally interesting was that the 2 groups showed no statistically significant differences on the secondary outcome measure of treatment-emergent affective switch (ie, iatrogenic mania) up to 26 weeks into treatment.

FDA-approved medication regimens for bipolar depression are limited to quetiapine,[34–37] olanzapine-fluoxetine,[38] and lurasidone.[39,40] Quetiapine is particularly appealing as a first-line agent given it is also effective in acute mania. Tohen and colleagues[38] found superiority of both olanzapine and olanzapine-fluoxetine over placebo, but, notably, the combination showed a more robust response without increasing the risk for treatment-emergent affective switch. The added benefit provided by fluoxetine initially comes across as at odds with the Systematic Treatment Enhancement Program for Bipolar Disorder finding cited above,[30] but in Sachs and colleagues, most mood stabilizer regimens among enrolled patients (ie, >85%) did not include an antipsychotic, and the combination of an atypical with fluoxetine may afford a unique pharmacologic effect. It is also important to note that results obtained with olanzapine-fluoxetine are not necessarily generalizable to alternative atypical antipsychotic–selective serotonin reuptake inhibitor combinations, as demonstrated by the comparatively modest effects generated in a separate study examining combinations of a nonantipsychotic mood stabilizer with risperidone, paroxetine, or risperidone-paroxetine.[41] Lurasidone is the most recently approved medication (both as monotherapy and, alternatively, in combination with lithium or valproate) for bipolar depression and is dosed at 20 to 120 mg/d. It is significant that all 3 of these options entail use of atypical antipsychotics, the long-term risks of which have already been discussed above.

Table 8
Mood stabilizers and guidelines for dosing and monitoring

Medication	Dosing	Monitoring Guidelines	Side Effects	Additional Notes
Atypical antipsychotics		Monitoring guidelines for metabolic indices are nicely summarized in a review by Hasnain and colleagues[62], some of these recommendations include obtaining baseline weight, waist circumference, blood pressure, fasting glucose, fasting lipids; repeat at 3 mo, then fasting glucose Q y & fasting lipids Q 5 y.	Sedation, orthostatic hypotension, extrapyramidal side effects, neuroleptic malignant syndrome, metabolic syndrome, hyperprolactinemia, sexual side effects	Recent literature suggests that some of the metabolic risks may be mitigated by concurrent use of metformin,[63-66] even without a diagnosis of diabetes, and this intervention has been incorporated into the American Psychiatric Association (APA) practice guidelines[67]
Aripiprazole (ABILIFY)	15–30 mg/d		Lower metabolic risks	Partial dopamine (D₂) agonist; available as soluble tablet & Q 4-wk depot injection
Asenapine (SAPHRIS)	5–10 mg SL BID		Lower metabolic risks	Must be absorbed sublingually; oral ingestion reduces absorption
Lurasidone (LATUDA)	20–120 mg/d		Lower metabolic risks	
Olanzapine (Zyprexa)	5–20 mg/d		Higher metabolic risks	Available as a soluble tablet & Q 4-wk depot injection
Olanzapine-fluoxetine (Symbyax)	6/25–18/75 mg/d		Higher metabolic risks	
Paliperidone (INVEGA)	6–12 mg/d		Moderate metabolic risks	Available as Q 4-wk depot injection
Quetiapine (SEROQUEL)	300–800 mg/d		Moderate metabolic risks	
Risperidone (RISPERDAL)	1–6 mg/d		Moderate metabolic risks	Available as soluble tablet & Q 2-wk depot injection

(continued on next page)

Table 8
(continued)

Medication	Dosing	Monitoring Guidelines	Side Effects	Additional Notes
Ziprasidone (GEODON)	40–80 mg BID		Lower metabolic risks; EKG at baseline and with dose adjustments if patient has preexisting cardiac issues (given possible QTc prolongation)	Administer with food to maximize absorption
Typical antipsychotics				
Haloperidol (Haldol)	0.5–10 mg/d	Check prolactin if clinically indicated	Sedation, extrapyramidal side effects, neuroleptic malignant syndrome, hyperprolactinemia	
Antiepileptic drugs				
Carbamazepine extended release (Tegretol XR)	200–1600 mg/d	Check for HLA-B1502 before starting in East Asian patients because of Stevens-Johnson syndrome risk;[68] adjust to target serum level of 4–12 µg/mL (more for limiting toxicity than for any correlation with therapeutic benefit[69]), including 1 mo after initiation because of auto-induction of CYP3A4	Agranulocytosis, Stevens-Johnson syndrome	Concurrent antipsychotics (as well as carbamazepine itself) may require dose increase after about 1 mo given CYP3A4 induction
Lamotrigine (Lamictal)	200 mg/d		Stevens-Johnson syndrome	Slow titration (ie, Q 2 wks for each step, starting with 25 mg orally Q morning) to minimize Stevens-Johnson syndrome risk; doses should be halved if there is concurrent valproic acid, which can cause a drug-drug interaction[70]; best to avoid if there is a concurrent estrogen-based oral contraceptive with variable dosing caused by drug-drug interaction

Valproate (Depakote)	500–2500 mg/d	Adjust to target serum level of 50–120 µg/mL,[71] although the default convention of aiming for the higher end of this range (ie, levels >75 or 80) does not appear to have a clear correlation with greater therapeutic effect[72]	Alopecia, sedation, polycystic ovarian syndrome (young females), thrombocytopenia, transaminitis, tremor, weight gain	Typically prescribed in its divalproex formulation; may have superiority to lithium in mixed presentations[73] and in mania when there is an additional history of a substance use disorder;[74] caution with this agent is appropriate in women of reproductive age (given teratogenicity, eg, up to 5%–10% of first trimester exposures result in neural tube defects, and associations with polycystic ovarian syndrome)[75,76] and in patients with preexisting hepatic issues.
Other				
Lithium	900–1200 mg/d	Check baseline and then Q 6 mo TSH, Cr; adjust to target serum level of 0.6–1.2 mEq/L	Diabetes insipidus, diarrhea, nausea, hypothyroidism, polyuria, renal failure (chronic), sedation, thirst	Often favored among available options because of its broader spectrum of activity and low cost but does have a narrow therapeutic window and should generally be avoided in patients in whom the potential for renal impairment is prohibitive; avoid combining with NSAIDs (aspirin and sulindac safer)

Abbreviations: BID, twice a day; Cr, creatinine; CYP, cytochrome P450; EKG, electrocardiogram; HLA, human leukocyte antigen; NSAID, non-steroidal anti-inflammatory drug; Q, each/every; SL, sublingual; TSH, thyroid stimulating hormone.
   Data from Refs.[59–62]

In the event of treatment failure in bipolar depression, there is also the option of electroconvulsive therapy (ECT). Comparative efficacy studies of ECT versus pharmacologic strategies in bipolar depression are lacking, but ECT is found to be as effective in bipolar depression as it is in unipolar depression, with an 80% response rate (ie, 50% reduction in symptom burden, as measured on the Hamilton Depression Rating Scale[42]) and at least a 60% remission rate in a recently published study.[43] Although ECT is underutilized because of misconceptions and negative stereotypes, it remains a safe and viable treatment choice, although it is typically only available at tertiary medical facilities given the need for general anesthesia.

Outcomes for treatment of bipolar depression are best tracked with many of the same instruments used for unipolar depression, and we favor the Patient Health Questionnaire-9[44] or Quick Inventory of Depressive Symptomatology,[45] both because they are freely available and can be completed rapidly.

Maintenance refers to strategies for maintaining euthymia and, thus, preventing mood episode relapses. Despite its episodic course, BD requires long-term maintenance to most effectively reduce episode frequency and severity and associated morbidity and mortality. Maintenance can be difficult to persuade patients to accept given both the side effects of long-term medication use and the episodic course of the illness.

Clinical trials of maintenance strategies are complicated by design issues (eg, inconsistent definitions of when maintenance begins; inadequate standardization of whether the last mood episode was manic, hypomanic, or depressed; and a belated realization by investigators that dramatic dose reductions or medication substitutions to fit patients into particular study arms can themselves be quite destabilizing[31]). Mood stabilizing drugs are found to have different profiles regarding how well they prevent relapse and along which pole (ie, mania or depression). Whether to use monotherapy or combination therapy in maintenance is another question, and the combinatorial possibilities substantially outnumber what has already been tested. Ultimately, providers should aim for the minimum effective burden of medication(s) to both enhance compliance and reduce toxicity and should also consider whether there is a manic or depressive predominance (or neither) in a patient's history. An excellent summary of the bipolar maintenance literature can be found in Gitlin and Frye,[46] but, in brief, the more favored agents for maintenance include lithium, lamotrigine, olanzapine, and quetiapine—or combinations thereof, sometimes incorporating valproate (which is not generally viewed as effective in monotherapy for maintenance). Among all mood stabilizers, lithium has the best evidence base for reducing suicide risk,[47,48] although a careful risk-benefit analysis is warranted given how lethal this agent can be in an overdose. Lamotrigine occupies a unique niche, given its demonstrated efficacy in maintenance[46] but not in acute bipolar mania and inconsistently (or at least more modestly) in acute bipolar depression.[31,49] Quetiapine's FDA approval in maintenance is as an adjunct to either lithium or valproate.[50,51]

Pregnancy can complicate management of BD, particularly because of concerns of teratogenicity with the use of mood-stabilizing medications in the first trimester (during fetal organogenesis). Clinical considerations in pregnancy are summarized in **Table 9**, and can guide a careful discussion with patients of risks and benefits of the various treatment options.

PSYCHOTHERAPEUTIC AND PSYCHOSOCIAL MANAGEMENT

Even with pharmacotherapy, about half of BD patients will have another mood episode within 2 years and often spend a significant portion of time with ongoing impairment

Table 9
Pregnancy and BD

	Teratogenic Concerns
Antipsychotics	Although not comprehensively studied to date, atypical antipsychotics have not generated data to suggest higher rates of teratogenicity[77] and are thus cautiously used in pregnancy, although they are sometimes substituted by high-potency typical antipsychotics during the first trimester when treating mania or psychosis
Carbamazepine	Noted to pose a risk for neural tube defects (about 1%), although less than with valproate[69]
Lamotrigine	Has generated mixed data, with sources like Holmes and colleagues[78] pointing to a modest increase in oral cleft malformations and others like Cunnington and Ternis[79] finding malformation rates similar to those in the unexposed general population
Lithium	Although originally associated with a 400-fold increased risk of Ebstein's anomaly (a cardiac defect),[80] this was based on retrospective data and subject to significant recall bias; more recent estimates have placed the increase in risk at about 10-fold, but it is important to keep in perspective that this still translates to a generally favorable absolute risk of about 1 in 1000–2000 and that prospective studies have failed to find a difference with general population rates[81,82]
Valproate	First trimester exposure is associated with significantly higher rates of congenital malformations, including neural tube defects (absolute risk as high as 5%–10%) and craniofacial abnormalities, with the former showing poor rescue with folic acid supplementation[83]
ECT	American Psychiatric Association guidelines endorse the use of ECT in pregnancy[84] when there is medication resistance or prohibitive concern about medication-related teratogenicity; this recommendation rests on several hundred psychiatric case reports (not just of BD) but no prospective or controlled studies; complications such as fetal cardiac arrhythmias, vaginal bleeding, and uterine contractions have been documented, but not necessarily established to have been caused by ECT; also important to note is that untreated psychiatric illness is not benign for fetal development or longer-term outcomes in the children of BD patients

(mostly from depressive symptoms). Difficulties maintaining relationships and employment are common, and resulting stressors can trigger further episodes. Adjunctive psychosocial treatments, whether delivered individually, in a group, or in a family context, have been found to help symptoms, prevent recurrence, and improve functioning and are summarized in **Table 10**. All of these approaches have a role in helping patients and

Table 10 Psychosocial treatments for BD	
	General Description and Evidence Base
Psychoeducation	• Includes basic teaching about the natural history and different presentations of BD and how to develop relapse prevention plans; also covers topics such as medication adherence, maintaining a regular sleep schedule (with sensitivity to seasonal changes, disruptions from travel across time zones), and reducing stressors • One small RCT of BD2 patients found that a 6-mo manual-based group psychoeducation class added to standard pharmacotherapy had better 5-y outcomes than pharmacotherapy alone as far as time to relapse, duration of mood episodes, and level of functioning[85]
Family-focused therapy	• Involves psychotherapy with a patient and a family member with a focus not only on psychoeducation but also improving communication and problem solving[86] • Studies found that 20–30 sessions of family-focused therapy over 9–12 mo can lead to faster recovery from bipolar depression, fewer mood episodes, improved medication adherence, and improved functioning[87]
Cognitive behavioral therapy	• Focuses on the interplay between an individual's thoughts, behaviors, and emotions; recognition of thought distortions and maladaptive behaviors can help the patient make these less automatic • Most effective when initiated during a period of depression or minimal active symptoms and has efficacy in promoting faster recovery from a depressive episode, increasing time to next relapse and severity of depressive symptoms, and reducing functional impairment[88] • Adding 12–30 individual cognitive behavioral therapy sessions over 6–9 mo may be especially helpful for BD with more recurrent or treatment-resistant bipolar depression[87] • Cognitive behavioral therapy focused on active psychotic symptoms (including hallucinations and delusions) is an evidence-based treatment in chronic psychotic disorders, and this treatment could be considered for individuals with BD with more severe and prolonged psychosis[89]
Interpersonal and social rhythm therapy	• Focuses on teaching social skills to improve interpersonal communication and to stabilize social rhythms by promoting best practices for regular sleep, exercise, activity, and socialization • Most effective when initiated after an acute decompensation[88] • Has shown efficacy in promoting faster recovery from a bipolar depressive episode, increasing time to relapse, and decreasing functional impairment[88]

These interventions can complement and augment pharmacotherapies discussed earlier in the management of BD.

their families identify possible precipitants for mood episodes and in emphasizing the importance of rapidly obtaining help with early signs of decompensation—before insight and judgment become further impaired. In many instances, patients should be prepared to consider the need for a temporary increase in mood-stabilizing medication to reduce the risk of a full mood episode. Proactive efforts to anticipate potential side effects can aid with medication adherence. Discussion of the risks of BD should be balanced with hope about the prospects for symptom control, and, in the context of ongoing maintenance treatment, high functioning and quality of life.

SYSTEMS OF CARE

Ten percent to 38% of BD patients receive all mental health care in a primary care office.[52] Primary care physicians (PCP) often diagnose and treat BD without the help of psychiatrists or other mental health specialists, but access to a consulting psychiatrist (either onsite or offsite) can be helpful in confirming diagnosis or crafting a treatment plan. Collaborative care teams already have a body of compelling evidence for better outcomes in the management of MDD in primary care and could reasonably be considered for managing BD in this setting, too.[53] A collaborative care model in cludes a care manager dedicated to tracking mental health measures in the primary care office and serving as a liaison to a psychiatric consultant (who may be offsite). The care manager is tasked with assessing the patient frequently, monitoring symptoms and medication tolerance, and providing brief therapy and social interventions when needed. In effect, the care manager serves as the main link between the PCP and the psychiatrist. In this model, the PCP provides an initial assessment and referral to the designated care manager and prescribes psychiatric medications with the input of the care manager and consulting psychiatrist. An alternative to this is referral to an outside community mental health clinic, although data suggest that there is significant attrition both in patients reaching their first psychiatric appointment and in maintaining follow-up visits through resolution of their original symptoms. **Table 11** summarizes a few scenarios in which outside psychiatric help may be indicated.

CONTROVERSIES

Manic switch, defined above under Diagnosis and Screening, is now preferentially referred to as treatment-emergent affective switch because it is ambiguous as to whether mood agents (particularly antidepressants) are actually etiologic in conversions to acute mania from earlier bipolar depression or if such cycling would have occurred anyway in the natural history of a given patient's illness. In addition to the Sachs and colleagues[30] study cited above, it is worth noting that a paroxetine monotherapy group in EMBOLDEN II, a study that validated the use of Seroquel for bipolar depressed patients, did not find an increased switch risk compared with placebo.[34] Although the controversy over whether reuptake blockers actually pose such a danger continues, it may be a moot point given the limited support in the literature for their efficacy in bipolar patients.[54] Nevertheless, there appears to be modest support for greater susceptibility in BD1 than in BD2 patients[55] and for greater risk with tricyclic antidepressants and serotonin-norepinephrine reuptake inhibitors than for selective serotonin reuptake inhibitors or bupropion.[56]

Treatment-emergent suicidality, a hot-button issue in major depressive disorder with the use of selective serotonin reuptake inhibitors, has been raised in BD as well. Specifically, in 2009, the FDA issued an advisory that the use of antiepileptic drugs (AEDs) for any indication can increase the risk of suicidal behavior or ideation, based on a meta-analysis of 199 RCTs yielding an odds ratio of 1.87 for patients on

Table 11 When to get additional help	
	Circumstances for Which a PCP May Wish to Make an Outside Referral
Consulting psychiatrist	• Refractory symptoms • Difficult-to-manage side effects • Overly complex medication regimen
Community mental health clinic	• Heavy need for social work/case management (eg, assistance with applying for state or federal benefits, disability, coordination of psychiatric care, support and problem solving) • Frequently hospitalized for psychiatric decompensations and requires more frequent provider contact (eg, multiple times a month to daily) • Requires provider outreach to place of residence • Difficulty managing own medications (eg, overdose risk, cognitive difficulties) • Needs a payee to manage funds • Homeless, needs more structured living situation or support in current housing • Would benefit from vocational rehabilitation • Would benefit from group therapy and increased social support • Requires complex medication management or depot injections

Psychiatric consultation can be accessed either in a collaborative care model or an outside referral. Community mental health centers are a system of care implemented in the public sector for patients with severe functional impairment from mental illness.

AEDs compared with patients on placebo.[57] Countering this is a reassuring 30-year prospective observational study that found no evidence for increased suicide attempts or completions for bipolar patients while they were taking AEDs compared with these same patients during intervals when they were not.[58] As the authors of this observational study note, their findings do not necessarily contradict the FDA meta-analysis, which examined a larger patient population (ie, not just bipolar patients), incorporated data on suicidal ideation (Leon and colleagues[58] only focused on suicide attempts and completions), and compared use of AEDs with placebo. It should also be noted that the number needed to harm in the FDA study was estimated at approximately 769 and that two-thirds of the adverse events were suicidal ideation only.

SUMMARY

BD is an inherently more complicated disorder to detect than MDD because of its varied presentations and sometimes very subtle distinguishing characteristics (if any) early in its natural history. Despite substantially lower prevalence in the general population, it is important to remember that it can be overrepresented among patients in primary care seeking treatment for depressive symptoms. Having a systematic approach to mood disorder patients and screening for BD can avert misdiagnosis and significant morbidity, and greater command of appropriate mood stabilizers for specific types of presentations can empower primary care providers to make a significant difference in outcomes for this patient subpopulation. Recognition that patient stigma has a significant impact on follow through with specialty referral in mental health makes a strong case for newer, more integrated models of delivery of psychiatric care, such as the collaborative care model.

REFERENCES

1. Weissman MM, Bland RC, Canino GJ, et al. Cross-national epidemiology of major depression and bipolar disorder. JAMA 1996;276(4):293–9.
2. Kupfer DJ. The increasing medical burden in bipolar disorder. JAMA 2005; 293(20):2528–30. http://dx.doi.org/10.1001/jama.293.20.2528.
3. American Psychiatric Association. Diagnostic and statistical manual of mental disorders: DSM-5. 5th edition. Washington, DC: American Psychiatric Publishing; 2013.
4. Das AK, Olfson M, Gameroff MJ, et al. Screening for bipolar disorder in a primary care practice. JAMA 2005;293(8):956–63. http://dx.doi.org/10.1001/jama.293.8.956.
5. Manning JS, Haykal RF, Connor PD, et al. On the nature of depressive and anxious states in a family practice setting: the high prevalence of bipolar II and related disorders in a cohort followed longitudinally. Compr Psychiatry 1997;38(2):102–8.
6. Judd LL, Akiskal HS, Schettler PJ, et al. The long-term natural history of the weekly symptomatic status of bipolar I disorder. Arch Gen Psychiatry 2002; 59(6):530–7.
7. Judd LL, Akiskal HS, Schettler PJ, et al. A prospective investigation of the natural history of the long-term weekly symptomatic status of bipolar II disorder. Arch Gen Psychiatry 2003;60(3):261–9.
8. Barondes SH. Mood genes: hunting for origins of mania and depression. New York: W.H. Freeman; 1998.
9. Kelsoe JR, Ginns EI, Egeland JA, et al. Re-evaluation of the linkage relationship between chromosome 11p loci and the gene for bipolar affective disorder in the Old Order Amish. Nature 1989;342(6247):238–43. http://dx.doi.org/10.1038/342238a0.
10. Psychiatric GWAS Consortium Bipolar Disorder Working Group. Large-scale genome-wide association analysis of bipolar disorder identifies a new susceptibility locus near ODZ4. Nat Genet 2011;43(10):977–83. http://dx.doi.org/10.1038/ng.943.
11. Cross-Disorder Group of the Psychiatric Genomics Consortium, Lee SH, Ripke S, Neale BM, et al. Genetic relationship between five psychiatric disorders estimated from genome-wide SNPs. Nat Genet 2013;45(9):984–94. http://dx.doi.org/10.1038/ng.2711.
12. Guze SB, Robins E. Suicide and primary affective disorders. Br J Psychiatry 1970;117(539):437–8.
13. Goodwin FK, Jamison KR, Ghaemi S. Manic-depressive illness: bipolar disorders and recurrent depression. 2nd edition. New York: Oxford University Press; 2007.
14. Rihmer Z, Kiss K. Bipolar disorders and suicidal behaviour. Bipolar Disord 2002; 4(Suppl 1):21–5.
15. Valtonen HM, Suominen K, Mantere O, et al. Suicidal behaviour during different phases of bipolar disorder. J Affect Disord 2007;97(1–3):101–7. http://dx.doi.org/10.1016/j.jad.2006.05.033.
16. Elizabeth Sublette M, Carballo JJ, Moreno C, et al. Substance use disorders and suicide attempts in bipolar subtypes. J Psychiatr Res 2009;43(3):230–8. http://dx.doi.org/10.1016/j.jpsychires.2008.05.001.
17. Roshanaei-Moghaddam B, Katon W. Premature mortality from general medical illnesses among persons with bipolar disorder: a review. Psychiatr Serv 2009; 60(2):147–56. http://dx.doi.org/10.1176/appi.ps.60.2.147.

18. Crump C, Sundquist K, Winkleby MA, et al. Comorbidities and mortality in bipolar disorder: a Swedish national cohort study. JAMA Psychiatry 2013;70(9): 931–9. http://dx.doi.org/10.1001/jamapsychiatry.2013.1394.

19. Chwastiak LA, Rosenheck RA, Kazis LE. Utilization of primary care by veterans with psychiatric illness in the National Department of Veterans Affairs Health Care System. J Gen Intern Med 2008;23(11):1835–40. http://dx.doi.org/10. 1007/s11606-008-0786-7.

20. American Psychiatric Association, Task Force on DSM-IV. Diagnostic and statistical manual of mental disorders DSM-IV-TR. 4th edition, text revision. Washington, DC: American Psychiatric Association; 2000.

21. FDA Public Health Advisory. Information by drug class - antidepressant use in children, adolescents, and adults. 2010. Available at: http://www.fda.gov/ Drugs/DrugSafety/InformationbyDrugClass/UCM096273. Accessed October 9, 2013.

22. Unützer J, Park M. Strategies to improve the management of depression in primary care. Prim Care 2012;39(2):415–31. http://dx.doi.org/10.1016/j.pop. 2012.03.010.

23. Hirschfeld RM, Williams JB, Spitzer RL, et al. Development and validation of a screening instrument for bipolar spectrum disorder: the Mood Disorder Questionnaire. Am J Psychiatry 2000;157(11):1873–5.

24. Nassir Ghaemi S, Miller CJ, Berv DA, et al. Sensitivity and specificity of a new bipolar spectrum diagnostic scale. J Affect Disord 2005;84(2–3):273–7. http:// dx.doi.org/10.1016/S0165-0327(03)00196-4.

25. Phelps JR, Ghaemi SN. Improving the diagnosis of bipolar disorder: predictive value of screening tests. J Affect Disord 2006;92(2–3):141–8. http://dx.doi.org/ 10.1016/j.jad.2006.01.029.

26. Manning JS. Tools to improve differential diagnosis of bipolar disorder in primary care. Prim Care Companion J Clin Psychiatry 2010;12(Suppl 1):17–22. http://dx. doi.org/10.4088/PCC.9064su1c.03.

27. Salloum IM, Thase ME. Impact of substance abuse on the course and treatment of bipolar disorder. Bipolar Disord 2000;2(3 Pt 2):269–80.

28. Parikh SV, LeBlanc SR, Ovanessian MM. Advancing bipolar disorder: key lessons from the Systematic Treatment Enhancement Program for Bipolar Disorder (STEP-BD). Can J Psychiatry 2010;55(3):136–43.

29. Baldessarini RJ, Leahy L, Arcona S, et al. Patterns of psychotropic drug prescription for U.S. patients with diagnoses of bipolar disorders. Psychiatr Serv 2007;58(1):85–91. http://dx.doi.org/10.1176/appi.ps.58.1.85-a.

30. Sachs GS, Nierenberg AA, Calabrese JR, et al. Effectiveness of adjunctive antidepressant treatment for bipolar depression. N Engl J Med 2007;356(17): 1711–22. http://dx.doi.org/10.1056/NEJMoa064135.

31. Sachs GS, Dupuy JM, Wittmann CW. The pharmacologic treatment of bipolar disorder. J Clin Psychiatry 2011;72(5):704–15. http://dx.doi.org/10.4088/JCP. 10m06523.

32. Kane JM. Tardive dyskinesia rates with atypical antipsychotics in adults: prevalence and incidence. J Clin Psychiatry 2004;65(Suppl 9):16–20.

33. Young RC, Biggs JT, Ziegler VE, et al. A rating scale for mania: reliability, validity and sensitivity. Br J Psychiatry 1978;133:429–35.

34. McElroy SL, Weisler RH, Chang W, et al. A double-blind, placebo-controlled study of quetiapine and paroxetine as monotherapy in adults with bipolar depression (EMBOLDEN II). J Clin Psychiatry 2010;71(2):163–74. http://dx. doi.org/10.4088/JCP.08m04942gre.

35. Young AH, McElroy SL, Bauer M, et al. A double-blind, placebo-controlled study of quetiapine and lithium monotherapy in adults in the acute phase of bipolar depression (EMBOLDEN I). J Clin Psychiatry 2010;71(2):150–62. http://dx.doi.org/10.4088/JCP.08m04995gre.

36. Calabrese JR, Keck PE Jr, Macfadden W, et al. A randomized, double-blind, placebo-controlled trial of quetiapine in the treatment of bipolar I or II depression. Am J Psychiatry 2005;162(7):1351–60. http://dx.doi.org/10.1176/appi.ajp.162.7.1351.

37. Thase ME, Macfadden W, Weisler RH, et al. Efficacy of quetiapine monotherapy in bipolar I and II depression: a double-blind, placebo-controlled study (the BOLDER II study). J Clin Psychopharmacol 2006;26(6):600–9. http://dx.doi.org/10.1097/01.jcp.0000248603.76231.b7.

38. Tohen M, Vieta E, Calabrese J, et al. Efficacy of olanzapine and olanzapine-fluoxetine combination in the treatment of bipolar I depression. Arch Gen Psychiatry 2003,60(11):1079–88. http://dx.doi.org/10.1001/archpsyc.60.11.1079.

39. Loebel A, Cucchiaro J, Silva R, et al. Lurasidone monotherapy in the treatment of bipolar I depression: a randomized, double-blind, placebo-controlled study. Am J Psychiatry 2013. http://dx.doi.org/10.1176/appi.ajp.2013.13070984.

40. Loebel A, Cucchiaro J, Silva R, et al. Lurasidone as adjunctive therapy with lithium or valproate for the treatment of bipolar I depression: a randomized, double-blind, placebo-controlled study. Am J Psychiatry 2013. http://dx.doi.org/10.1176/appi.ajp.2013.13070985.

41. Shelton RC, Stahl SM. Risperidone and paroxetine given singly and in combination for bipolar depression. J Clin Psychiatry 2004;65(12):1715–9.

42. Hamilton M. A rating scale for depression. J Neurol Neurosurg Psychiatry 1960; 23:56–62.

43. Bailine S, Fink M, Knapp R, et al. Electroconvulsive therapy is equally effective in unipolar and bipolar depression. Acta Psychiatr Scand 2010;121(6):431–6. http://dx.doi.org/10.1111/j.1600-0447.2009.01493.x.

44. Kroenke K, Spitzer RL, Williams JB. The PHQ-9: validity of a brief depression severity measure. J Gen Intern Med 2001;16(9):606–13.

45. Rush AJ, Trivedi MH, Ibrahim HM, et al. The 16-item quick inventory of depressive symptomatology (QIDS), clinician rating (QIDS-C), and self-report (QIDS-SR): a psychometric evaluation in patients with chronic major depression. Biol Psychiatry 2003;54(5):573–83.

46. Gitlin M, Frye MA. Maintenance therapies in bipolar disorders. Bipolar Disord 2012;14(Suppl 2):51–65. http://dx.doi.org/10.1111/j.1399-5618.2012.00992.x.

47. Baldessarini RJ, Tondo L, Davis P, et al. Decreased risk of suicides and attempts during long-term lithium treatment: a meta-analytic review. Bipolar Disord 2006; 8(5 Pt 2):625–39. http://dx.doi.org/10.1111/j.1399-5618.2006.00344.x.

48. Cipriani A, Hawton K, Stockton S, et al. Lithium in the prevention of suicide in mood disorders: updated systematic review and meta-analysis. BMJ 2013; 346:f3646.

49. Geddes JR, Calabrese JR, Goodwin GM. Lamotrigine for treatment of bipolar depression: independent meta-analysis and meta-regression of individual patient data from five randomised trials. Br J Psychiatry 2009;194(1):4–9. http://dx.doi.org/10.1192/bjp.bp.107.048504.

50. Vieta E, Suppes T, Eggens I, et al. Efficacy and safety of quetiapine in combination with lithium or divalproex for maintenance of patients with bipolar I disorder (international trial 126). J Affect Disord 2008;109(3):251–63. http://dx.doi.org/10.1016/j.jad.2008.06.001.

51. Suppes T, Vieta E, Liu S, et al, Trial 127 Investigators. Maintenance treatment for patients with bipolar I disorder: results from a north american study of quetiapine in combination with lithium or divalproex (trial 127). Am J Psychiatry 2009;166(4):476–88. http://dx.doi.org/10.1176/appi.ajp.2008.08020189.

52. Kilbourne AM, Goodrich DE, O'Donnell AN, et al. Integrating bipolar disorder management in primary care. Curr Psychiatry Rep 2012;14(6):687–95. http://dx.doi.org/10.1007/s11920-012-0325-4.

53. Miller CJ, Grogan-Kaylor A, Perron BE, et al. Collaborative chronic care models for mental health conditions: cumulative meta-analysis and metaregression to guide future research and implementation. Med Care 2013;51(10):922–30. http://dx.doi.org/10.1097/MLR.0b013e3182a3e4c4.

54. Pacchiarotti I, Bond DJ, Baldessarini RJ, et al. The International Society for Bipolar Disorders (ISBD) task force report on antidepressant use in bipolar disorders. Am J Psychiatry 2013;170(11):1249–62. http://dx.doi.org/10.1176/appi.ajp.2013.13020185.

55. Altshuler LL, Suppes T, Black DO, et al. Lower switch rate in depressed patients with bipolar II than bipolar I disorder treated adjunctively with second-generation antidepressants. Am J Psychiatry 2006;163(2):313–5. http://dx.doi.org/10.1176/appi.ajp.163.2.313.

56. Leverich GS, Altshuler LL, Frye MA, et al. Risk of switch in mood polarity to hypomania or mania in patients with bipolar depression during acute and continuation trials of venlafaxine, sertraline, and bupropion as adjuncts to mood stabilizers. Am J Psychiatry 2006;163(2):232–9. http://dx.doi.org/10.1176/appi.ajp.163.2.232.

57. Postmarket Drug Safety Information for Patients and Providers. Suicidal behavior and ideation and antiepileptic drugs. Available at: http://www.fda.gov/Drugs/DrugSafety/PostmarketDrugSafetyInformationforPatientsandProviders/ucm100190.htm. Accessed November 18, 2013.

58. Leon AC, Solomon DA, Li C, et al. Antiepileptic drugs for bipolar disorder and the risk of suicidal behavior: a 30-year observational study. Am J Psychiatry 2012;169(3):285–91. http://dx.doi.org/10.1176/appi.ajp.2011.11060948.

59. Brunton LL. Goodman & Gilman's the pharmacological basis of therapeutics. New York: McGraw-Hill Medical; 2011.

60. Citrome L, Ketter TA, Cucchiaro J, et al. Clinical assessment of lurasidone benefit and risk in the treatment of bipolar I depression using number needed to treat, number needed to harm, and likelihood to be helped or harmed. J Affect Disord 2013. http://dx.doi.org/10.1016/j.jad.2013.10.040.

61. Dols A, Sienaert P, van Gerven H, et al. The prevalence and management of side effects of lithium and anticonvulsants as mood stabilizers in bipolar disorder from a clinical perspective: a review. Int Clin Psychopharmacol 2013;28(6):287–96. http://dx.doi.org/10.1097/YIC.0b013e32836435e2.

62. Hasnain M, Vieweg WV, Fredrickson SK, et al. Clinical monitoring and management of the metabolic syndrome in patients receiving atypical antipsychotic medications. Prim Care Diabetes 2009;3(1):5–15. http://dx.doi.org/10.1016/j.pcd.2008.10.005.

63. Wu RR, Zhao JP, Jin H, et al. Lifestyle intervention and metformin for treatment of antipsychotic-induced weight gain: a randomized controlled trial. JAMA 2008;299(2):185–93. http://dx.doi.org/10.1001/jama.2007.56-b.

64. Wu RR, Zhao JP, Guo XF, et al. Metformin addition attenuates olanzapine-induced weight gain in drug-naive first-episode schizophrenia patients: a double-blind, placebo-controlled study. Am J Psychiatry 2008;165(3):352–8. http://dx.doi.org/10.1176/appi.ajp.2007.07010079.

65. Klein DJ, Cottingham EM, Sorter M, et al. A randomized, double-blind, placebo-controlled trial of metformin treatment of weight gain associated with initiation of atypical antipsychotic therapy in children and adolescents. Am J Psychiatry 2006;163(12):2072–9. http://dx.doi.org/10.1176/appi.ajp.163.12.2072.

66. Baptista T, Rangel N, Fernández V, et al. Metformin as an adjunctive treatment to control body weight and metabolic dysfunction during olanzapine administration: a multicentric, double-blind, placebo-controlled trial. Schizophr Res 2007;93(1–3):99–108. http://dx.doi.org/10.1016/j.schres.2007.03.029.

67. Dixon L, Perkins D, Calmes C. Guideline watch (September 2009): practice guideline for the treatment of patients with schizophrenia. 2009. Available at: http://psychiatryonline.org/content.aspx?bookid=28&sectionid=1682213. Accessed December, 2013.

68. Locharernkul C, Shotelersuk V, Hirankarn N. Pharmacogenetic screening of carbamazepine-induced severe cutaneous allergic reactions. J Clin Neurosci 2011;18(10):1289–94. http://dx.doi.org/10.1016/j.jocn.2010.12.054.

69. Post RM, Ketter TA, Uhde T, et al. Thirty years of clinical experience with carbamazepine in the treatment of bipolar illness: principles and practice. CNS Drugs 2007;21(1):47–71.

70. Anderson GD, Yau MK, Gidal BE, et al. Bidirectional interaction of valproate and lamotrigine in healthy subjects. Clin Pharmacol Ther 1996;60(2):145–56. http://dx.doi.org/10.1016/S0009-9236(96)90130-7

71. Hirschfeld RM, Allen MH, McEvoy JP, et al. Relation of serum valproate concentration to response in mania. Am J Psychiatry 1996;153(6):765–70.

72. Haymond J, Ensom MH. Does valproic acid warrant therapeutic drug monitoring in bipolar affective disorder? Ther Drug Monit 2010;32(1):19–20. http://dx.doi.org/10.1097/FTD.0b013e3181c13a30.

73. Freeman TW, Clothier JL, Pazzaglia P, et al. A double-blind comparison of valproate and lithium in the treatment of acute mania. Am J Psychiatry 1992;149(1):108–11.

74. Goldberg JF, Garno JL, Leon AC, et al. A history of substance abuse complicates remission from acute mania in bipolar disorder. J Clin Psychiatry 1999; 60(11):733–40.

75. Reynolds MF, Sisk EC, Rasgon NL. Valproate and neuroendocrine changes in relation to women treated for epilepsy and bipolar disorder: a review. Curr Med Chem 2007;14(26):2799–812.

76. Verrotti A, D'Egidio C, Mohn A, et al. Antiepileptic drugs, sex hormones, and PCOS. Epilepsia 2011;52(2):199–211. http://dx.doi.org/10.1111/j.1528-1167.2010.02897.x.

77. McKenna K, Koren G, Tetelbaum M, et al. Pregnancy outcome of women using atypical antipsychotic drugs: a prospective comparative study. J Clin Psychiatry 2005;66(4):444–9 [quiz: 546].

78. Holmes LB, Baldwin EJ, Smith CR, et al. Increased frequency of isolated cleft palate in infants exposed to lamotrigine during pregnancy. Neurology 2008; 70(22 Pt 2):2152–8. http://dx.doi.org/10.1212/01.wnl.0000304343.45104.d6.

79. Cunnington M, Tennis P, International Lamotrigine Pregnancy Registry Scientific Advisory Committee. Lamotrigine and the risk of malformations in pregnancy. Neurology 2005;64(6):955–60. http://dx.doi.org/10.1212/01.WNL.0000154515.94346.89.

80. Nora JJ, Nora AH, Toews WH. Letter: Lithium, Ebstein's anomaly, and other congenital heart defects. Lancet 1974;2(7880):594–5.

81. Cohen LS, Friedman JM, Jefferson JW, et al. A reevaluation of risk of in utero exposure to lithium. JAMA 1994;271(2):146–50.

82. Yacobi S, Ornoy A. Is lithium a real teratogen? What can we conclude from the prospective versus retrospective studies? A review. Isr J Psychiatry Relat Sci 2008;45(2):95–106.

83. Wyszynski DF, Nambisan M, Surve T, et al. Increased rate of major malformations in offspring exposed to valproate during pregnancy. Neurology 2005; 64(6):961–5. http://dx.doi.org/10.1212/01.WNL.0000154516.43630.C5.

84. American Psychiatric Association, Committee on Electroconvulsive Therapy, Weiner RD. The practice of electroconvulsive therapy: recommendations for treatment, training, and privileging: a task force report of the American Psychiatric Association. Washington, DC: American Psychiatric Association; 2001.

85. Colom F, Vieta E, Sánchez-Moreno J, et al. Psychoeducation for bipolar II disorder: an exploratory, 5-year outcome subanalysis. J Affect Disord 2009;112(1–3): 30–5. http://dx.doi.org/10.1016/j.jad.2008.03.023.

86. Morris CD, Miklowitz DJ, Waxmonsky JA. Family-focused treatment for bipolar disorder in adults and youth. J Clin Psychol 2007;63(5):433–45. http://dx.doi.org/10.1002/jclp.20359.

87. Miklowitz DJ, Otto MW, Frank E, et al. Psychosocial treatments for bipolar depression: a 1-year randomized trial from the Systematic Treatment Enhancement Program. Arch Gen Psychiatry 2007;64(4):419–26. http://dx.doi.org/10.1001/archpsyc.64.4.419.

88. Miklowitz DJ. Adjunctive psychotherapy for bipolar disorder: state of the evidence. Am J Psychiatry 2008;165(11):1408–19. http://dx.doi.org/10.1176/appi.ajp.2008.08040488.

89. Rathod S, Kingdon D, Weiden P, et al. Cognitive-behavioral therapy for medication-resistant schizophrenia: a review. J Psychiatr Pract 2008;14(1): 22–33. http://dx.doi.org/10.1097/01.pra.0000308492.93003.db.

Borderline Personality Disorder in the Primary Care Setting

Amelia N. Dubovsky, MD[a,*], Meghan M. Kiefer, MD[b]

KEYWORDS

- Borderline personality disorder • Primary care • Psychopharmacology
- Behavioral problems • Personality disorder
- Management of borderline personality disorder

KEY POINTS

- Borderline personality disorder is a commonly encountered problem in primary care settings.
- The disorder is characterized by interpersonal problems, which often play out in the relationship between doctor and patient.
- The underlying cause of the disorder is multifactorial, and includes both brain abnormalities, genetics, and experiences early in life.
- The doctor–patient relationship can be greatly improved by better physician understanding of the disorder, good communication with all involved providers, minimization of polypharmacy, and learning how to respond to commonly encountered behavioral problems.

CASE

The first person on the morning's clinic schedule is a 27-year-old woman, Jane, who arrives 10 minutes late, accompanied by her boyfriend. She unfolds a piece of paper with jotted notes and tells you that, "I am really sick, Doc," and proceeds to relay an array of complaints ranging from migraine disorder, chronic back pain, and urinary incontinence. When you attempt to orient yourself by asking what prompted her transition in care, she laughs and tells you she has moved from another state for her boyfriend. She smokes cigarettes and reports taking sertraline, olanzapine, topiramate, and clonazepam, all of she tells you require refills today: "I'm out of everything."

Disclosure: The authors have nothing to disclose.
[a] Department of Psychiatry and Behavioral Sciences, Harborview Medical Center, University of Washington School of Medicine, 325 9th Avenue, Box 359896, Seattle, WA 98104, USA;
[b] Division of General Internal Medicine, University of Washington General Internal Medicine Center, University of Washington School of Medicine, Box 354760, Seattle, WA 98195-4750, USA
* Corresponding author.
E-mail address: ameliand@uw.edu

http://dx.doi.org/10.1016/j.mcna.2014.06.005
0025-7125/14/$ – see front matter © 2014 Elsevier Inc. All rights reserved.
medical.theclinics.com

When you inquire about the indications for her medications, she abruptly becomes tearful, telling you, "I need them to live after my sister died. I think about dying to be with her, but I have to stay." She endorses prior history of suicide attempt with acetaminophen, which required hospitalization, and reports she began cutting herself beginning in the 8th grade "to relieve stress." She then returns to discussing her migraine disorder and tells you, "My doctor in Arizona was really good, she knew all about this stuff," and requests an urgent referral to neurology.

EPIDEMIOLOGY

- Borderline personality disorder (BPD) is common in the primary care setting.
- Higher rates are documented in specific illnesses (chronic pain, migraine).

Estimates of the prevalence of BPD vary significantly based on the setting. BPD has a lifetime prevalence of up to 6% in the US population[1] with a 12-month period prevalence of approximately 1.6%,[2] and affects men and women equally overall. Prevalence is higher in younger adults, those with lower incomes and education, and shows racial and ethnic variability (higher in Native American men, lower in Asian women and Hispanic persons.)

Both life experience and genetics are thought to play a role in this disorder, and a family history of BPD is often present.[3,4] The majority of persons with BPD report a history of some type of childhood abuse, including sexual abuse and/or neglect.[5] However, although common, a history of trauma is not always present in patients with BPD.

In the primary care setting, BPD prevalence is estimated at 6%,[6] with a prevalence of nearly 10% in the outpatient psychiatry setting.[7] However, this disorder often goes undiagnosed by primary care providers, and those with BPD are less likely to be recognized as suffering from emotional or psychiatric problems by their providers than those with other psychiatric disorders.

BPD prevalence has been shown to be higher among certain populations, affecting an estimated 18% of chronic pain patients and 26% of depressed primary care patients.[8,9] In 1 study of patients diagnosed with BPD presenting for psychiatric care, the prevalence rate of severe headache was 60%, with half of women and nearly one quarter of men reporting a diagnosis of migraine, a rate several times that found in the general population.[10] Given the complexities of the patient–provider relationship with BPD, managing these medical conditions in this frequently encountered setting can be challenging. Further, management of physical health in persons with BPD can be made more challenging by higher rates of unhealthy behaviors, such as smoking, excess alcohol intake, and increased risk taking.[11] Illustrating the dilemma, in 1 study, 27% of outpatients who met criteria for BPD self-reported misuse/abuse of prescription drugs.

BPD is associated with increased medical and psychiatric utilization and health care expenditures.[12] However, a significant proportion of the costs associated with BPD are owing to the significant financial burden of decreased productivity.[13,14] The unhealthy and risky behaviors noted are likely to be a factor in both medical and nonmedical costs.

REMISSION

- Remission rates are high, but relapse can occur.
- Remission of diagnostic criteria does not always indicate functional improvement.

Consistent with the decreasing prevalence with age noted, many patients initially diagnosed with BPD are found to improve symptomatically, with many no longer meeting criteria over time.[15] In contrast with mood disorders, which may remit rapidly but often recur, it seems that BPD is relatively slow to remit but recurrence is less common.[5]

Estimates of BPD remission are variable and reflect the heterogeneity of the patient population and remission criteria; however, several studies suggest that at 2 years' follow-up, 35% to 45% of BPD patients will no longer meet criteria, and the majority of patients will be in remission by 10 years' follow-up.[5,16,17] Relapse rates also vary by follow-up time, but estimates range from 6% to 15%. Not surprisingly, those patients who have been in remission for a longer period of time are more likely to maintain it.[18] It is important to note that remission by diagnostic criteria does not necessarily indicate increased functioning; rates of recovery/improvement of global function are low even among those who have achieved remission, with 75% lacking full-time employment and approximately 40% receiving disability payments.[19] However, patients who have achieved remission from BPD are more likely to report improved health status and healthier behaviors.[11]

In 1 inpatient study, 7 variables were noted to be significant predictors of successful remission when adjusting for other factors: Younger age, absence of childhood sexual abuse, no family history of substance use disorder, good vocational record, absence of an anxious cluster personality disorder, low neuroticism, and high agreeableness.[17] In another cohort of 100 patients, remission was estimated at 75% by 15 years follow-up, and 93% by 27 years follow-up, although nearly 20% of the cohort was deceased by that time, over half by suicide.[15]

SUICIDE

- Although much of the suicidal behavior in BPD does not lead to completed suicide, suicide remains a major cause of death for this population.

Suicidal behavior (defined as any action that could potentially cause one to die) is found in approximately 80% of BPD patients, a substantial increase from the general population, with 60% to 70% of patients engaging in suicide attempts.[20,21] A history of self-injurious behavior doubles the risk for suicide[22] among BPD patients, but affective instability is also associated with increased suicide attempts.[23] The risk of suicide for persons diagnosed with BPD is estimated at 8% to 10%.[24,25] This suicide rate is 50 times higher than that of the general population[26]; it is estimated that BPD may account for 18% of all US suicides.[27]

CRITERIA AND CLINICAL CHARACTERISTICS

- Definition and characteristics of BPD.

BPD is characterized by a longstanding, pervasive pattern of instability in interpersonal relationships, identity, impulsivity, and affect.[28] The criteria for the diagnosis of BPD can be found in the *Diagnostic and Statistical Manual of Mental Disorders*, fifth edition.[28] One of the most useful ways to make the diagnosis is by asking patients if they believe the criteria characterize them.[19] Repeated suicidal threats or acts, unstable relationships, and fear of abandonment are highly associated with the diagnosis.[29] Nonsuicidal self-injurious behavior is common in these patients.

There are 4 categories into which the features of BPD can be classified: Interpersonal hypersensitivity and unstable relationships, affective dysregulation, impulsivity, and disturbed cognition.[19,30] Interpersonal hypersensitivity and unstable relationships are a hallmark of BPD. Patients with this condition tend to be extremely sensitive to rejection and have a preoccupation with abandonment.[31] They often have unrealistic expectations of others in relationships (especially professional relationships, as with doctors and therapists), and develop increased emotional instability when the relationship inevitably disappoints them or when rejection is perceived. In the primary care setting, this disappointment can take the form of the physician being unavailable when the patient expects (eg, for last-minute appointments, unscheduled refills of medications, or after-hour phone calls). This can be confusing for the primary care provider, who previously was idealized by the patient as "the only person who understands me," and now is devalued as "the worst doctor I've ever had" after a perceived minor disappointment.

Affective dysregulation is characterized by a range of intense emotions including rage, shame, sorrow, panic, emptiness, and loneliness, often all experienced multiple times within a single day.[32] Although such episodes seem unpredictable and out of the blue, they are often preceded by interpersonal conflict.

Impulsivity can take the form of impulsive suicidal behaviors, as well as impulsive substance use, binge eating, spending sprees, verbal outbursts, and reckless driving. This type of impulsivity is different from the impulsive behavior exhibited during manic episodes, which is more prolonged and are accompanied by other symptoms of mania, such as grandiosity, pressured speech, and lack of need for sleep.

Disturbed cognition can be further divided into three categories[33]: (1) Disturbed but nonpsychotic thoughts, such as dissociation, depersonalization, derealization, and intense feelings of guilt or shame, (2) transitory, loosely reality-based delusions and hallucinations (such as thinking others are talking about them in a malicious way), and (3) frank hallucinations and delusions. Some form of disturbed thinking is experienced by almost all individuals with BPD; outright psychosis is much less common and transitory, when it does occur.

COMORBIDITY

- Associated with other psychiatric disorders.
- Associated with worse outcomes in Axis I disorders.

Individuals with BPD have a high comorbidity with Axis I and II psychiatric disorders: 84.5% meet criteria for an Axis I disorder in the past 12 months and 73.9% meet criteria for another lifetime Axis II disorder.[2] BPD is most highly associated with mood disorders, anxiety disorders, and substance misuse disorders.[1,2,34] In addition, patients with BPD are often misdiagnosed with bipolar disorder or major depressive disorder.[35] In contrast with the mood episodes associated with major depression and bipolar disorder, mood episodes with BPD are often short lived (several episodes of dysphoria and euthymia occurring in 1 day), without sustained periods of mania or elation.[30] Mood swings are common with interpersonal difficulty or rejection. It was previously thought that trauma was among the most significant predictors for the development of BPD. However BPD has an approximate 30% comorbidity with posttraumatic stress disorder,[36] and it is now known that BPD often develops without a history of trauma.

Unfortunately, patients with BPD often have worse outcomes with their comorbid psychiatric disorders. BPD patients are twice as likely to have ongoing substance use disorders at 3 years' follow-up when adjusting for other risk factors,[37] and patients with BPD and comorbid substance use have an increased mortality risk compared with others with substance use disorders. BPD may also be a risk factor for major depression persistence.[8,38]

As is true of mood and anxiety disorders, BPD is associated with increased morbidity and mortality of medical disorders, such as cardiovascular disease and diabetes.[39,40] Frankenburg and Zanarini[11] compared patients with remitted and nonremitted BPD and found that patients with nonremitted illness were more likely to have fibromyalgia, chronic fatigue, and temporomandibular joint syndrome, as well as a history of obesity, osteoarthritis, diabetes, hypertension, back pain, and urinary incontinence. These findings were consistent with a 10-year follow-up study.[41] El-Gabalawy and colleagues[42] used the National Epidemiologic Survey on Alcohol and Related Conditions Wave 2 to look at the comorbidity of medical disorders in a large number of individuals (2231) suffering from BPD. The authors found that the presence of BPD (after controlling for other Axis I and II disorders as well as socioeconomic variables) was significantly associated with arteriosclerosis or hypertension, hepatic disease, cardiovascular disease, gastrointestinal disease, arthritis, and sexually transmitted infections. The authors also found that individuals with BPD and cardiovascular disease, sexually transmitted infections, and "any assessed physical health condition" have a greater likelihood of attempting suicide compared with those with BPD alone. Obesity and the metabolic syndrome have also been found to have an increased incidence in individuals with BPD, especially women.[43] This could be partially explained by side effects of atypical antipsychotics prescribed in this population compounded by poor self-care and unhealthy behaviors.

PATHOPHYSIOLOGY

- Multiple contributing factors.

Although the exact cause of BPD is unknown, the origins of the illness are likely multifactorial and can be divided into putative genetic causes, brain abnormalities, neurohormonal factors, and environmental influences.

Genetics

Previously, it was thought that environmental factors such as early adverse childhood experiences were the sole cause of BPD; however, it is now known that the cause of BPD also involves genetic factors. Although no specific genes have been identified, BPD is significantly inheritable: Iorgensen and colleagues[44] found that BPD has 68% heritability. Additional twin studies have shown heritability ranges from 0.65 to 0.75.[45]

Brain Abnormalities

Although results have been inconsistent, individuals with BPD have shown reduced volume in the amygdala on magnetic resonance imaging.[46,47] They also exhibit varied (some studies indicate increased,[48] some decreased[49]) amygdala activation on functional magnetic resonance imaging when processing negative emotions. Despite inconsistent data, it is likely that the amygdala is somehow altered in patients with BPD, indicating that the limbic system processes emotional information differently than patients without BPD. Evidence has also been found that there is altered metabolism in prefrontal regions, including the anterior cingulate cortex,[50,51] which could partially explain these individuals' propensity toward impulsivity.

Neurohormones

There has been evidence that altered activity of neuropeptides, including oxytocin and opioids, may play a role in mediating some of the symptoms of BPD, including affective reactivity and anger outbursts.[52]

Environmental Factors

Negative events during childhood, such as trauma, abuse, or neglect, in addition to insecure attachment, can contribute to the development of BPD,[53,54] although they are usually not the sole reason for developing BPD. It seems more likely that an interaction between negative childhood experiences, genetics, and brain function abnormalities lead to the development of BPD. What is clear is that it is not helpful to conceptualize these patients simply as "victims" of trauma.

TREATMENT

- Psychotherapy is the mainstay of treatment.
- Manualized, structured forms of therapy are more effective.
- Psychopharmacology can be used to treat symptoms, but polypharmacy should be avoided if possible.

In the past, BPD has been viewed as a disorder that is largely untreatable, but it is now becoming apparent that it has a better than expected prognosis and has even been referred to "the good-prognosis diagnosis" by Zanarini after studying the patient population over 10 years.[16,55,56]

The primary treatment for BPD is psychotherapy, although not all forms of psychotherapy are equally effective.[57] Traditional psychoanalytic therapy can even be harmful to the patient, so it is important to help the patient find the appropriate treatment.[19,58] Psychopharmacology should be seen as an adjunctive treatment, rather than the primary treatment.

Psychotherapy

There are 4 types of empirically studied treatments for BPD: Dialectic behavior therapy (DBT), mentalization-based therapy, transference-focused psychotherapy, and general psychiatric management, which are all manualized (meaning the therapy has been tested, is highly structured, and the therapist and patient closely follow a manual throughout the treatment), making it easier to assess therapists' adherence to the treatment.[19] Although these treatments are becoming more available than in the past, they require therapists to undergo extensive training and are not always easily accessible by patients. These treatments also require therapists to be self-aware and have access to consultation by other colleagues to avoid burnout. DBT, a manual-based 1-year outpatient treatment involving group and individual therapy[59] is perhaps among the most well-known and effective treatments for BPD. DBT focuses on teaching the patient how to manage self-destructive feelings and behaviors. Additionally, the DBT therapist helps the patient to regulate emotion, and develop reality testing and interpersonal effectiveness through various techniques, including distress tolerance, acceptance, and mindfulness. It has been found to reduce self-harm and suicidality in addition to lowering health care costs and utilization of emergency department and inpatient admission.[60] Mentalization-based therapy is another group and individual manualized therapy.[61] Treatment is focused on helping the patient to "mentalize" or understand the mental state of oneself and others and to think before reacting. Transference-focused psychotherapy is an individual, twice-weekly therapy derived from psychoanalysis. It is focused on transference (feelings of the patient projected onto the therapist), and is among the more difficult techniques to learn. General psychiatric management is a once-weekly psychodynamic therapy. It focuses on the patient's interpersonal relationships and can also include pharmacotherapy and family therapy. This is the most available and easiest to learn, although is also the least well-validated. In general, effective treatment requires the patient's active involvement and commitment (**Table 1**).

Psychopharmacology

Polypharmacy is a common problem encountered in patients with BPD. In a study by Zanarini and colleagues,[62] 80% of patients with the disorder were taking medications regularly, and over 40% were taking 3 or more standing medications. However, evidence for psychopharmacology in this population is scant. Selective serotonin reuptake inhibitors are commonly prescribed to patients with BPD, but have little benefit over placebo in randomized, controlled trials.[63] However, they can be helpful if comorbid depression is present. Of all antidepressants, there has only been 1 study that showed a positive effect for amitriptyline in the reduction of depressive symptoms.[64] Caution should be taken with patients who are prone to suicide attempts, because tricyclic antidepressants like amitriptyline can be lethal in overdose. The use of benzodiazepines in BPD is controversial. Although there are no data to support the use of benzodiazepines in the treatment of BPD, these medications are commonly used to treat anxiety and emotional lability. However, they have not been shown to be effective for reducing the hallmarks of BPD, particularly self-harm behavior, and have not been shown to improve outcomes. Benzodiazepines are also commonly used in overdose. The limited data available suggest that benzodiazepines can be associated with increased emotional lability and suicidality in patients with BPD.[65] If deemed necessary, benzodiazepines should only be used with great care, in low doses, and ideally in conjunction with psychotherapy. Of the anticonvulsants, beneficial effects have been found for valproate, lamotrigine, and topiramate. Valproate has been shown to decrease interpersonal problems and depression.[66,67] Lamotrigine is commonly used for augmentation of depression treatment in clinical practice, but has only

Table 1			
Psychotherapy strategies for borderline personality disorder			
Therapy	**Structure**	**Advantages**	**Disadvantages**
Dialectic behavior therapy	Yearlong outpatient treatment Group and individual therapy Manual-based Focus on distress tolerance, emotional regulation, mindfulness	Well-studied Documented efficacy More widely available than MBT	Requires specialized training
Mentalized behavior therapy	Group and individual therapy Manual-based Focus on understanding the mental state of self and others, reflection before reaction	Documented efficacy	Requires specialized training Less widely available
Transference focused	Focuses on individual's feelings projected onto therapist		Difficult to learn
Psychodynamic therapy	Weekly individual sessions Focus on interpersonal relationships	Most widely available	Least well validated

been shown to improve impulsivity in long-term follow-up.[68,69] Antipsychotics are also frequently used in patients with BPD both for psychotic symptoms and management of mood instability, although it is important to take into consideration the risk of obesity and the metabolic syndrome associated, especially with second-generation antipsychotics. In comparison with placebo, haloperidol has been shown to reduce symptoms of anger.[64,70] Olanzapine has been shown to reduce affective instability, anger, and psychotic symptoms.[71] In a study of 52 patients, aripiprazole was found to significantly reduce symptoms of anger, psychosis, impulsivity, and interpersonal problems as well as depression and anxiety.[72] Ziprasidone has not been shown to have any beneficial effect (**Table 2**).[73]

MANAGEMENT IN THE PRIMARY CARE SETTING

- Setting clear boundaries is critical.
- Set regular scheduled appointments for check-ins, rather than only seeing the patient during crises.
- Communicate with all providers involved.

BPD is associated with use of greater numbers of primary care physicians, increased use of medical office visits, telephone calls to medical offices, and medication prescriptions.[74,75] Often this increased utilization of services represents patients seeking dependent relationships as substitutes for poor parenting. Although treating patients with BPD in the outpatient primary care setting can be extremely challenging, providers can often feel much less frustrated if they have a better understanding of BPD.[6] It is important to recognize that "difficult" behavior is often driven by underlying fears of abandonment. Treatment of these patients is best done in the context of a team of providers, including an individual therapist, group therapist, and psychiatrist, if possible. However, many patients refuse psychiatric referral or even consultation

Table 2 Pharmacologic therapies for borderline personality disorder		
Pharmacologic Class	**Specific Agents**	**Advantage/Disadvantages**
Antipsychotics	**Haloperidol**: ↓ anger symptoms **Olanzapine**: ↓ mood instability, ↓ anger **Ariprazole**: ↓ anger, impulsivity, interpersonal problems, ↓ depression/anxiety **Ziprasidone**: no demonstrated effect	Can reduce psychotic symptoms and/or act as mood stabilizer Increased risk of obesity, metabolic syndrome
Anticonvulsants	**Valproate**: ↓ interpersonal problems, depression **Lamotrigine**: ↓depression (added to other prescription), ↓impulsivity	Can help with mood stabilization Valproate requires monitoring Lamotrigine carries risk of Stevens–Johnson syndrome
SSRIs/SNRIs	No SSRI or SNRI has been proven more effective than another	Limited evidence for benefit Useful if comorbid depression present
TCAs	**Amitriptyline**: ↓ depressive symptoms	Caution with patients at risk of overdose

Abbreviations: SNRI, serotonin and norepinephrine reuptake inhibitor; SSRI, selective serotonin reuptake inhibitor; TCA, tricyclic antidepressant.

because they experience the suggestion as rejection. Consultation may be facilitated by reassuring the patient that the primary physician will continue treatment. Communication between providers (especially those prescribing medications) is crucial, especially in minimizing overprescribing of potentially dangerous medications in light of the frequency of suicidal behaviors.

One of the most important factors in treating patients with BPD is setting clear boundaries and expectations for all parties involved at the beginning of a treatment relationship. This serves to minimize the amount of perceived abandonment that occurs, although will likely still occur. Clear boundaries provide a holding environment for the patient and reduce physician burnout. It is important to set up regular, scheduled appointments to reassure the patient that even if he or she becomes "well," the physician will not abandon the patient, which is often the motivation behind treatment resistance.[76] Although participation of patients in a highly structured treatment such as DBT or mentalization-based therapy is ideal, this is not always feasible owing to cost, availability of such specialized treatments in the area, and patient willingness to participate. Regardless of the type of treatment the patient is participating in, it is crucial for the primary care physician to not be the sole provider of all medical and psychiatric care. **Box 1** contains tips on how to manage patients with BPD in the primary care setting. Although patients with BPD have been found to display an increased propensity toward disruptive behaviors in the clinical setting, primarily resulting from impulsive anger, they do not have an increased incidence of violent behavior.[77]

It is important to remember when treating patients with BPD that the disorder is extremely stigmatized, even among mental health providers. This is primarily owing to lack of education about the disorder, limited empirical data on treatment, and the lack of adequate resources to treat these individuals.[58] It is important to remember that manipulative behavior often occurs in response to expected abandonment and

---

Box 1
Tips for the management of borderline personality disorder in the primary care setting

1. Learn about common clinical presentations and causes of undesirable behavior.
2. Validate the patient's feelings by naming the emotion you suspect, such as fear of abandonment, anger, shame, and so on, before addressing the "facts" of the situation and acknowledge the real stresses in the patient's situation.
3. Avoid responding to provocative behavior.
4. Schedule regular, time-limited visits that are not contingent on the patient being "sick."
5. Set clear boundaries at the beginning of the treatment relationship and do not respond to attempts to operate outside of these boundaries unless it is a true emergency.
6. Make open communication with all other providers a condition of treatment.
7. Avoid polypharmacy and large-volume prescriptions of potentially toxic medications (including tricyclic antidepressants, cardiac medications, and benzodiazepines).
8. Avoid prescribing potentially addicting medications such as benzodiazepines, opiates, or other controlled substances. Inform patients of your policies regarding these medications early in the treatment relationship so they are aware of your limits.
9. Set firm limits on manipulative behavior while avoiding being judgmental.
10. Do not reward difficult behavior with more contact and attention. Provide attention based on a regular schedule rather than being contingent on behavior.

Table 3
Common behavioral problems associated with borderline personality disorder encountered in the primary care setting and their management

Clinical Scenario	Management Strategy
Follow-up with patient "Jane"	With the patient's help, pick the most urgent matter and address only that today.
	Review clinic policy requiring review of outside records before providing refills of psychoactive substances such as benzodiazepines.
	Set up a follow-up appointment for next week to address additional concerns.
	If patient's use of suicidal statements increase, refer to the emergency room because she is an unfamiliar patient to you.
The patient has called the clinic 7 times in 1 d demanding to speak to the doctor, and refusing to specify the reason for calling. She has a regularly scheduled appointment for the next day. She has engaged in abusive and threatening language with the staff when they inquire her reason for calling.	Remind the patient that you will see her the next day for her appointment.
	Speak in a calm and even tone; do not engage in arguing or admonishing her over the phone. Cut off contact if patient escalates.
	During her appointment remind her of the clinic policies about abusive language toward staff; remind her that abusive behavior in the future will result in her termination from the clinic.
	Move on to discuss medical problems without further judgment or scolding tone.
The patient requests a refill for Adderall "just this one time" that her psychiatrist normally prescribes because he is out of town and the hard copy of the prescription was stolen by a friend.	Do not refill the prescription because this will set a precedent for further boundary limit testing in the future.
	Tell patient it is a clinic policy that you do not refill prescriptions written by another doctor no matter what the circumstances, and that she will need to contact her psychiatrist when he is back in town.

The patient has received a prescription for oxycodone after a visit to the emergency department for a migraine. She comes to the office in tears requesting a refill for the medication because "this is the only medication that has ever helped my pain."	Do not refill the prescription. Acknowledge the patient's distress ("you are very upset right now"). Firmly state that it is against your policy to prescribe opioids for migraines.
The patient presents with symptoms she feels indicate a serious illness, despite a pattern of similar complaints leading to repeated evaluations without evidence of significant pathology. When you attempt reassurance, she demands elaborate testing to confirm "I know there's something wrong."	Briefly see and evaluate the patient and provide reassurance that there is no infection present. Validate the patient that she is suffering and uncomfortable, and that you will continue to follow her symptoms. Schedule a regular follow-up appointment. Remind her ahead of time that you will only be available to her only during regularly scheduled appointments. Do not acquiesce to requests to repeat invasive medical tests or provide treatment that is not indicated.
You have secured an outpatient psychiatry consultation for the patient, but she refuses to go "because they won't understand me like you do."	Discuss fears about seeing the psychiatrist including fear of abandonment by you (the primary care provider); provide reassurance that you will continue to treat her despite another physician being involved. If recurrent maladaptive behavior continues to disrupt the doctor–patient relationship, tell the patient that consultation is necessary if treatment is to continue

may be managed by strict limit setting and consistent availability that is not contingent on expressions of distress.

Referral to emergency psychiatric services (emergency room or psychiatric crisis center) should be considered if the patient has new or changing thoughts about suicide, or if these thoughts increase in intensity or frequency, and/or if the patient expresses desire or intent to act on impulses rather than having fleeting thoughts of suicide (**Table 3**).

FUTURE DIRECTIONS

BPD is a commonly encountered disorder in the primary care setting. Despite the difficulty in the management of these patients, with a good understanding of the illness, support from other providers, and clear boundaries, relationships can be extremely rewarding to both parties involved, and the primary care physician can make a significant impact in these patients' lives. With the implementation of the Affordable Care Act, it is possible that more patients will be able to obtain access to specialized psychiatric services, including structured therapy, which can result in not only a reduction in symptoms, but a remittance of the disorder altogether.

REFERENCES

1. Grant BF, Chou SP, Goldstein RB, et al. Prevalence, correlates, disability, and comorbidity of DSM-IV borderline personality disorder: results from the Wave 2 National Epidemiologic Survey on Alcohol and Related Conditions. J Clin Psychiatry 2008;69:533–45.
2. Lenzenweger MF, Lane MC, Lorganger AW, et al. DSM-IV personality disorders in the National Comorbidity Survey Replication. Biol Psychiatry 2007;62:553–64.
3. Distel MA, Willemsen G, Ligthart L, et al. Genetic covariance structure of the four main features of borderline personality disorder. J Pers Disord 2010;24(4):427–44.
4. Gunderson JG, Zanarini MC, Choi-Kain LW, et al. Family study of borderline personality disorder and its sectors of psychopathology. Arch Gen Psychiatry 2011;68(7):753–62.
5. Zanarini MC, Frankenburg FR, Hennen J, et al. The McLean Study of Adult Development (MSAD): overview and implications of the first six years of prospective follow-up. J Pers Disord 2005;19(5):505–23.
6. Gross R, Olfson M, Gameroff M, et al. Borderline personality disorder in primary care. Arch Intern Med 2002;162:53–60.
7. Zimmerman M, Rothschild L, Chelminski I. The prevalence of DSM-IV personality disorders in psychiatric outpatients. Am J Psychiatry 2005;162(10):1911–8.
8. Riihimäkia K, Vuorilehtoa M, Isometsä E. Borderline personality disorder among primary care depressive patients: a five-year study. J Affect Disord 2014;155:303–6.
9. Sansone RA, Whitecar P, Meier BP, et al. The prevalence of borderline personality among primary care patients with chronic pain. Gen Hosp Psychiatry 2001;23(4):193–7.
10. Hegarty AM. The prevalence of migraine in borderline personality disorder. Headache 1993;33:271.
11. Frankenburg FR, Zanarini MC. The association between borderline personality disorder and chronic medical illnesses, poor health-related lifestyle choices, and costly forms of health care utilization. J Clin Psychiatry 2004;65:1660–5.

12. Bender DS, Dolan RT, Skodol AE, et al. Treatment utilization by patients with personality disorders. Am J Psychiatry 2001;158(2):295–302.
13. van Asselt AD, Dirksen CD, Arntz A, et al. The cost of borderline personality disorder: societal cost of illness in BPD-patients. Eur Psychiatry 2007;22(6):354–61.
14. Soeteman DI, Hakkaart-van Roijen L, Verheul R, et al. The economic burden of personality disorders in mental health care. J Clin Psychiatry 2008;69(2): 259–65.
15. Paris J, Zweig-Frank HA. 27-year follow-up of patients with borderline personality disorder. Compr Psychiatry 2001;42(6):482–7.
16. Gunderson JG, Stout RL, McGlashan TH, et al. Ten-year course of borderline personality disorder: psychopathology and function from the Collaborative Longitudinal Personality Disorders study. Arch Gen Psychiatry 2011;68:827–37.
17. Zanarini MC, Frankenburg FR, Hennen J, et al. Prediction of the 10-year course of borderline personality disorder. Am J Psychiatry 2006;163(5):827–32.
18. Zanarini MC, Frankenburg FR, Reich DB, et al. Attainment and stability of sustained symptomatic remission and recovery among patients with borderline personality disorder and axis II comparison subjects: a 16 year prospective follow-up study. Am J Psychiatry 2012;169(5):476–83.
19. Gunderson JG. Borderline personality disorder. N Engl J Med 2011;364: 2037–42.
20. Linehan MM, Comtois KA, Murray AM, et al. Two-year randomized controlled trial and follow-up of dialectical behavior therapy vs therapy by experts for suicidal behaviors and borderline personality disorder. Arch Gen Psychiatry 2006; 63(7):757–66.
21. Gunderson JG. Borderline personality disorder: a clinical guide. Washington, DC: American Psychiatric Press; 2001.
22. Gunderson JG, Ridolfi ME. Borderline personality disorder. Suicidality and self-mutilation. Ann N Y Acad Sci 2001;932:61–73 [discussion: 73–7].
23. Yen S, Shea MT, Pagano M, et al. Axis I and axis II disorders as predictors of prospective suicide attempts: findings from the collaborative longitudinal personality disorders study. J Abnorm Psychol 2003;112(3):375–81.
24. Black DW, Blum N, Pfohl B, et al. Suicidal behavior in borderline personality disorder: prevalence, risk factors, prediction, and prevention. J Pers Disord 2004; 18(3):226–39.
25. Oldham JM. Borderline personality disorder and suicidality. Am J Psychiatry 2006;163(1):20–6.
26. Leichsenring F, Leibing E, Kruse J, et al. Borderline personality disorder. Lancet 2011;377(9759):74–84.
27. Bolton JM, Robinson J. Population-attributable fractions of axis I and axis II mental disorders for suicide attempts: findings from a representative sample of the adult, noninstitutionalized US population. Am J Public Health 2010; 100(12):2473–80.
28. American Psychiatric Association. Diagnostic and statistical manual of mental disorders. 5th edition. Washington, DC: American Psychiatric Association; 2013.
29. Grilo CM, Sanislow CA, Skodol AE, et al. Longitudinal diagnostic efficiency of DSM-IV criteria for borderline personality disorder: a 2-year prospective study. Can J Psychiatry 2007;52:357–62.
30. Lieb K, Zanarini MC, Schmahl C, et al. Borderline personality disorder. Lancet 2004;364:453–61.
31. Gunderson JG, Lyons-Ruth K. BPD's interpersonal hypersensitivity phenotype: a gene-environment-development model. J Pers Disord 2008;22:22–41.

32. Koenigsberg HW, Harvey PD, Mitropoulou V, et al. Characterizing affective insta-bility in borderline personality disorder. Am J Psychiatry 2002;159:784–8.
33. Zanarini MC, Gunderson JG, Frankenberg FR. Cognitive features of borderline personality disorder. Am J Psychiatry 1990;147:57–63.
34. Skodol AE, Gunderson JG, Shea MT, et al. The Collaborative Longitudinal Per-sonality Disorders Study (CLPS): overview and implications. J Pers Disord 2005;19:487–504.
35. Zimmerman M, Ruggero CJ, Chleminski I, et al. Psychiatric diagnoses in patients previously overdiagnosed with bipolar disorder. J Clin Psychiatry 2010;71:26–31.
36. Swartz M, Blazer D, George L, et al. Estimating the prevalence of borderline per-sonality disorder in the community. J Pers Disord 1990;4:257–72.
37. Hasin D, Fenton MC, Skodol A, et al. Personality disorders and the 3-year course of alcohol, drug, and nicotine use disorders. Arch Gen Psychiatry 2011;68(11):1158–67.
38. Skodol AE, Grilo CM, Keyes KM, et al. Relationship of personality disorders to the course of major depressive disorder in a nationally representative sample. Am J Psychiatry 2011;168(3):257–64.
39. Park M, Katon WJ, Wolf FM. Depression and risk of mortality in individuals with diabetes: a meta-analysis and systematic review. Gen Hosp Psychiatry 2013;35:217–25.
40. Pan A, Sun Q, Okereke OI, et al. Depression and risk of stroke morbidity and mortality: a meta-analysis and systematic review. JAMA 2011;306:1241–9.
41. Keuroghlian AS, Frankenberg FR, Zanarini MC. The relationship of chronic med-ical illnesses, poor health-related lifestyle choices, and health care utilization to recovery status in borderline patients over a decade of prospective follow-up. J Psychiatr Res 2013;47:1499–506.
42. El-Gabalawy R, Katz LY, Sareen J. Comorbidity and associated severity of borderline personality disorder and physical health conditions in a nationally representative sample. Psychosom Med 2010;72:641–7.
43. Kahl KG, Greggersen W, Schweiger U, et al. Prevalence of the metabolic syn-drome in patients with borderline personality disorder: results from a cross-sectional study. Eur Arch Psychiatry Clin Neurosci 2013;263:205–13.
44. Torgensen S, Lygren S, Ojen PA, et al. A twin study of personality disorders. Compr Psychiatry 2000;41:416–25.
45. New AS, Goodman M, Triebwasser J, et al. Recent advances in the biological study of personality disorders. Psychiatr Clin North Am 2008;31:441–61.
46. Schmahl CG, Vermetten E, Elzinga BM, et al. Magnetic resonance imaging of hippocampal and amygdala volume in women with childhood abuse and borderline personality disorder. Psychiatry Res 2003;122:193–8.
47. Weniger G, Lange C, Sachsse U, et al. Reduced amygdala and hippocampus size in trauma-exposed women with borderline personality disorder and without posttraumatic stress disorder. J Psychiatry Neurosci 2009;34:383–8.
48. Koenigsberg HW, Siever LJ, Lee H, et al. Neural correlates of emotion process-ing in borderline personality disorder. Psychiatry Res 2009;172:192–9.
49. Ruocco AC, Amirthavasagam S, Choi-Kain LW, et al. Neural correlates of nega-tive emotionality in borderline personality disorder: an activation-likelihood-estimation meta-analysis. Biol Psychiatry 2013;73:153–60.
50. Soloff PH, Meltzer CC, Becker C, et al. Impulsivity and prefrontal hypometabo-lism in borderline personality disorder. Psychiatry Res 2003;123:153–63.
51. Juengling FD, Schmahl C, Hesslinger B, et al. Positron emission tomography in fe-male patients with borderline personality disorder. J Psychiatr Res 2003;37:109–15.

52. Stanley B, Siever LJ. The interpersonal dimension of borderline personality disorder: toward a neuropeptide model. Am J Psychiatry 2010;167:24–39.
53. Zanarini MC, Gunderson JG, Marino MF, et al. Childhood experiences of borderline patients. Compr Psychiatry 1989;30:18–25.
54. Zanarini MC, Williams AA, Lewis RE, et al. Reported pathological childhood experiences associated with the development of borderline personality disorder. Am J Psychiatry 1997;154:1101–6.
55. Zanarini MC, Frankenberg FR, Hennen J, et al. The longitudinal course of borderline psychopathology: 6-year prospective follow-up of the phenomenology of borderline personality disorder. Am J Psychiatry 2003;160: 274–83.
56. Zanarini MC, Frankenberg FR, Reich DB, et al. The subsyndromal phenomenology of borderline personality disorder: a 10-year follow-up study. Am J Psychiatry 2007;164:929–35.
57. Tucker L, Bauer SF, Wagner SC, et al. Long-term hospital treatment of borderline patients: a descriptive outcome study. Am J Psychiatry 1987;144:1443–8.
58. Gunderson JG. Borderline personality disorder: ontogeny of a diagnosis. Am J Psychiatry 2009;166:530–9.
59. Linehan MM. Skills training manual for treating borderline personality disorder. New York: Guilford; 1993.
60. Linehan MM, Armstrong HE, Suarez A, et al. Cognitive-behavioral treatment of chronically parasuicidal borderline patients. Arch Gen Psychiatry 1991;48: 1060 4.
61. Bateman AW, Fonagy P. Mentalization-based treatment of BPD. J Pers Disord 2004;18:36–51.
62. Zanarini MC, Frankenburg FR, Hennen J, et al. Mental health service utilization by borderline personality disorder patients and axis II comparison subjects followed prospectively for 6 years. J Clin Psychiatry 2004;65:28 36.
63. Lieb K, Völlm B, Rücker G, et al. Pharmacotherapy for borderline personality disorder: cochrane systematic review of randomised trials. Br J Psychiatry 2010; 196:4–12.
64. Soloff PH, George L, Nathan S, et al. Amitriptyline versus haloperidol in borderlines: final outcomes and predictors of response. J Clin Psychopharmacol 1989; 9:238–46.
65. Cowdry RW, Gardner DL. Pharmacotherapy of borderline personality disorder. Alprazolam, carbamazepine, trifluoperazine, and tranylcypromine. Arch Gen Psychiatry 1988;45(2):111–9.
66. Frankenburg FR, Zanarini MC. Divalproex sodium treatment of women with borderline personality disorder and bipolar II disorder: a double-blind placebo-controlled pilot study. J Clin Psychiatry 2002;63:442–6.
67. Hollander E, Allen A, Lopez RP, et al. A preliminary double-blind, placebo-controlled trial of divalproex sodium in borderline personality disorder. J Clin Psychiatry 2001;62:199–203.
68. Tritt K, Nickel C, Lahmann C, et al. Lamotrigine treatment of aggression in female borderline-patients: a randomized, double-blind, placebo-controlled study. J Psychopharmacol 2005;19:287–91.
69. Leiberich P, Nickel MK, Tritt K, et al. Lamotrigine treatment of aggression in female borderline patients, part II: an 18-month follow-up. J Psychopharmacol 2008;22:805–8.
70. Soloff PH, Cornelius JR, George A, et al. Efficacy of phenelzine and haloperidol in borderline personality disorder. Arch Gen Psychiatry 1993;50:377–85.

71. Bogenschutz MP, Nurnberg HG. Olanzapine versus placebo in the treatment of borderline personality disorder. J Clin Psychiatry 2004;65:104–9.
72. Nickel MK, Muehlbacher M, Nickel C, et al. Aripiprazole in the treatment of patients with borderline personality disorder: a double-blind, placebo-controlled study. Am J Psychiatry 2006;163(5):833–8.
73. Pascual JC, Soler J, Puigdemont D, et al. Ziprasidone in the treatment of borderline personality disorder: a double-blind, placebo-controlled, randomized study. J Clin Psychiatry 2008;69:603–8.
74. Sansone RA, Farukhi S, Widerman MW. Utilization of primary care physicians in borderline personality. Gen Hosp Psychiatry 2011;33:343–6.
75. Sansone RA, Widerman MW, Sansone LA. Borderline personality symptomatology, experience of multiple types of trauma, and health care utilization among women in a primary care setting. J Clin Psychiatry 1998;59:108–11.
76. Ricke AK, Lee MJ, Chambers JE. The difficult patient: borderline personality disorder in the obstetrical and gynecological patient. Obstet Gynecol Surv 2012;67:495–502.
77. Sansone RA, Farukhi S, Wiederman MW. Disruptive behaviors in the medical setting and borderline personality. Int J Psychiatry Med 2011;41:355–63.

Seasonal Affective Disorder, Grief Reaction, and Adjustment Disorder

 CrossMark

Justin Osborn, MD[a,*], Jacqueline Raetz, MD[a], Amanda Kost, MD[b,*]

KEYWORDS

- Adjustment disorder • Grief reaction • Complex grief • Seasonal affective disorder
- Diagnosis • Treatment

KEY POINTS

- Patients with seasonal affective disorder meet criteria for major depressive disorder or bipolar disorder, with symptoms occurring seasonally and with spontaneous remission that can be treated with phototherapy or antidepressants.
- Grief is a normal response to loss; complex grief affects 7% of patients and is characterized by more severe symptoms that may require pharmacotherapy
- Adjustment disorder is an abnormal response to a stress that is time-limited and is best treated with psychotherapy.
- Referrals for psychotherapy for counseling or to psychiatry for severe symptoms for all 3 disorders may be indicated.

INTRODUCTION

Primary care providers (PCPs) are on the front line for patients experiencing affective disorders and normal or abnormal responses to loss or stressors. Identifying which patients with affective disorders such as major depressive disorder (MDD) or bipolar disorder have seasonality to their symptoms can allow the PCPs to guide the patient to the most appropriate care, including light therapy that is not typically used in other affective disorders. For patients who experience loss or stress, knowing normal and abnormal responses, including the typical temporal course of emotions, can help the PCP design an appropriate treatment plan depending on the severity of symptoms. Most patients with seasonal affective disorder (SAD), grief reactions, or adjustment disorder can be managed in the primary care setting, possibly in conjunction with a therapist.

[a] Department of Family Medicine, University of Washington, 331 Northeast Thornton Place, Box 358732, Seattle, WA 98125, USA; [b] Department of Family Medicine, University of Washington, Box 356390, Seattle, WA 98195, USA
* Corresponding authors.
E-mail addresses: josborn@fammed.washington.edu; akost@uw.edu

Med Clin N Am 98 (2014) 1065–1077
http://dx.doi.org/10.1016/j.mcna.2014.06.006   medical.theclinics.com

SEASONAL AFFECTIVE DISORDER
Symptoms

SAD is not a separate mood disorder from MDD, bipolar 1 disorder, or bipolar 2 disorders. Instead the *Diagnostic and Statistical Manual of Mental Disorders*, 5th edition (DSM-5) classified SAD as a subtype of these mood disorders with a seasonality of onset and remission.[1] Affective symptoms occur during a particular time of year and then spontaneously remit. Two types of SAD have been described.[2] Winter-onset SAD is more common and frequently presents with increased appetite, weight, and sleep. Spring/summer SAD is less common and is characterized more often with poor appetite, weight loss, and insomnia. Patients need to meet criteria for MDD (**Fig. 1**) with full remission as the season progresses.

Diagnostic Tests

Several screening tools can assist in identifying patients with SAD. The Patient Health Questionnaire 2 can identify patients who need additional evaluation for a depressive disorder. The Seasonal Pattern Assessment Questionnaire (SPAQ) is an older instrument that can be used to screen but not diagnose patients who may have SAD.[3,4] The SPAQ includes changes of mood, appetite, sleep, weight, and social activities across seasons, a rating of how much the changes are a problem to the individual, and consideration of months during which the symptoms are worse (December, January, February for winter SAD; June, July, August for summer SAD). The Seasonal Health Questionnaire (SHQ) is a newer instrument that has improved sensitivity and specificity.[5] This questionnaire is divided into 6 sections, and probes for the number of times a person has had depression symptoms over the past 10 years lasting more than 2 weeks and the seasonality of the symptoms. Patients who do not screen positive for depression on the initial sections do not complete the remainder of the instrument that assesses for seasonality.

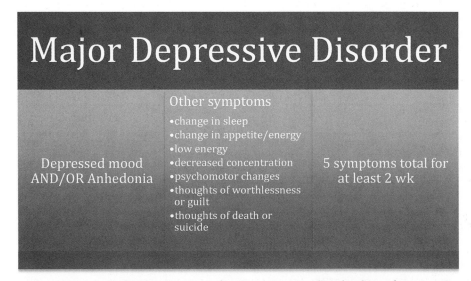

Fig. 1. DSM-5 criteria for the diagnosis of major depressive disorder. (*Data from* American Psychiatric Association. Diagnostic and statistical manual of mental disorders. 5th edition. Arlington, VA: American Psychiatric Publishing; 2013.)

Who Is at Risk for Developing SAD?

Approximately 5% to 10% of the population in the United States suffers from SAD. The higher measure was based on the SPAQ, which may have overestimated the incidence. Using the SHQ, approximately 5% of patients in primary care practices have SAD.[6] The disorder is more common in women and tends to affect younger adults. Several pathophysiologic mechanisms have been proposed. Those who develop SAD may have certain genetic factors, neurotransmitter differences, or circadian rhythm abnormalities including improper release of melatonin or problems with phase shifting.[7] A notable risk factor for the development of SAD is implicit in individuals who live at or move to higher latitudes, where there are more extreme differences between daylight and nighttime durations with respect to the seasons (**Table 1**).[8]

Differential Diagnosis

Highest on the differential diagnosis for SAD are other affective disorders that do not have a seasonal component, which include MDD, bipolar 1 and bipolar 2 disorders, and dysthymia. PCPs need to consider the possibility of underlying medical disease such as thyroid disorders, and should also assess patients for substance abuse.

Treatment

Different treatment options allow PCPs to tailor recommendations to each specific patient. Treatment choices include light therapy, antidepressants, psychotherapy, and complementary and alternative therapies.

Light therapy is the most studied treatment of SAD

Light therapy involves exposure of the patient to artificial light on a daily basis.[9,10] Lights that are bright (more than 6000 lux) and blue may be more effective than dim to medium lights or red lights. Ultraviolet lights should be avoided because of the increased risk of skin cancer. Patients should use the lights for 30 to 90 minutes daily, with their eyes open, but should avoid staring directly into the light to avoid possible retinal injury. Light therapy used in the morning may be more effective and can avoid problems with insomnia in comparison with light used in the evening. The mechanism of action of light therapy is thought be due to melatonin suppression and shifting of circadian rhythms to address the underlying pathophysiology of phase shifting.[11] Patients usually experience an improvement in symptoms within 3 weeks, and treatment should continue throughout the season until the time when symptoms typically spontaneously resolve. Light therapy can be used prophylactically before the onset of symptoms. Side effects are typically mild, and include vision issues such as blurry vision, photophobia, or headache. Patients and PCPs should be aware that light therapy might induce mania in patients with unrecognized or undertreated bipolar disorder. Multiple commercially produced light sources or boxes are available. Lights for the treatment of SAD provide continuous bright light and are different from daylight

Table 1 Risk factors for developing SAD	
Demographic	**Pathophysiologic**
Women	Genetic factors
Young adults	Neurotransmitter differences
Moving to or living at higher latitudes	Circadian rhythm abnormalities

simulators that are designed to reproduce the gradual lightening at sunrise. Daylight simulators have not been studied for SAD (**Box 1**).

Antidepressants offer another treatment option for SAD

Placebo-controlled studies indicate that several second-generation antidepressants are effective for the treatment of SAD, including sertraline, fluoxetine, duloxetine, and escitalopram.[12] Buproprion XL in doses of 150mg to 300mg have been studied and approved for the prevention of MDD symptoms in patients with SAD.[13] Comparison of light therapy with fluoxetine showed that they were equally beneficial.[14] Because no drug is clearly superior to another, decisions on treatment should be made based on prior successful treatment, potential drug interactions, or adverse effects.

Cognitive-behavioral therapy can be used to augment light therapy

A single study indicated that cognitive-behavioral therapy (CBT) in combination with light therapy improved SAD symptoms; however, CBT alone was less efficacious.[15] Adding CBT to light therapy may be particularly useful in preventing relapse in subsequent years.

Several complementary and alternative treatments have been suggested for SAD

St John's wort at a total daily dose of 900 mg is effective in treating SAD.[16,17] Small trials involving fewer than 20 patients each indicate that melatonin improves sleep in patients with subsyndromal SAD and that tryptophan has efficacy similar to that of light therapy.[18,19] High-dose vitamin D supplementation (100,000 IU one-time dose) also decreased depressive symptoms.[20] However, the small number of patients involved in these studies makes it difficult to generalize results.

There is scant evidence comparing available treatments or their use in combination

Therapies may be used in conjunction with one another, but with the exception of CBT there is little evidence to guide combination therapy. Adding light therapy to St. John's wort therapy did not result in significant improvements when compared with pharmacotherapy alone.[16,17]

The duration of treatment should last at least the typical SAD season

Most studies have used seasonal treatment of less than 8 weeks to assess response. For patients with mild to moderate episodes seasonal therapy is likely an appropriate choice, and treatment should continue until symptoms usually remit on their own. Because most individuals with SAD are at risk for yearly recurrences, starting treatment a few weeks before the time of typical symptom onset is a reasonable approach. Continuous therapy may be considered for patients with severe symptoms such as suicidal ideation or psychosis.

Box 1
Pearls for light therapy treatment of SAD

Light should be bright (6000 lux or more)

Blue light may be more effective than others

Avoid ultraviolet light

Use for 30 to 90 minutes in the morning

Face the light with open eyes but do not stare into the light

Management

Patients do not require a prescription to obtain a light box, although PCPs should offer patients information about the kind of box to obtain and how to use it. The medications used to treat SAD are familiar to most PCPs because of their use in nonseasonal affective disorders, and include selective serotonin reuptake inhibitors, serotonin norepinephrine reuptake inhibitors, and tricyclic antidepressants. Referral to psychotherapy is indicated if a patient desires CBT to augment his or her therapy. For patients with severe symptoms, such as psychosis and a plan to harm themselves or others, emergency evaluation by a psychiatrist is needed. Psychiatric consultation could also be considered in patients with less severe symptoms who fail to respond to appropriate treatments (**Box 2**).

GRIEF REACTION
Symptoms

Grief, a normal emotional reaction to loss, may be from loss of a person or from significant change in function, community, or social position.[21] It is an entity distinct from depression and may manifest itself physically, emotionally, cognitively, behaviorally, and spiritually.[22] Individuals may experience grief in anticipation of losing a loved one or in anticipation of one's own death. This concept is sometimes referred to as anticipatory grief or mourning. Bereavement is grief experienced after the death of a loved one. Complex grief is also referred to in the literature as complicated grief and prolonged grief disorder, and in the DSM-5 as persistent complex bereavement disorder. It is defined as grief with clinically significant symptoms that has persisted longer than 12 months and causes impairment in function.

Healthy Grieving Is a Normal Process

Grief may produce feelings of shock, denial, anger, disbelief, yearning, anxiety, sadness, or helplessness. It is normal for grief to cause problems with sleep and appetite, significant fatigue, and social withdrawal.[22] It is also normal for grief to disrupt daily life and to make it difficult to manage for weeks to months after a loss.[22] Grief often occurs in waves. Triggers may be difficult to establish, but may include holidays and anniversaries. As time passes the waves become less intense. There are defined phases of grief, but they may occur in a different order in different individuals.[21]

Bereavement has long been described to occur in stages, as first formally described by Bowlby and Parks.[23] These stages have been described as shock-numbness, yearning-searching, disorganization-despair, and reorganization.[23] Jacobs described them as disbelief, yearning, anger, depression, and acceptance.[23]

With anticipatory grief, patients may reflect on their life, friends, and family, and begin to imagine a future without their loved one.[21] Kubler-Ross identified 5 stages: denial-dissociation-isolation, anger, bargaining, depression, and acceptance.[23]

Box 2
Pearls for effective treatment of SAD

Light therapy with bright blue light used 30 to 90 minutes in the morning

Antidepressants including sertraline, fluoxetine, duloxetine, escitalopram, and bupropion

Complementary therapies include St. John's wort, vitamin D, tryptophan, and melatonin

Cognitive-behavioral therapy can be used adjunctively with medication or light therapy

---

People vary in how long they experience grief.[21] Hypothesized theories have often suggested the normal grieving process lasts about 6 months, but recent empirical evidence suggests that most symptoms of grief are only just peaking at or near 6 months. In one study, yearning peaked near 4 months, anger near 5 months, and depression near 6 months after loss of a close family member.[23]

Differential Diagnosis

Approximately 7% of grieving people experience complex grief.[24] The DSM-5 defines Persistent Complex Bereavement Disorder if 1 or more of the following symptoms significantly persists on more days than not beyond 12 months: yearning or longing for the deceased, intense sorrow or emotional pain, and preoccupation with the deceased or circumstances of death. In addition, at least 6 of the following symptoms must persist on more days than not: difficulty accepting the death, disbelief or numbness, difficulty with positive reminiscing about the deceased, bitterness or anger, self-blame, excessive avoidance of reminders of the loss, a desire to die to be with the deceased, difficulty trusting others, feeling alone or detached from others, feeling that life is meaningless or that one cannot function without the deceased, diminished self-identity, and reluctance to pursue interests or plan for the future. The distress must cause clinically significant distress or impair function, and be out of proportion to cultural norms.

Several Risk Factors Exist for Complex Grief

Women are more at risk than men of complex grief. Individuals with preexisting mental health and substance abuse disorders are at higher risk. A history of trauma (particularly childhood), recent or multiple prior losses, insecure attachment, little social support, or a caretaking role also increases the risk of complex grief. Complex grief is also more likely to occur from a sudden, violent, unexpected death, or a death of which the circumstances are unclear.[24] Not knowing, acknowledging, or preparing for death may impede normal anticipatory grief.[21]

Diagnostic Tests

Getting stuck in one phase of the grieving process may signal complex grief.[21] It is important for primary care physicians to ask about symptoms of complex grief, particularly in patients at higher risk. The Brief Grief Questionnaire is a 5-question screening tool that may be practical for primary care physicians to use in the outpatient setting. It asks participants to rate symptoms as not at all, somewhat, and a lot. The questionnaire asks about how much the patient is having trouble accepting the death of a loved one, how much grief still interferes with the patient's life, how much he or she is having images or thoughts of their loved one when he or she died or other thoughts about the death that are bothersome, avoidance of activities that used to be done with the person who died or avoiding looking at pictures or talking about him or her, and how much the patient is feeling cut off from others.[24]

Distinguishing Between Grief and Depression

Many symptoms between grief and depression overlap, and can occur together. A change between the DSM-IV and DSM-5 is that the *Diagnostic and Statistical Manual of Mental Disorders*, 4th edition (DSM-IV) criteria for a major depressive episode that stated "the symptoms are not better accounted for by bereavement" was removed. In the DSM-IV, to qualify for depression symptoms had to be present at least 2 months, and either lead to marked loss of function or include symptoms of suicidality, morbid preoccupation with worthlessness, psychotic symptoms, or psychomotor retardation.

Instead a note is made that clinical judgment must be used to distinguish between a major depressive episode and the normal response to loss. These changes were made in response to evidence suggesting that response to treatment and short-term prognosis is similar for bereavement-related and non–bereavement-related depression.[25]

As suggested in the DSM-IV bereavement exemption, a key element distinguishing grief from depression is a lack of self-worth. Depressed patients are also more likely to have feelings of pervasive hopelessness, helplessness, guilt, lack of pleasure, and suicidal ideation.[22] It is important for primary care physicians to assess for and treat coexisting depression.[21]

Treatment

Pharmacologic treatment is not indicated for uncomplicated grief, and many patients do not seek professional assistance.[22]

Physicians should offer empathy and encourage expression of emotions. It may be beneficial to help patients identify and seek support within their own network of family, friends, and community. Physicians should actively listen.[22] To assist patients in talking about the grief they are experiencing it can be helpful to ask patients open-ended questions, such as "how you are managing?" and "what is going through your mind?"[21]

Psychotherapy and consideration of antidepressants is indicated for the treatment of complex grief. Patients are at higher risk for suicidality, and should be screened accordingly. Complex grief is associated with several negative outcomes.[24] Patients with complex grief have higher rates of cardiovascular disease and cancer.[24] Identification and treatment of complex grief may improve the quality of life, functional status, and sleep problems.[24]

Management

As most people cope with grief without seeking medical attention, PCPs play a supportive role when their patients are grieving. Interdisciplinary teams including nurses, social workers and other types of primary care providers can assist in supporting patients their families with grief. Nurses, social workers, psychologists, and chaplains may all be of assistance.[21] The Medicare hospice benefit includes bereavement services for surviving family members.

PCPs should seek referral to specialists when initial therapy for grief, complex grief, concurrent depression, or substance abuse extends beyond the scope or comfort of their practice (**Box 3**).

ADJUSTMENT DISORDER
Symptoms

Adjustment disorders are amplified stress responses that impair daily function and occur within 3 months of a distressing event or events. The event(s) may have been traumatic or nontraumatic, and symptoms must resolve within 6 months after the event or cessation of the stressor(s). Because of the short duration of this diagnosis, PCPs diagnose and treat most cases of adjustment disorder. Examples include breakup of a relationship, marital or business distress, natural disasters, or life changes such as school, an illness, marriage, divorce, retirement, or having a new baby or an ill parent.[26] Triggering stressors may be a single event, ongoing events, collective experiences, or continuous events. Adjustment disorder first appeared in DSM-III in 1980, and the 2013 DSM-5 has evolved to take into account cultural factors and external context. Adjustment disorder is a common psychiatric diagnosis, but there has been

---

Box 3
Pearls for grief reaction

Grief is a normal response to loss of a person or a significant change in function, community, or social position

Self-worth is more often preserved in grief then in depression. Depressed patients are also more likely to have feelings of pervasive hopelessness, helplessness, guilt, lack of pleasure, and suicidal ideation

Grief is an entity distinct from depression. Clinical judgment must be used to distinguish between grief and major depression

PCPs, nurses, social workers, psychologists, and chaplains may be of assistance

Grief may manifest itself physically, emotionally, cognitively, behaviorally, and spiritually. There are defined phases of grief

People may grieve in very different ways. Different phases may occur in a different order in different individuals

Persistent complex bereavement disorder may be diagnosed if symptoms of grief cause significant distress and impairment of function for more than 12 months, and should be treated

It is normal for symptoms of grief to come in waves and peak near 6 months

---

limited research into its causes, treatments, and outcomes. The limited duration of the disorder and symptom overlap with subclinical depression may contribute to the lack of research on adjustment disorder. The spectrum of responses to a stressful life event ranges from normal adaptive reactions to adjustment disorder, and if persistent beyond 6 months a different diagnosis, such as MDD or posttraumatic stress disorder (PTSD), should be considered.

Risk Factors for Adjustment Disorder Depend on the Patient or the Stressor

Acute stress from a loss, event, or new medical diagnosis is the most common trigger. Limited coping skills may also result in a higher degree of distress. Patients with cancer or severe burns have high rates of adjustment disorder.[27,28] High-stress situations such as war can trigger adjustment disorder. The best studies on risk factors come from the military. Military recruits diagnosed with adjustment disorder had personality characteristics showing less skill in self-transcendence (the ability to see beyond oneself and be a part of an interconnected larger universe), self-directedness, and cooperativeness when compared with controls. Those who had adjustment disorder with depressed mood also had higher scores on harm avoidance.[29] During the Iraq War, adjustment disorder was the most common psychiatric reason for military personnel to be extracted from the theater of operations. Similar findings from prior studies showed that adjustment disorder was the most common psychiatric problem in the armed forces.[30,31] Other risks include alexithymia, the subclinical inability to identify and describe one's own emotions. Alexithymia can lead to less empathy, and this can predispose one to develop adjustment disorder.[32] Natural disasters may also trigger adjustment disorder.[33]

Diagnostic Tests

There is no validated screening tool solely for adjustment disorder in the general population. Clinical studies on adjustment disorder often use semistructured interview tools such as the Structured Clinical Interview for DSM disorders (SCID), which uses open-ended questions, takes 30 to 120 minutes to administer, and has a validated guide on interpretation. The SCID is rarely used in primary care, and the questions on adjustment disorder are at the end of the test, which does not lend itself to use in isolation.[34]

In patients with cancer, the One Question interview, Distress Thermometer, and Hospital Anxiety and Depression Score have similar sensitivity (0.8–0.92) and specificity (0.57–0.62) for diagnosing adjustment disorder and depression.[35,36]

Studies have not shown distinct identifiable risk factors or predictors that are able to separate adjustment disorder from a depressive episode, so the timing and duration of symptoms discriminate it from acute stress reaction and major depression.[37]

Fig. 2 shows an algorithmic approach to the diagnosis of adjustment disorder. Adjustment disorder can have subtypes, including with depressed mood, with anxiety, with mixed anxiety and depressed mood, with disturbance of conduct, with mixed disturbance of emotions and conduct, and unspecified.

Differential Diagnosis

Differential diagnoses may include a normal stress response, acute stress reaction that develops within 3 days of the stressor and resolves by 1 month, subclinical depression that does not fit the diagnostic criteria of major depression, persistent complex bereavement disorder, personality disorders, anxiety, and PTSD whereby effects persist at least 1 month after an event. Hypothyroidism should also be considered.

Many Other Disorders Can Co-Occur with Adjustment Disorder

Substance use disorder was the most common reported comorbid condition during hospitalizations for adjustment disorder. In one study, 76% of patients with

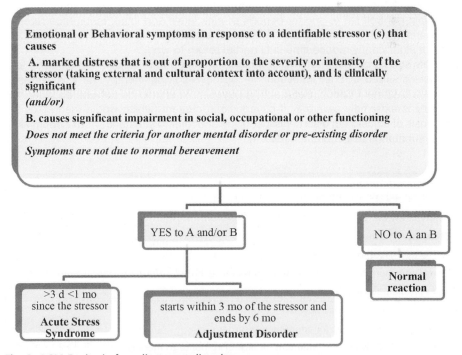

Fig. 2. DSM-5 criteria for adjustment disorder.

adjustment disorder had substance use disorder as either a primary or secondary diagnosis at the time of discharge.[38] Personality disorders, anxiety, and PTSD were also noted.

Incidence of suicidality is higher in major depression, but may occur in adjustment disorder, particularly if coupled with substance abuse. Therefore the assessment of suicide risk and comorbid diagnoses is important. The suicidality dissipates more rapidly in adjustment disorder than in major depression.[38]

Treatment

Primary care practitioners can and do manage most adjustment disorders. Psychotherapy is the best treatment choice at present. Brief problem-solving therapy that combines interpersonal therapy with solution-focused goals has helped patients with adjustment disorder. There are no reliable pharmacotherapy studies to suggest that treatment with medication is better than psychotherapy. However, because studies show similar regional brain changes in adjustment disorder and MDD, medications used in depression might be helpful in severe adjustment disorder.[39]

A 5-year follow-up study showed that 71% of patients diagnosed with adjustment disorder had no active psychiatric diagnosis, 13% had major depression with or without alcoholism, and 8% had antisocial personality disorder.[40]

Management

Evidence of moderate quality shows that problem-solving therapy significantly enhances partial return to work at 1-year follow-up compared with non–guideline-based care, but did not significantly enhance the time to full return to work at 1-year follow-up.[41] Treatment with a medication slowed the return to work. A randomized controlled trial on psychotherapy for those on sick leave for adjustment disorder showed that "activating intervention" (consisting of acquisition of coping skills and helping patients to regain control) led to shorter periods of sick leave and lower recurrence rates in comparison with a control group.[42] There was moderate-quality evidence that CBT did not significantly reduce time until partial return to work.

PCPs should consider referral of patients suffering from adjustment disorder to a counselor skilled in brief interventional problem-solving therapy, as it is currently the best treatment option. Referral to a psychiatrist should be considered when the severity is extremely severe or if psychosis is present (which would mean that the diagnosis of adjustment disorder is incorrect) and refer to substance abuse counseling when substance use is present (**Box 4**).

Box 4
Pearls for adjustment disorder

Amplified stress response that impairs daily function

Starts within 3 months of onset of stressor and resolves within 6 months of end of stressor

PCP often makes the diagnosis

Consider comorbid conditions (ie, substance abuse), but most have no other diagnoses

Brief problem-solving psychotherapy is the best treatment

Medication treatment may slow the return to work

No specific validated test for adjustment disorder

Refer for suicidality, severe symptoms, or lack of response to therapy

SUMMARY

SAD, grief reaction, and adjustment disorder are common conditions that PCPs can successfully diagnose and manage in the ambulatory setting. For SAD, light therapy is the best studied intervention, although antidepressants can also be used. Supportive care is indicated for most cases of grief reaction because it is considered a normal process. Referral for counseling or pharmacotherapy may be appropriate for patients with complex grief. Adjustment disorder is best treated with problem-solving psychotherapy, and symptoms should resolve within 6 months. If symptoms persist, another diagnosis and treatment plan should be considered.

REFERENCES

1. American Psychiatric Association. Diagnostic and statistical manual of mental disorders. 5th Edition. Arlington, VA: American Psychiatric Publishing; 2013.
2. Faedda GL, Tondo L, Teicher MH, et al. Seasonal mood disorders: patterns of seasonal recurrence in mania and depression. Arch Gen Psychiatry 1993;50(1):17.
3. Thompson C, Stinson D, Fernandez M, et al. A comparison of normal, bipolar and seasonal affective disorder subjects using the seasonal pattern assessment questionnaire. J Affect Disord 1988;14(3):257–64.
4. Mersch PP, Vastenburg NC, Meesters Y, et al. The reliability and validity of the seasonal pattern assessment questionnaire: a comparison between patient groups. J Affect Disord 2004;80(2–3):209–19.
5. Thompson C, Cowan A. The seasonal health questionnaire: a preliminary validation of a new instrument to screen for seasonal affective disorder. J Affect Disord 2001;64(1):89–98.
6. Thompson C, Thompson S, Smith R. Prevalence of seasonal affective disorder in primary care; a comparison of the seasonal health questionnaire and the seasonal pattern assessment questionnaire. J Affect Disord 2004;78(3):219–26.
7. Miller AL. Epidemiology, etiology, and natural treatment of seasonal affective disorder. Altern Med Rev 2005;10(1):5–13.
8. Rosen LN, Targum SD, Terman M, et al. Prevalence of seasonal affective disorder at four latitudes. Psychiatry Res 1990;31(2):131–44.
9. Eastman CI, Young MA, Fogg LF, et al. Bright light treatment of winter depression: a placebo-controlled trial. Arch Gen Psychiatry 1998;55(10):883.
10. Golden RN, Gaynes BN, Ekstrom RD, et al. The efficacy of light therapy in the treatment of mood disorders: a review and meta-analysis of the evidence. Am J Psychiatry 2005;162(4):656–62.
11. Murray G, Michalak EE, Levitt AJ, et al. Therapeutic mechanism in seasonal affective disorder: do fluoxetine and light operate through advancing circadian phase? Chronobiol Int 2005;22(5):937–43.
12. Thaler K, Delivuk M, Chapman A, et al. Second-generation antidepressants for seasonal affective disorder. Cochrane Database Syst Rev 2011;(12):CD008591.
13. Modell JG, Rosenthal NE, Harriett AE, et al. Seasonal affective disorder and its prevention by anticipatory treatment with bupropion XL. Biol Psychiatry 2005; 58(8):658–67.
14. Lam R, Levitt A, Levitan R, et al. The can-SAD study: a randomized controlled trial of the effectiveness of light therapy and fluoxetine in patients with winter seasonal affective disorder. Am J Psychiatry 2006;163(5):805–12.
15. Rohan KJ, Roecklein KA, Tierney Lindsey K, et al. A randomized controlled trial of cognitive-behavioral therapy, light therapy, and their combination for seasonal affective disorder. J Consult Clin Psychol 2007;75(3):489.

16. Martinez B, Kasper S, Ruhrmann S, et al. Hypericum in the treatment of seasonal affective disorders. J Geriatr Psychiatry Neurol 1994;7(1):S29–33.

17. Wheatley D. Hypericum in seasonal affective disorder (SAD). Curr Med Res Opin 1999;15(1):33–7.

18. McGrath RE, Buckwald B, Resnick EV. The effect of L-tryptophan on seasonal affective disorder. J Clin Psychiatry 1990;51(4):162–3.

19. Lewy AJ, Bauer VK, Cutler NL, et al. Melatonin treatment of winter depression: a pilot study. Psychiatry Res 1998;77(1):57–61.

20. Gloth FM 3rd, Alam W, Hollis B. Vitamin D vs broad spectrum phototherapy in the treatment of seasonal affective disorder. J Nutr Health Aging 1999;3(1):5–7.

21. Hallenbeck J. Grief and bereavement. 2nd edition. Fast facts and concepts [Internet]. 2005. [cited January 7, 2014]. 32. January 7, 2014. Available at: http://www.eperc.mcw.edu/EPERC/FastFactsIndex/ff_032.htm.

22. Widera EW, Block SD. Managing grief and depression at the end of life. Am Fam Physician 2012;86(3):259–64.

23. Maciejewski PK, Zhang B, Block SD, et al. An empirical examination of the stage theory of grief. JAMA 2007;297(7):716–23.

24. Simon NM. Treating complicated grief. JAMA 2013;310(4):416–23.

25. Uher R, Payne JL, Pavlova B, et al. Major depressive disorder in DSM-5: Implications for clinical practice and research of changes from DSM-IV. Depress Anxiety 2014;31(6):459–71.

26. Strain JJ, Friedman MJ. Considering adjustment disorders as stress response syndromes for DSM-5. Depress Anxiety 2011;28(9):818–23.

27. de Vries M, Steifel F. Psycho-oncological interventions and psychotherapy in the oncological setting. In: Ute, Goerling, editors. Psycho-Oncology (Recent Results Cancer Research). Springer-Verlag Berlin Heidelberg. 2014. p. 121–35.

28. Vera I, Ferrando E, Vidal I, et al. Burns and mental disorder. Rev Psiquiatr Salud Ment 2010;3(1):19–22.

29. Na K, Oh S, Jung H, et al. Temperament and character of young male conscripts with adjustment disorder: a case-control study. J Nerv Ment Dis 2012;200(11):973–7.

30. Hansen-Schwartz J, Kijne B, Johnsen A, et al. The course of adjustment disorder in Danish male conscripts. Nord J Psychiatry 2005;59(3):193–7.

31. Rundell JR. Demographics of and diagnoses in Operation Enduring Freedom and Operation Iraqi Freedom personnel who were psychiatrically evacuated from the theater of operations. Gen Hosp Psychiatry 2006;28(4):352–6.

32. Chen P, Chen C, Chen C. Alexithymia as a screening index for male conscripts with adjustment disorder. Psychiatr Q 2011;82(2):139–50.

33. North CS, Pfefferbaum B. Mental health response to community disasters: a systematic review. JAMA 2013;310(5):507–18.

34. First MB, Spitzer RL, Gibbon M, et al. Structured Clinical Interview for the DSM-IV Axis I Disorders, (SCID-I), Clinician Version. Administration Booklet. Washington, DC: American Psychiatric Press, Inc; 2012.

35. Akizuki N, Akechi T, Nakanishi T, et al. Development of a brief screening interview for adjustment disorders and major depression in patients with cancer. Cancer 2003;97(10):2605–13.

36. Adjustment to cancer: Anxiety and distress (PDQ) - National Cancer Institute [Internet]. [cited January 3, 2014]. Available at: http://www.cancer.gov/cancer topics/pdq/supportivecare/adjustment/HealthProfessional/page4.   Accessed January 3, 2014.

37. Casey P, Maracy M, Kelly BD, et al. Can adjustment disorder and depressive episode be distinguished? Results from ODIN. J Affect Disord 2006;92(2):291–7.

38. Greenberg WM, Rosenfeld DN, Ortega EA. Adjustment disorder as an admission diagnosis. Am J Psychiatry 1995;152(3):459–61.
39. Kumano H, Ida I, Oshima A, et al. Brain metabolic changes associated with predisposition to onset of major depressive disorder and adjustment disorder in cancer patients–a preliminary PET study. J Psychiatr Res 2007;41(7):591–9.
40. Andreasen NC, Hoenck P. The predictive value of adjustment disorders: a follow-up. Alcohol Treat Quart 1982;9(17):6.
41. Arends I, Bruinvels DJ, Rebergen DS, et al. Interventions to facilitate return to work in adults with adjustment disorders. Cochrane Database Syst Rev 2012;(12):CD006389.
42. Van der Klink J, Blonk R, Schene A, et al. Reducing long term sickness absence by an activating intervention in adjustment disorders: a cluster randomised controlled design. Occup Environ Med 2003;60(6):429–37.

Approach to the Patient with Multiple Somatic Symptoms

Carmen Croicu, MD[a],*, Lydia Chwastiak, MD, MPH[a],
Wayne Katon, MD[b]

KEYWORDS

- Somatic symptoms • Somatization • Depression • Anxiety • Collaborative care

KEY POINTS

- Patients with multiple and persistent physical symptoms are common in primary care.
- Collaboration with the patient is critical for effective management. Patients should be actively involved in setting treatment goals and deciding among therapeutic options.
- Screening and treatment of depression and anxiety disorders is a key component of management. Patients should be educated about how psychosocial stressors and somatic symptoms interact.
- Somatization can occur among patients with chronic medical conditions, such as cardiovascular disease or chronic obstructive pulmonary disease. Providers should avoid setting up a dichotomy between mental health and physical causation of symptoms.
- Twenty percent to 25% of patients with multiple somatic symptoms develop a chronic course of illness. Management should focus on improving functional status and avoiding unnecessary or invasive diagnostic tests and use of potentially addictive medications that increase the risk of iatrogenic complications.
- Patients with persistent somatic symptoms should have regular follow-up. Somatic symptom burden can be followed with a validated instrument, such as the 8-item Somatic Symptoms Scale.

INTRODUCTION

Patients with multiple somatic symptoms are common in primary care settings, in which more than half of all visits are for somatic complaints.[1] For some of the most common symptoms in primary care, such as chest pain, fatigue, dizziness, headache,

Disclosures: None of the other authors has conflicts of interest to report.
[a] Department of Psychiatry and Behavioral Sciences, University of Washington School of Medicine, Box 359911, 325 Ninth Avenue, Seattle, WA 98104, USA; [b] Division of Health Services and Psychiatric Epidemiology, Department of Psychiatry and Behavioral Sciences, University of Washington School of Medicine, Box 356560, 1959 Northeast Pacific, Seattle, WA 98195, USA
* Corresponding author.
E-mail address: croicu@u.washington.edu

and dyspnea, a medical diagnosis is not found in up to half of cases.[2] Patients with chronic and severe somatic symptoms have high levels of role impairment and spend more days in bed per month than patients with several major medical disorders.[3,4] Patients with multiple and persistent somatic symptoms are also at risk for extensive investigations and referrals to specialists. Several studies have shown a strong relationship between somatization and excess health care costs resulting from high numbers of health care visits, repeated diagnostic testing, and costly treatments.[5]

Many patients with multiple somatic symptoms receive unnecessary and invasive somatic investigations, whereas psychological factors are insufficiently explored.[6] In primary care settings, more than 70% of patients with major depression present with predominantly physical complaints rather than affective symptoms of depression.[7,8] Kirmayer and Robbins[5] found that most (73%) primary care patients with depressive or anxiety disorders presented exclusively with somatic symptoms. Compared with patients without psychiatric illness, those with anxiety and depressive disorders tend to have more somatic symptoms without identified disease and are more likely to be high users of health care resources.[3,9–12]

There is also a strong correlation between the number of somatic symptoms and the likelihood of a depression or anxiety diagnosis.[13] The higher number of somatic complaints in patients with comorbid depression or anxiety and chronic medical illness (compared with those with medical illness alone) might explain the increased diagnostic testing and higher medical costs that these patients incur.[13] In addition to depression and anxiety, other risk factors for a chronic high number of somatic symptoms include childhood psychological abuse, education, being unmarried or widowed, and severity of medical illness.[14]

The category of somatoform disorders has been highly controversial since its introduction in the *Diagnostic and Statistical Manual of Mental Disorders, Third Edition* (DSM-III) 30 years ago. These disorders, such as somatization disorder and hypochondriasis, were difficult to diagnosis, and the diagnoses were not useful to primary care physicians and rarely used clinically. In DSM-IV, a key feature of somatoform disorders was the concept of medically unexplained symptoms. This concept was not well accepted by patients, and also ignored the fact that many cases of somatization occur in patients with comorbid psychiatric disorders and medical disorders. The comorbid psychiatric disorders often lead to amplification of medical symptoms in these patients.[15]

One of the most substantive changes in DSM-5 involves the replacement of several somatoform disorders, including somatization disorder, pain disorder and hypochondriasis, with somatic symptom disorder (SSD) (**Fig. 1**).

SSD is a category of disorders characterized by somatic symptoms that either are distressing or result in significant disruption of functioning, as well as excessive and disproportionate thoughts, feelings, and behaviors regarding those symptoms.[16] To be diagnosed with SSD, the individual must be persistently symptomatic for at least 6 months. Moreover, the DSM-IV requirement that these somatic symptoms be medically unexplained has been eliminated, so individuals who meet criteria for SSD may or may not have a medically diagnosed condition. Rather, the diagnosis of SSD is based on the reporting of bothersome and persistent somatic symptoms accompanied by excessive psychological responses (**Box 1**). Hypochondriasis has also been eliminated as a disorder. Most patients with hypochondriasis now receive a DSM-5 diagnosis of SSD. Those with high health anxiety and minimal to no somatic symptoms are diagnosed with illness anxiety disorder (**Box 2**).

Primary care providers have a crucial role in the recognition and adequate treatment of patients with multiple somatic complaints. These patients can elicit powerful

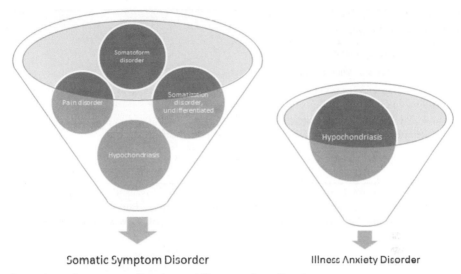

Fig. 1. Somatic symptom disorder and illness anxiety disorder.

emotional reactions in physicians,[17,18] which may result in less than optimal clinical care. Physicians often feel frustrated by patients' frequent complaints and dissatisfaction with treatment.[19] Although physicians may think that their competence is challenged by their inability to find a medical cause for the symptoms, the patients may think that they are discredited and accused of fabricating their symptoms.

One of the biggest challenges in the primary care settings is to simultaneously address potential medical causes for physical symptoms while considering an associated mental health diagnosis. A major aim of this article is to enhance recognition of somatization and to describe treatment and management options that can lead to improvement in patient care.

SPECTRUM OF SEVERITY OF SOMATIC SYMPTOMS: A BIOPSYCHOSOCIAL APPROACH TO DIAGNOSIS AND MANAGEMENT

The 3 common types of somatization seen in primary care and management approaches to patients with these varying types of somatization are described in **Box 3**.

1. In primary care settings, it is common for patients to present with somatic symptoms related to temporary stressors. For example, symptoms such as headache or back pain could be triggered or amplified in the context of a job loss, divorce,

---

Box 1
Somatic symptom disorder

- One or more somatic symptoms associated with distress and impairment

- Excessive thoughts, feelings, and behaviors in response to somatic symptoms

- Somatic symptom does not have to always be present but must be persistent (at least 6 months)

Adapted from American Psychiatric Association. Diagnostic and statistical manual of mental disorders. 5th edition. American Psychiatric Association; 2013. p. 309–27.

Box 2
Illness anxiety disorder

- Persistent preoccupation with having a serious illness (at least 6 months)
- Very high levels of health anxiety
- Complete absence of somatic symptoms, or if any somatic symptoms are present, they are very mild
- Excessive health-related behaviors (eg, constantly checking for signs of illness) or maladaptive avoidance (eg, avoids a visit to the doctor's office)

Adapted from American Psychiatric Association. Diagnostic and statistical manual of mental disorders. 5th edition. American Psychiatric Association; 2013. p. 309–27.

---

or interpersonal difficulties. Resolution of these acute somatic symptoms requires minimal treatment or occurs after stressors resolve, and there are typically no long-term adverse consequences and minimal functional impairment. According to Kroenke and Jackson,[20] in patients presenting to a general medicine clinic with physical symptoms, 70% of patients reported improvement within 2 weeks. The few patients who fail to improve often have even more severe symptoms at 3 months, and in 1 study[20] were twice as likely to be fearful about the prospect of an undiagnosed severe medical illness.

2. Although most patients with stress-related somatic symptoms improve within several weeks of seeing a health care provider, approximately 20% to 25% of patients suffer from chronic or recurrent symptoms that are often present at 5-year follow-up.[21–23] Patients with a longer duration of symptoms are likely to fall into the other 2 common types of somatization: relapsing/remitting episodes of somatization associated with acute or recurrent anxiety and depressive episodes or chronic somatization, which is largely covered by the DSM-5 term somatic symptom disorder. The relapsing/remitting form of somatization is characterized by episodes of somatic symptoms associated with repetitive psychosocial stressors (eg, marital conflicts, job difficulties), anxiety and depression episodes, and substantial impairment in daily functioning (**Box 4**).

Early accurate diagnosis is important to prevent progressive negative consequences such as job loss, marital problems, and financial problems. Delays in diagnosis and intervention for this condition can lead to worsening affective and anxiety symptoms and high medical costs as a result of multiple specialist visits and medical testing. The case outlined in **Box 5** shows some of the key features of relapsing/remitting somatization associated with an anxiety disorder.

Box 3
Subtypes of somatization

1. Acute somatization
   - Temporary production of physical symptoms associated with transient stressors
2. Relapsing somatization
   - Repeated episodes of physical symptoms associated with repetitive stressors and anxiety or depressive episodes
3. Chronic somatization
   - Nearly continuous somatic focus, perception of ill health, development of disability

---

Box 4		
A comparison between relapse/remitting and chronic somatization		
	Acute	Chronic
	Anxiety/Depression	Anxiety/Depression
	Somatization	Somatization
Childhood history	Normal	Neglect, abuse
		Multiple losses
Job history	Stable	Poor to unstable
Intimate relationships	Stable, long-term	Unstable, abusive
		Multiple partners

3. The chronic subtype of somatization is often characterized by a history of multiple and persistent somatic symptoms associated with a high level of functional impairment. When diagnostic evaluations fail to fully show the cause for their suffering, these patients often seek additional diagnostic assessment and studies or self-medicate with alcohol, illicit drugs, or chronic opioid pain medications. Extensive diagnostic testing and medical/surgical procedures may also increase the risk of iatrogenic injury, further increasing the costs associated with chronic and persistent somatic symptoms.

Several risk factors have been associated with chronic and severe somatic symptoms, including childhood neglect or sexual abuse, chaotic lifestyle, a history of alcohol and substance use, poor work history, and tumultuous relationships. In addition to higher rates of comorbid chronic medical illness and psychiatric disorders, chronic and severe somatization has also been associated with the presence of axis II disorders. According to Rost and colleagues,[24] avoidant, paranoid, self-defeating, and obsessive-compulsive are the most common personality disorders identified. Among personality traits, high levels of neuroticism and harm avoidance are associated with a higher number of somatic symptoms as well with axis II personality disorders.[25,26]

The case described in **Box 6** shows some of the key features of chronic somatization.

Complex biological, psychological, and environmental factors play a significant role in patients with multiple somatic symptoms. The identification of factors that contribute to the initiation, maintenance, or exacerbation of symptoms can help the physician understand the patient as a person and enhance the therapeutic alliance

Box 5
Key features of relapsing/remitting somatization associated with an anxiety disorder
Mrs S, a 35-year-old woman, married with 2 children, presented with an 8-week history of muscle tension, intermittent heart palpitations, and dizziness. Over the previous 2 weeks, Mrs S had presented twice to the emergency room with chest pain, palpitations, sweating, and shortness of breath. Workup over the last 2 months, including routine blood chemistries, blood cell count, calcium concentration, thyroid-stimulating hormone, electrocardiography, treadmill, and Holter monitor, had shown no signs of cardiovascular abnormalities. In the last week, she had had to leave work twice when the anxiety became intolerable. Physical examination showed a healthy, tense woman with normal vital signs. She took no medications and denied using alcohol or drugs. She reported that she had been under a lot of stress because of marital problems since her husband had lost his job 2 months previously.

> **Box 6**
> **Case showing some of the key features of chronic somatization**
>
> Ms T was a 42-year-old divorced woman with recurrent severe abdominal pain, fatigue, and disturbed sleep. After a viral respiratory infection, she presented with worsening fatigue and nausea. Her multiple physical complaints began after a litigious divorce when she began suffering from tension headaches and legs that became "weak" at times. In the last 2 months, she had gone to the emergency room (ER) 3 times for acute pain and was hospitalized once. Over the previous 2 years, she had undergone extensive investigations, including abdominal radiography, abdominal ultrasonography, esophagogastroduodenoscopy, and colonoscopy, all of which were normal. Past medical history showed negative exploratory laparotomy 1 year previously, multiple previous ER visits for migraines, and 2 back surgeries. She had a history of recurrent depressive symptoms, for which she had never been prescribed antidepressant medication or been referred for psychotherapy. She also had a history of domestic violence. She was on disability for chronic back pain. In the last year, she had received care from 3 different physicians. When you refused to prescribe opioids, she started yelling at you "You think that it is all in my head… you're fired."

with the patient. When health care providers use this approach, patients are not set up to perceive their problems as either physical or mental, and the pitfall of assuming that symptoms have only a psychological basis is avoided. A biopsychosocial approach is also consistent with the new DSM-5 diagnosis of SSD, a multidimensional descriptive system that underlines the patient's difficulties coping with distressing somatic symptoms and emphasizes the contribution of biological and psychosocial factors in the development of somatic symptoms.[27,28]

There is some evidence that genetic factors play a role in the development of somatic symptoms, and that SSD reflects complex relationships among genetic factors, somatic symptoms, anxiety, and depression.[29–31] The history of SSD can start in early life. A childhood history of chronic illness or abnormal illness behavior, or the presence of a family member with a chronic illness seems to predispose to somatization later in life.[32,33] Childhood adversity, such as neglect and sexual and physical abuse has been associated with a greater risk of both psychological and somatic problems as an adult. Several studies have suggested an association between childhood and adult trauma experiences and increased somatic symptom reporting in adults.[34–37]

The model proposed by Walker and colleagues (the P-P-P [predisposing, precipitating, perpetuating] model) is a valuable tool to understanding and guiding management of these challenging patients.[38] This 3-stage model includes biological, psychological, and social factors with a role in the initiation, maintenance, or exacerbation of symptoms (**Table 1**).

- Predisposing factors make individuals more vulnerable to disease. Examples of predisposing factors for SSD include chronic illness during childhood, childhood adversity, family of origin modeling of abnormal illness behavior, poor coping ability, comorbid medical illness, and psychiatric illness.

Table 1
Predisposing, precipitating, and perpetuating factors

Predisposing	Precipitating Factors	Perpetuating
Chronic childhood illnesses	Medical illness	Chronic stressors
Childhood adversities	Psychiatric disorder	Maladaptive coping skills
Comorbid medical illness	Social and occupational stress	Negative health habits
Lifetime psychiatric diagnosis	Changes in social support	Disability payments
Poor coping ability		

- Precipitating factors are stressors or elements of a patient's life that have a chronologic relationship with the onset of the symptoms or precipitate a crisis. They can include medical illness, psychiatric disorder, losses or changes in important relationships, change in employment or financial status, traumatic events for the individual or community, and changes in social support.
- Perpetuating factors that maintain the patient's current difficulties include medical illness, maladaptive coping strategies, lack of social support, social isolation, ongoing financial problems, opiate medication dependence, and legal issues related to the symptoms. Katon and colleagues[8] have labeled psychosocial factors that perpetuate illness "illness maintenance systems."

PSYCHIATRIC DISORDERS AMONG PATIENTS WITH SOMATIC SYMPTOMS

Up to 20% of patients presenting for a primary care visit report significant depressive symptoms, and 5% to 10% meet diagnostic criteria for major depression.[39] Depression is characterized by changes in mood accompanied by somatic and cognitive changes.[16] When patients with depression seek care from their health care provider, their chief complaint is often somatic rather than emotional.[40] In an international multicenter study of more than 1000 patients,[7] 69% of patients with depression reported only somatic symptoms as the reason for their visit. In addition to fatigue and sleep disturbances, nonspecific musculoskeletal complaints and gastrointestinal problems can be the presenting symptoms of depression. Depressed patients with general aches and pains make 20% more visits to their health care provider each year than those without such aches and pains.[7] The presence of multiple pain symptoms (eg, back pain, headache, abdominal pain) increases the risk for comorbid depression by at least 2 fold.[41,42]

Primary care providers do not recognize depression in about 50% of depressed patients.[43] In particular, a diagnosis of depression can be missed when the physician is focused on finding a cause for the physical symptoms and the patient is not asked questions that could show psychiatric comorbidity. Despite high rates of depression in primary care, making an accurate diagnosis is complicated by several factors. Stigma regarding mental illness and mental health treatment can make patients reticent about expressing feelings of sadness and more comfortable reporting somatic symptoms. In addition, a somatic presentation of depression is more common in patients who do not have an ongoing relationship with the physician.[7] Without a trusting relationship, self-disclosure of psychological complaints is less likely. Another barrier to an accurate diagnosis is that depression, anxiety, and medical conditions often coexist, complicating the clinical picture. A cross-sectional survey of the associations among depression, anxiety, and multiple somatic symptoms in 15 primary care centers found considerable overlap.

75% of depressed patients had comorbid anxiety, somatization or both; 57% of the patients with anxiety had comorbid depression, somatization; or both and 54% of the patients with somatization had comorbid depression, anxiety or both.[44]

Among primary care patients with chronic medical conditions, depression has been associated with decreased self-care, poor adherence to medical treatment, and also amplification of somatic symptoms.[45] In a review of 31 studies involving 16,922 patients, Katon and colleagues[13] evaluated the impact of depression and anxiety on somatic symptom reporting in patients with chronic medical conditions, such as diabetes, pulmonary disease, heart disease, and arthritis. In patients with chronic medical illness, those with comorbid depression or anxiety reported more medical symptoms, even after controlling for the severity of the medical disorder. Other studies[46] have suggested that among patients with diabetes, the severity of diabetic symptoms is more strongly associated with depressed mood than with glycosylated hemoglobin levels or number of diabetes complications.

Anxiety disorders are the most common mental disorders in the general population and occur at least as commonly among primary care patients as depression. As many as one-third of primary care patients have significant anxiety symptoms; and anxiety disorders can be as disabling as depression.[47] Moreover, depression and anxiety co-occur up to 50% of the time.[48] Anxiety disorders can be difficult to diagnose, because anxiety can be a symptom of another psychiatric disorder, an expression of the patient's response to a medical illness, a medication side effect or secondary to a general medical condition, withdrawal from alcohol, or a symptom of drug use.[49] For example, patients with generalized anxiety disorder (GAD), one of the most common mental disorders in primary care, typically present with nonspecific somatic symptoms, such as headaches, muscle aches, fatigue, and gastrointestinal symptoms. A myriad of somatic symptoms are also present in patients with panic attacks (eg, palpitations, chest pain, dizziness, and diaphoresis). Anxiety disorders can confuse the clinical picture, and multiple anxiety disorders can occur in the same patient (panic disorder and posttraumatic stress disorder [PTSD]). Sometimes, the physical manifestations of anxiety can lead to multiple diagnostic procedures, including invasive procedures, and iatrogenic complications.

Psychiatric comorbidity in patients presenting with somatic complaints should be suspected in the following scenarios:

- The number of physical symptoms is a powerful predictor of psychiatric comorbidity, because the likelihood of coexisting depression or anxiety increases with the number of physical symptoms.[12]
- The risk for coexisting depression is doubled when patients present with 2 or more pain symptoms.[50]
- When somatic symptoms remain unexplained after a thorough medical workup, there is an increased probability of a psychiatric comorbidity.[21,51]
- Frequent clinic visits and high use of health care services is a predictor of psychological distress.[37]

Several investigators have identified important clinical factors that predict depression and anxiety disorders in primary care patients presenting with physical complaints.[3,4,52] In a study of 500 patients presenting to a general medicine walk-in clinic with physical symptoms as the main complaint,[3] 4 clinical predictors significantly increased the possibility of a depressive or anxiety disorder: recent stress, total number of somatic symptoms (with or without explained cause), poor self-reported health status, and symptom severity. A follow-up study[52] supported these findings, suggesting that the strongest predictors of an underlying mental disorder were recent stress, 5 or more physical symptoms, or poor health.

The S4 model (symptom count, stress, severity, and self-rated health) proposed by Jackson and Kroenke may help the physician recognize the need for exploration of psychological symptoms by acting as an excellent tool for identification of patients who might be at risk for an underlying mental health disorders. The model can also improve patient care by helping a busy family practitioner to target those high-risk patients and come to an accurate diagnosis.

Items in the S4 model include:

1. Stress recently (last week) (yes/no)
2. Symptom count (checklist of 15 common somatic symptoms); scored as positive if more than 5 symptoms

3. Self-rated overall health poor or fair on a 5-point scale (excellent, very good, good, fair, poor); scored as positive for fair or poor responses
4. Self-rated severity of symptoms from 0 (none at all) to 10 (unbearable) scale; scored as positive for responses greater than 5

The presence of any of these 4 predictors seems to increase the likelihood of an underlying depressive or anxiety disorder at least 2-fold to 3-fold.

MANAGEMENT RECOMMENDATIONS

Our approach to management of patients with somatic symptoms is based on the effective methods supported by published evidence and also on our experience working with primary care providers. First, an overview is presented of general strategies, and then, specific recommendations tailored to the severity of the patient's symptoms and comorbidities are made.

General Principles of Management

Engagement and building a sound therapeutic alliance with the patient

In the management of the patient presenting with somatic complaints, empathy is essential for the development of a strong therapeutic relationship with the patient.[53] This alliance is strengthened when the physician listens carefully, encourages the patient to describe their symptoms, and explores the meaning of each symptom for the patient.[54] The patient not only feels understood but also feels reassured that their concerns are taken seriously. As described by Coulehan and colleagues,[55] building empathy entails asking patients to tell you more about their problem (such as "What has this been like for you?," "How has all of this made you feel?"), clarifying (such as "Let me see if I've gotten this right..."), and communicating your understanding to the patient ("I can imagine that must be...").

Biopsychosocial history and physical examination

In the first phase of clinical assessment, a detailed history and physical examination are powerful tools to enhance engagement, to rule out serious or treatable medical conditions, and to guide test selection and treatment. However, when doctors focus primarily on physical symptom relief, they can miss clues about the reason for the visit and miss the opportunity to explore the patient's perspective of the symptoms and associated psychosocial stressors.[56,57] The BATHE technique is an excellent tool for engaging a patient while simultaneously assessing psychosocial factors. This technique consists of asking 4 specific questions: the patient's background, affect (the feeling state), the most troubling problem, and how the patient is handling the situation (**Box 7**). The questions are followed by an empathic response.[58]

It is also important to elicit the patient's exploratory model of their illness.[53] This process includes what the patient thinks might be causing the symptoms, how the illness

---

Box 7
The BATHE technique

B: Background: "What is going on in your life?" and "What brings you in today?"

A: Affect: "How do you feel about that?"

T: Trouble: "What bothers you the most about this situation?"

H: Handling: "How are you handling that?"

E: Empathy: "That must be very difficult for you"

or symptoms have affected their lives and their family, what their expectations are for investigations, and what they expect from treatment.[59]

Diagnostic evaluation to rule out medical illness

Diagnostic tests are selected based on the history and physical examination. However useful diagnostic tests are, they seldom have 100% sensitivity and specificity in identifying the cause of a disease, and uncertainty often remains, with negative results. As more tests are performed, finding a chance abnormality is always a possibility, and the doctor's fear of angering the patient or missing a serious condition can trigger unnecessary extensive investigations.

Although care must be taken to provide appropriate investigation for signs or symptoms, a recent meta-analysis[60] suggested that physicians overestimate the value of diagnostic testing on reassurance. Moreover, in this meta-analysis, tests for symptoms with a low risk of serious illness had no impact on decreasing illness anxiety. Although it is important to provide reassurance that a serious illness is unlikely, explaining the results and acknowledging the patient's frustration at not finding a specific cause for their symptoms may be more important. When doctors reassure patients without providing a clear explanation for symptoms, these symptoms may even be exacerbated.[61]

Educate patients how psychosocial stressors and symptoms interact

Instead of performing an exhaustive search for a mysterious illness, it may be helpful to gradually move from investigating somatic symptoms to exploring social or psychological distress, which may amplify or prolong the symptoms. However, premature inquiry about depression or anxiety can trigger negative reactions in some patients and may damage rapport. In patients with a higher risk based on your objective elements, including psychiatric disorders in the primary differential diagnosis often makes for an easier transition to a more detailed discussion when a reasonable workup is negative. A useful strategy is to explain how stress and symptoms interact and how physical illness and emotional problems often co-occur. Addressing the connection between how the brain and body interact can help restore hope in an individual who is suffering and feels powerless to control them.

Specific Management Strategies

For patients with recurrent somatic symptoms in whom acute anxiety and depression are the likely cause or a major contributor to the somatic presentation, screening for psychiatric comorbidity is recommended.

Screening for depression and anxiety

Considering the well-documented overlap of depression, anxiety, and somatic symptoms (SAD triad), one of the most important steps in the evaluation of patients with SSD is screening for psychiatric disorders, especially depression and anxiety. The Patient Health Questionnaire-9 (PHQ-9) can be used as a diagnostic tool for major depressive disorder, to monitor response to treatment, or to guide treatment.[62] The 7-item GAD scale (GAD-7) is a reliable, valid, and easy-to-use self-report questionnaire for evaluating the presence and severity of 1 of 4 anxiety disorders: panic, generalized anxiety, social phobia, and PTSD. Once a patient scores 10 or more on the GAD-7, follow-up questions are needed to diagnose which of these specific disorders are present.

Evaluate somatic symptom burden

The 8-item Somatic Symptoms Scale (SSS-8), an abbreviated version of the PHQ-9, was recently developed as a brief, patient-reported measure of the severity of somatic symptoms. The SSS-8 may facilitate the diagnosis of SSD and may be helpful to monitor somatic symptom burden and guide treatment.[63]

Treatment of comorbid psychiatric disorders

A comprehensive discussion of effective treatment of depression and anxiety is beyond the scope of this article. However, it is important for physicians treating patients with SSD to be aware that both medication and cognitive-behavioral therapy (CBT) have proven effectiveness in treating depression and many anxiety disorders.[64] Therefore, when a depressive or anxiety disorder is diagnosed, the physician should consider both psychopharmacologic treatment and psychotherapy as treatment options.

There is increasing evidence that both antidepressant and CBT are valuable treatment modalities for patients who present with multiple somatic complaints, whether the symptom has a medical explanation or not.[65–67] Antidepressants may be helpful in relieving chronic pain symptoms, independent of the presence of a comorbid psychiatric disease.[65] The serotonin-norepinephrine reuptake inhibitors, such as venlafaxine and duloxetine, have been found mostly effective in treating neuropathic pain.[68] There is increasing evidence that dual-acting antidepressants that modulate both norepinephrine and serotonin receptors may ameliorate other somatic symptoms as well.[69–71] It is important to optimize the management of pain that commonly co-occurs with depression, because this can improve treatment outcomes and quality of life.[72] Some studies have shown that although the burden of physical symptoms diminishes significantly in the first month of selective serotonin reuptake inhibitor (SSRI) treatment, patients with moderately severe pain at the start of treatment are 2-fold less likely to respond to antidepressant treatment.[73,74] Given the negative consequences associated with opioid therapy, physicians should avoid prescribing opioid analgesics. Some of the problems related to opioid therapy include frequent visits to the emergency room for opioid prescriptions, misuse to self-medicate, and development of tolerance and addiction.

CBT has the strongest and most consistent evidence for its efficacy among different psychotherapeutic modalities.[66,75] In a review of 13 randomized controlled trials (RCTs) of treatment modalities for somatoform disorders, Kroenke showed that CBT was effective in most studies (supported by 11 of 13 RCTs).[75] A recent meta-analysis including 10 randomized and 6 nonrandomized trials suggested that psychotherapy for more severe forms of somatoform disorder that were treated in secondary and tertiary care was more effective than usual treatment with respect to reduction of physical symptoms and functional impairment (eg, life satisfaction, interpersonal problems, maladaptive cognitions and behavior).[76] One of the cases described earlier shows this clinical approach.

In treating patients with chronic somatic symptoms, the main goal is not to cure the disease but to improve function and help the patient cope more effectively with symptoms. It is also important to convey that the primary care provider will continue to collaborate with the patient to alleviate suffering and distress from their symptoms (**Box 8**).

The second clinical vignette shows some of these familiar problems encountered by primary care providers (**Box 9**).

In addition to the guidelines discussed earlier, the following strategies are recommended[77–80]:

- Schedule time-limited regular appointments (eg, every 4–6 weeks) rather than erratic appointments to address complaints

---

Box 8
Treatment: essential concepts and goals

- Collaborate with patient to help reduce distress from symptoms
- Explain that although there may not be a reason for their symptoms, you will work together to improve their functioning as much as possible
- Educate patients how psychosocial stressors and symptoms interact
- Avoid comments like "Your symptoms are all psychological" or "There is nothing wrong with you medically"
- Avoid the temptation to order unnecessary, repetitive, or invasive investigations
- Educate the patient on how to cope with their symptoms instead of focusing on a cure
- Involve and collaborate with the patient in setting treatment goals.

- Perform a brief physical examination at each visit to address new symptoms or health concerns
- Avoid unnecessary diagnostic tests unless objective evidence of a disease is present
- Treat comorbid psychiatric disorders and alcohol and substance abuse problems
- Minimize polypharmacy, tapering and discontinuing medications with high potential for abuse (eg, narcotic agents, sedatives)
- Prescribe regular dosing of pain medications and avoid as needed analgesics (especially opiates)
- Encourage mobility to prevent physical deconditioning (eg, physical therapy, regular exercise)

Psychiatric consultation and the role of collaborative care model

Referral to a psychiatrist consultant can be perceived as abandonment by the patient or invalidation of their symptoms. Patients are more likely to accept a referral when the provider underscores how the consultation will help both the patient and the doctor to find other ways to alleviate suffering and improve coping with illness. A follow-up visit with the primary care physician after the psychiatric consultation is recommended to discuss recommendations for further treatment. Patients with more severe somatization, or those who have not responded to trials of 1 or 2 medications, who require combination therapy, or who have had intolerable side effects, may benefit from a psychiatric referral.

Box 9
Familiar problems encountered by primary care providers

Mrs S had symptoms typical of panic disorder. The initial evaluation of a patient presenting with somatic symptoms and anxiety should include a history and physical examination, an evaluation of the potential role of medications and substances, and screening diagnostic tests (eg, routine blood chemistries, thyroid-stimulating hormone [TSH] level, electrocardiogram). TSH level is recommended for patients with new-onset anxiety disorders. Because patients with panic disorder often present with somatic complaints, and most are fearful of having a serious condition, such as a heart attack, an important step after the clinical diagnosis is made is to discuss with the patient their fears of medical illness and expectations of medical testing and treatment. Mrs T felt relieved when you reassured her that with appropriate treatment her symptoms could be controlled. You discussed that both CBT and antidepressant medication have been shown in controlled trials to be equally effective.[81] The patient agreed to a trial of an SSRI and her anxiety symptoms improved when she returned 2 weeks later.

Patients are more likely to accept mental health treatment when it is provided as part of primary care treatment. There is an increasing body of research on how to integrate mental health treatment into primary care as a collaborative care model of treatment, in which mental health professionals work together with providers in the primary care setting. A meta-analysis of 79 randomized trials of collaborative care depression and anxiety interventions in primary care[81] found that depression and anxiety outcomes were improved for up to 2 years compared with usual care approaches. Integration of mental health treatment into primary care may improve the care of patients with somatic symptoms and increase physician satisfaction.

SUMMARY

In primary care settings, patients frequently present with multiple somatic complaints, which can be associated with significant distress and functional impairment. When these somatic complaints are related to acute psychosocial stressors, the somatic symptoms resolve relatively rapidly in most cases, usually without any specific treatment. However, in 20% to 25% of cases, these symptoms can recur or become chronic and can be associated with high use of medical services and increased risk of iatrogenic complications. Risk factors for chronic multiple somatic symptoms include childhood abuse and neglect, childhood illness, and co occurring psychiatric illness.

These conditions can be effectively managed in primary care, and primary care providers should use a biopsychosocial approach. Collaboration and education are key at every point in management, and patients should be actively involved in setting treatment goals. Patients should also be screened with brief validated instruments for current depression or anxiety disorders, because these frequently occur in patients with multiple somatic complaints. It is critical for primary care providers to remember that somatization can also occur among patients with chronic medical conditions. Distinctions between physical and mental phenomena can make patients feel the need to choose one or the other explanation, and often interfere with the therapeutic alliance. It is more helpful to educate patients about how psychosocial stressors and somatic symptoms interact. Education and regular scheduled visits are central to the management of these patients. Evidence based treatments should be provided for depression or any anxiety disorder that is identified. There is also increasing evidence that these treatments (antidepressant medications, CBT, exercise, and collaborative care) are also effective for improving functioning and decreasing somatic symptom burden.

REFERENCES

1. Kroenke K, Mangelsdorff AD. Common symptoms in ambulatory care: incidence, evaluation, therapy, and outcome. Am J Med 1989;2:262–6.
2. Khan A, Harezlak J, Tu W, et al. Somatic symptoms in primary care: etiology and outcome. Psychosomatics 2003;44(6):471–8.
3. Kroenke K, Jackson JL, Chamberlin J. Depressive and anxiety disorders in patients presenting with physical complaints: clinical predictors and outcome. Am J Med 1997;103(5):339–47.
4. Jackson JL, O'Malley PG, Kroenke K. Clinical predictors of mental disorders among medical outpatients. Validation of the "S4" model. Psychosomatics 1998;39(5):431–6.
5. Kirmayer LJ, Robbins JM. Three forms of somatization in primary care: prevalence, co-occurrence, and socio-demographic characteristics. J Nerv Ment Dis 1991;179:647–55.

6. Smith RC, Lein C, Collins C, et al. Treating patients with medically unexplained symptoms. J Gen Intern Med 2003;18:478–89.

7. Simon G, Von Korff M, Piccinelli M, et al. An international study of the relation between somatic symptoms and depression. N Engl J Med 1999;341:1329–35.

8. Katon W, Kleinman A, Rosen G. Depression and somatization: a review. Part I. Am J Med 1982;72(2):241–7.

9. McLaughlin TP, Khandker RK, Kruzikas DT, et al. Overlap of anxiety and depression in a managed care population: prevalence and association with resource utilization. J Clin Psychiatry 2006;67:1187–93.

10. Simon GE, Von Korff M. Somatization and psychiatric disorder in the NIMH Epidemiologic Catchment Area study. Am J Psychiatry 1991;148:1494–500.

11. Katon W, Lin E, Von KM, et al. Somatization: a spectrum of severity. Am J Psychiatry 1991;148:34–40.

12. Kroenke K, Spitzer RL, Williams JB, et al. Physical symptoms in primary care: predictors of psychiatric disorders and functional impairment. Arch Fam Med 1994;3:774–9.

13. Katon W, Lin EH, Kroenke K, et al. The association of depression and anxiety with medical symptom burden in patients with chronic medical illness. Gen Hosp Psychiatry 2007;29(2):147–55.

14. Creed FH, Davies I, Jackson J, et al. The epidemiology of multiple somatic symptoms. J Psychosom Res 2012;72(4):311–7.

15. Dimsdale JE, Levenson J. Diagnosis of somatic symptom disorder requires clinical judgment. J Psychosom Res 2013;75(6):588.

16. American Psychiatric Association. Diagnostic and statistical manual of mental disorders. 5th edition. American Psychiatric Association; 2013.

17. Abbey SE, Wulsin L, Levenson JL. Somatization and somatoform disorders. In: Levenson JL, editor. Textbook of psychosomatic medicine. 2nd edition. American Psychiatric Publishing; 2011. p. 261–89.

18. Sharpe M, Mayou R, Seagroatt V, et al. Why do doctors find some patients difficult to help? Q J Med 1994;87:187–93.

19. Hahn SR. Physical symptoms and physician-experienced difficulty in the physician-patient relationship. Ann Intern Med 2001;134:897–904.

20. Kroenke K, Jackson JL. Outcome in general medical patients presenting with common symptoms: a prospective study with a 2-week and 3-month follow-up. Fam Pract 1998;15:398–403.

21. Kroenke K. Patients presenting with somatic complaints: epidemiology, psychiatric comorbidity and management. Int J Methods Psychiatr Res 2003;12: 34–43.

22. Jackson JL, Passamonti M. The outcomes among patients presenting in primary care with a physical symptom at 5 years. J Gen Intern Med 2005;20:1032–7.

23. Smith RC, Dwamena FC. Classification and diagnosis of patients with medically unexplained symptoms. J Gen Intern Med 2007;22(5):685–91.

24. Rost KM, Akins RN, Brown FW, et al. The comorbidity of DSM-III-R personality disorders in somatization disorder. Gen Hosp Psychiatry 1992;13(5):322–6.

25. Trull TJ. DSM-III-R personality disorders and the five-factor model of personality: an empirical comparison. J Abnorm Psychol 1992;101:553–60.

26. Larsen RJ, Ketelaar T. Personality and susceptibility to positive and negative emotional states. J Pers Soc Psychol 1991;61:132–40.

27. Dimsdale J, Creed F. The proposed diagnosis of somatic symptom disorders in DSM-V to replace somatoform disorders in DSM-IV–a preliminary report. J Psychosom Res 2009;66(6):473–6.

28. Dimsdale JE, Creed F, Escobar J, et al. Somatic symptom disorder: an important change in DSM. J Psychosom Res 2013;75(3):223–8.
29. Kato K, Sullivan PF, Evengård B, et al. A population-based twin study of functional somatic syndromes. Psychol Med 2009;39(3):497–505.
30. Holliday KL, Macfarlane GJ, Nicholl BI, et al. Genetic variation in neuroendocrine genes associates with somatic symptoms in the general population: results from the EPIFUND study. J Psychosom Res 2010;68(5):469–74.
31. Kendler KS, Walters EE, Truett KR, et al. A twin-family study of self-report symptoms of panic-phobia and somatization. Behav Genet 1995;25:499–515.
32. Rief W, Broadbent E. Explaining medically unexplained symptoms–models and mechanisms. Clin Psychol Rev 2007;27(7):821–41.
33. Craig T, Boardman A, Mills K, et al. The South London Somatisation Study. I. Longitudinal course and the influence of early life experiences. Br J Psychiatry 1993;163:579–88.
34. Walker EA, Gelfand A, Katon WJ, et al. Adult health status of women with histories of childhood abuse and neglect. Am J Med 1999;107(4):332–9.
35. Paras ML, Murad MH, Chen LP, et al. Sexual abuse and lifetime diagnosis of somatic disorders: a systematic review and meta-analysis. JAMA 2009;302:550–61.
36. Walker E, Katon W, Harrop-Griffiths J, et al. Relationship of chronic pelvic pain to psychiatric diagnoses and childhood sexual abuse. Am J Psychiatry 1988;145:75–80.
37. Katon W, Sullivan M, Walker E. Medical symptoms without identified pathology: relationship to psychiatric disorders, childhood and adult trauma, and personality traits. Ann Intern Med 2001;134:017–26.
38. Walker EA, Unutzer J, Katon WJ. Understanding and caring for the distressed patient with multiple medically unexplained symptoms. J Am Board Fam Pract 1998;11:347–56.
39. Katon WJ, Schulberg H. Epidemiology of depression in primary care. Gen Hosp Psychiatry 1992;14:237–47.
40. Kirmayer LJ, Robbins JM, Dworkind M, et al. Somatization and the recognition of depression and anxiety in primary care. Am J Psychiatry 1993;13:734–41.
41. Von Korff M, Dworkin SF, Le Resche L, et al. An epidemiologic comparison of pain complaints. Pain 1988;32:173–83.
42. Bair MJ, Robinson RL, Katon W, et al. Exploring depression and pain comorbidity: a literature review. Arch Intern Med 2003;163(20):2433–45.
43. Simon GE, Von Korff M. Recognition, management, and outcomes of depression in primary care. Arch Fam Med 1995;4:99–105.
44. Löwe B, Spitzer RL, Williams JB, et al. Depression, anxiety and somatization in primary care: syndrome overlap and functional impairment. Gen Hosp Psychiatry 2008;30(3):191–9.
45. Katon WJ. The effect of major depression on chronic medical illness. Semin Clin Neuropsychiatry 1998;3:82–6.
46. Ciechanowski PS, Katon WJ, Russo JE, et al. The relationship of depressive symptoms to symptom reporting, self-care and glucose control in diabetes. Gen Hosp Psychiatry 2003;25(4):246–52.
47. Stein MB, Roy-Byrne PP, Craske MG, et al. Functional impact and health utility of anxiety disorders in primary care outpatients. Med Care 2005;43:1164–70.
48. Toft T, Fink P, Oernboel E, et al. Mental disorders in primary care: prevalence and co-morbidity among disorders. Results from the functional illness in primary care (FIP) study. Psychol Med 2005;35:1175–84.

49. Löwe B, Gräfe K, Zipfel S, et al. Detecting panic disorder in medical and psychosomatic outpatients: comparative validation of the Hospital Anxiety and Depression Scale, the Patient Health Questionnaire, a screening question, and physicians' diagnosis. J Psychosom Res 2003;55(6):515–9.

50. Katon WJ, Walker EA. Medically unexplained symptoms in primary care. J Clin Psychiatry 1998;14(Suppl 20):15–21.

51. Kroenke K, Price RK. Symptoms in the community: prevalence, classification, and psychiatric comorbidity. Arch Intern Med 1993;153(21):2474–80.

52. Jackson JL, Houston JS, Hanling SR, et al. Clinical predictors of mental disorders among medical outpatients. Arch Intern Med 2001;161(6):875–9.

53. Rosen G, Kleinman A, Katon W. Somatization in family practice: a biopsychosocial approach. J Fam Pract 1982;14(3):493–502.

54. Heijmans M, Olde Hartman TC, van Weel-Baumgarten E, et al. Experts' opinions on the management of medically unexplained symptoms in primary care. A qualitative analysis of narrative reviews and scientific editorials. Fam Pract 2011;28(4):444–55.

55. Coulehan JL, Platt FW, Egener B, et al. "Let me see if I have this right...": words that help build empathy. Ann Intern Med 2001;135(3):221–7.

56. Nordin TA, Hartz AJ, Noyes R, et al. Empirically identified goals for the management of unexplained symptoms. Fam Med 2006;38:476–82.

57. Edwards TM, Stern A, Clarke DD, et al. The treatment of patients with medically unexplained symptoms in primary care: a review of the literature. Ment Health Fam Med 2010;7(4):209–21.

58. Stuart MR, Lieberman JA. The fifteen minute hour: applied psychotherapy for the primary care physician. New York: Praeger; 1986.

59. Barsky AJ. A comprehensive approach to the chronically somatizing patient. J Psychosom Res 1998;45:301–6.

60. Rolfe A, Burton C. Reassurance after diagnostic testing with a low pretest probability of serious disease systematic review and meta-analysis. JAMA Intern Med 2013;173:407–16.

61. Rief W, Heitmuller AM, Reisberg K, et al. Why reassurance fails in patients with unexplained symptoms: an experimental investigation of remembered probabilities. PLoS Med 2006;269:1266–72.

62. Löwe B, Unützer J, Callahan CM, et al. Monitoring depression treatment outcomes with the patient health questionnaire-9. Med Care 2004;42(12):1194–201.

63. Gierk B, Kohlmann S, Kroenke K, et al. The somatic symptom scale–8 (SSS-8): a brief measure of somatic symptom burden. JAMA Intern Med 2014;174(3):399–407.

64. Stanley MA, Wilson NL, Novy DM, et al. Cognitive behavior therapy for generalized anxiety disorder among older adults in primary care: a randomized clinical trial. JAMA 2009;301(14):1460–7.

65. O'Malley PG, Jackson JL, Santoro J, et al. Antidepressant therapy for unexplained symptoms and symptom syndromes. J Fam Pract 1999;48:980–90.

66. Kroenke K, Swindle R. Cognitive-behavioral therapy for somatization and symptom syndromes: a critical review of controlled clinical trials. Psychother Psychosom 2000;69:205–15.

67. Allen LA, Escobar JI, Lehrer PM, et al. Psychosocial treatments for multiple unexplained physical symptoms: a review of the literature. Psychosom Med 2002; 64(6):939–50.

68. Dworkin RH, Backonja M, Rowbotham MC, et al. Advances in neuropathic pain: diagnosis, mechanisms, and treatment recommendations. Arch Neurol 2003; 60(11):1524–34.

69. Stahl S. Antidepressants and somatic symptoms: therapeutic actions are expanding beyond affective spectrum disorders to functional somatic syndromes. J Clin Psychiatry 2003;64:745–6.
70. Brannan SK, Mallinckrodt CH, Detke MJ, et al. Onset of action for duloxetine 60 mg once daily: double-blind, placebo-controlled studies. J Psychiatr Res 2005; 39(2):161–72.
71. Goldstein DJ, Lu Y, Detke MJ, et al. Effects of duloxetine on painful physical symptoms associated with depression. Psychosomatics 2004;45(1):17–28.
72. Fava M, Mallinckrodt CH, Detke MJ, et al. The effect of duloxetine on painful physical symptoms in depressed patients: do improvements in these symptoms result in higher remission rates? J Clin Psychiatry 2004;13:521–30.
73. DeVeaugh-Geiss AM, West SL, Miller WC, et al. The adverse effects of comorbid pain on depression outcomes in primary care patients: results from the ARTIST trial. Pain Med 2010;11(5):732–41.
74. Bair MJ, Robinson RL, Eckert GJ, et al. Impact of pain on depression treatment response in primary care. Psychosom Med 2004;66(1):17–22.
75. Kroenke K. Efficacy of treatment for somatoform disorders: a review of randomized controlled trials. Psychosom Med 2007;13(9):881–8.
76. Koelen JA, Houtveen JH, Abbass A, et al. Effectiveness of psychotherapy for severe somatoform disorder: meta-analysis. Br J Psychiatry 2014;204:12–9.
77. Smith GR, Monson RA, Ray DC. Psychiatric consultation in somatization disorder. N Engl J Med 1986;314(22):1407–13.
78. Kashner TM, Rost K, Smith GR, et al. An analysis of panel data. The impact of a psychiatric consultation letter on the expenditures and outcomes of care for patients with somatization disorder. Med Care 1992;30:811–21.
79. Henningsen P, Zipfel S, Herzog W. Management of functional somatic syndromes. Lancet 2007;369(9565):946–55.
80. Archer J, Bower P, Gilbody S, et al. Collaborative care for depression and anxiety problems. Cochrane Database Syst Rev 2012;(10):CD006525.
81. Mitte K. A meta-analysis of the efficacy of psycho- and pharmacotherapy in panic disorder with and without agoraphobia. J Affect Disord 2005;88(1):27–45.

Addiction Disorders

Joseph O. Merrill, MD, MPH[a],*, Mark H. Duncan, MD[b]

KEYWORDS

- Substance use disorder • Addiction • Chemical dependency • Alcohol screening
- Brief intervention • Opioids • Chronic pain management

KEY POINTS

- Substance use disorders and risky substance use are common in primary care settings, although evidence-based screening, brief intervention, and pharmacotherapy are seldom provided.
- Primary care assessment of alcohol use disorders includes screening, followed by assessment for DSM-5 diagnosis, as appropriate treatment is based on whether a substance use disorder or risky drinking is present.
- Brief interventions are effective in reducing alcohol consumption and medical consequences among risky drinkers in primary care settings, whereas alcohol pharmacotherapy is appropriate for patients with moderate or severe alcohol use disorders.
- Patients on chronic opioid therapy for noncancer pain, particularly those on higher dose therapy, require routine monitoring for substance use disorders and safety problems.
- Opioid use disorders can be effectively treated with methadone in specially licensed and accredited programs or can be treated with buprenorphine by physicians in the primary care setting.

INTRODUCTION

Substance use disorders (SUD) are commonly found in primary care settings, although screening and assessment are often overlooked, and evidence-based treatments available to primary care providers are infrequently used. A study of more than 450,000 patients screened in a variety of health care settings found that 23% of patients had current alcohol or drug problems,[1] yet less than 20% of those with a substance use disorder nationally receive any treatment.[2] Although SUD are associated with a wide range of medical problems, historically the treatment of

The authors have no financial disclosures.
[a] Department of Medicine, Harborview Medical Center, University of Washington School of Medicine, 325 Ninth Avenue, Box 359780, Seattle, WA 98104, USA; [b] Department of Psychiatry & Behavioral Sciences, University of Washington, 1959 Northeast Pacific Street, Box 356560, Seattle, WA 98195-6560, USA
* Corresponding author.
E-mail address: joem@uw.edu

http://dx.doi.org/10.1016/j.mcna.2014.06.008
0025-7125/14/$ – see front matter © 2014 Elsevier Inc. All rights reserved.
medical.theclinics.com

SUD has been separate from medical care.[3] This separation has impeded care coordination for patients with multiple problems and adequate addiction medicine education for medical providers. This article focuses primarily on alcohol and opioid issues, including the overlap of SUD and opioid prescribing for chronic noncancer pain.

SUD ASSESSMENT AND DIAGNOSIS

Assessment of SUD in primary care can be challenging. The presentation of patients with SUD can be varied and may include obvious signs such as intoxication and withdrawal, or more subtle signs such as poor medication or appointment adherence, problems with sleep, unstable housing, or legal issues. To further complicate assessment, patients may see real or perceived consequences to disclosing their substance use problems, as may be seen in the patient prescribed opioids for pain, or they may have concerns that disclosure could affect their medical care or benefits. Provider vigilance and persistence are warranted because of the impact substances can have on a patient's overall health.

Approach to Assessing Patients for Substance Use

A nonjudgmental and compassionate approach to assessing patients for substance use disorder is essential to promote an open and honest dialogue. When patient attitudes and comfort in alcohol screening have been studied, most patients were comfortable with and in favor of screening and guidance about their use.[4,5] However, patients with positive alcohol screening or current problematic alcohol and drug use were more likely to feel embarrassed by alcohol questions or less comfortable talking about it, indicating the deeply vulnerable position these patients are likely experiencing around their substance use. Despite that, one study found that 75% of the primary care patients who screened positive for alcohol misuse show motivation to change, and motivation to change increased as the severity of alcohol misuse increased.[6] It can be less threatening to focus initially on past use and problems, because this allows the provider an opportunity to demonstrate empathy and understanding about the difficulty of behavior change before asking for disclosure about more recent use. Taking a supportive and motivational approach, and putting aside any negative assumptions when assessing patients for substance use problems, will support their readiness to make change.

Screening

The United States Preventive Services Task Force recommends that all adults aged 18 years or older be screened for alcohol misuse, with the goal of identifying both patients with alcohol use disorder and those who drink more than healthy limits.[7] Unhealthy alcohol use covers a spectrum of use from drinking more than the amount recommended (**Box 1**) to severe alcohol use disorders.[8] There is no specific recommended frequency around screening patients for alcohol use, but it can be done yearly, or as clinically indicated. Although there is no evidence supporting universal screening for problems with other drugs, it is generally recommended to screen all new patients and those with demographic or clinical risks, such as male sex, behavioral problems, family members with substance use problems, those with symptoms of a psychiatric disorder, or medical issues potentially related to drug use (**Box 2**). In pregnancy, expert opinion recommends universal screening for drug and alcohol use early in prenatal care. Because of the stigmatization associated with substance use in pregnancy, well-validated instruments for this population are necessary to assure

---

Box 1
Healthy drinking limits

Healthy men less than 65 years old

- ≤4 drinks in a day and
- ≤14 drinks in a week

All healthy women and healthy men older than 65 years old

- <3 drinks in a day and
- ≤7 drinks in a week

Abstinence for selected populations

- Pregnant
- Medication interactions
- Health conditions with contraindications
- Less than 18 years old

Data from National Institute on Alcohol Abuse and Alcoholism. Helping patients who drink too much: a practitioner's guide. 2005. Available at: http://pubs.niaaa.nih.gov/publications/Practitioner/CliniciansGuide2005/clinicians_guide.htm. Accessed June 27, 2014.

---

appropriate sensitivity (**Box 3**). The National Institute on Alcohol Abuse and Alcoholism (NIAAA) also recommends screening adolescents 14 to 18 by asking them questions about their used of substances and their friends' use of substances (see **Box 3**).

Assessing for SUD

In all cases, a positive screen for a substance demands further assessment. The main strategy for this in alcohol use disorders is to determine if a patient has unhealthy use or a mild use disorder versus a moderate to severe use disorder, because that will impact treatment decisions. Unfortunately, there is not a quick and comprehensive way to determine if a patient has a substance use disorder outside of reviewing the DSM-5 criteria with them (**Box 4**). Although scales like the AUDIT-C can measure severity, and higher scores are associated with alcohol dependence, it cannot make the formal diagnosis and may result in underdiagnosis.[9] In addition, there are no such scales appropriate for drug use. Although there are clinically significant time limitations in a primary care setting, obtaining the correct diagnosis is critical.

Drugs and alcohol use can affect every system of the body, so for all patients screening positive for unhealthy use or a substance use disorder, a physical examination, medical history, and psychiatric history are crucial (**Box 5**). Regular use of drugs or alcohol also carries with it several safety concerns, including suicide, which increased 10-fold in people with a substance use disorder and should be assessed.[10] Withdrawal syndromes are also common and have been defined for alcohol, cannabis, opioids, sedative-hypnotics, and stimulants, according to the DSM-5. Special attention should be given to alcohol, benzodiazepine, and barbiturate withdrawal symptoms, which can occur within hours after last use and can lead to seizures, delirium tremens, and death.

ALCOHOL USE DISORDERS

An initial approach to alcohol screening in primary care is outlined in **Fig. 1**. Once a person has screened positive and been found to have unhealthy drinking or an alcohol

---

Box 2
Screening tests for drug and alcohol use validated in primary care settings

Single-Item Alcohol Screener

"How many times in the past year have you had 5 (4 in women) or more drinks in a day?"

Scoring and Notes

- Positive response: any answer >0 or difficulty identifying how often
- Sensitivity: 82%, specificity: 79%[59]
- Easy to remember and quick.

AUDIT-C (Alcohol Use Disorders Identification Test-Consumption)

1. How often do you have a drink containing alcohol?

a: Never   b: Monthly or less   c: 2–4 times a month d: 2–3 times a week   e: 4 or more times per week

2. How many standard drinks containing alcohol do you have on a typical day?

a: 1 or 2   b: 3 or 4   c: 5 or 6   d: 7 or 9   e: 10 or more

3. How often do you have 6 or more drinks on one occasion?

a: Never   b: Less than monthly c: Monthly   d: Weekly   e: Daily or almost daily

Scoring and Notes

- Scoring: a = 0, b = 1, c = 2, d = 3, e = 4[60]
  - Positive response indicates unhealthy alcohol use
    - Men: >4, Sensitivity: 85%, specificity: 89%
    - Women: >3, Sensitivity: 73%, specificity: 91%[61]
  - Scores >7 suggest alcohol dependence[9]

Single-Item Drug Screener

"How many times in the past year have you used an illegal drug or used a prescription medication for nonmedical reasons?"

Scoring and Notes

- Positive response: any positive answer
- Sensitivity: 100%, specificity: 74%[45]

Other Screeners

- AUDIT: 10 items. Alcohol screener. Positive score: ≥8 for risky drinking. Sensitivity: 57%–97%, specificity: 78%–96%[62]
- CAGE: 4 items. Alcohol screener. Positive score: ≥2 affirmative answers. Not sensitive to risky drinking. Sensitivity: 77%, specificity: 79% for alcohol abuse and dependence.[62]
- DAST (Drug Abuse Screening Test): 10-, 20-, and 28-item varieties. Validated in addiction treatment centers. Positive 10-item score: ≥2 for risky drinking. Sensitivity: 80%, specificity: 88%[63]

Box 3
Screeners for special populations

Pregnancy

T-ACE (Tolerance, Annoyed, Cut-down, Eye opener)—Alcohol Screener[64–67]

4 items   Positive response: $\geq$2   Sensitivity: 69%–94.7%,
                                                               specificity: 40.4%–79%

- Recommended by the American College of Obstetrics and Gynecology.

- Asks about use in a more indirect way then the AUDIT–C, which may lead to more honest results.

AUDIT–C—Alcohol Screener[65]

3 items   Positive response: 3 or greater   Sensitivity: 95%, specificity: 85%

4P's Plus© (Parents, Partner, Past, Pregnancy)—Alcohol and Drug Screener[68]

5 items   Positive response: any   Sensitivity: 87.1%, specificity:
                 acknowledged use in pregnancy   76.1%

- Developed for pregnant women.

- This test is copyrighted and may not be reproduced in any form without permission.

CRAFFT (Car, Relax, Alone, Forget, Family/friends, Trouble)—Alcohol and Drug Screener for adolescents and young adults[69]

6 items   Positive response: $\geq$2   Positive predictive value: 90%

- Studied in pregnant young adults ages 17–25.

Teenagers

2-question drug and alcohol screener[70]

1. "In the past year, on how many days have you had more than a few sips of beer, wine, or any drink containing alcohol?"

2. "If your friends drink, how many drinks do they usually drink on an occasion?"

   - Any positive response requires further assessment.

   - Recommended by the NIAAA and the American Academy of Pediatrics.

   - Targets any use.

---

use disorder, there are several options for further treatment. Brief interventions are appropriate for all levels of alcohol use disorders, although additional treatment will likely be needed for those with a moderate to severe alcohol use disorder. Additional treatments in a primary care setting may include pharmacotherapy, motivational interviewing, and referrals to mutual help groups. Continuing to engage the patient through regular follow-up is important for patients who are both actively drinking and in recovery, as relapse is common.[11]

Brief Interventions

Brief intervention is an evidence-based approach to discussions of alcohol use in primary care and is recommended for all adults 18 years of age and old who engage in risky or hazardous drinking (see **Box 1**).[7] Lower levels of alcohol use are considered

---

Box 4
Assessing for substance use disorder in primary care

- After a positive screening test, begin the conversation with "tell me about your alcohol (or drug) use."

- Listen for statements indicating that the patient has or has had concerns about their substance use and reflect those concerns in order to encourage the patient to say more about possible problems.

- Listen especially for DSM-5 symptoms of a Substance Use Disorder, which include tolerance, withdrawal, using more than intended, failed efforts to cut down or quit, spending a lot of time related to use, craving, failure to fulfill important life roles, giving up important life activities, use in hazardous situations, and continued use in spite of either negative physical/ psychological problems, or social/interpersonal consequences. It is usually best to elicit these symptoms through a conversation that also allows providers to express empathy for the difficulty of dealing with addiction, rather than using a formal symptom checklist.

- If the patient seems to minimize current problems, more disclosure may be elicited by asking about past problems, even as a youth (including driving issues).

- If problems occurred, ask about prior treatment or AA/NA participation.

- Often a past or current diagnosis will become obvious with this approach. If a substance use disorder diagnosis is possible but not clearly present, it may be necessary to review DSM-5 criteria specifically.

- A DSM-5 Substance Use Disorder diagnosis requires that symptoms lead to clinically significant impairment and be present within a 12-month period. Severity of a Substance Use Disorder is estimated by the number of DSM-5 symptoms, with two or three representing a mild disorder, four or five a moderate disorder, and 6 or more a severe disorder. A moderate to severe disorder most closely approximates Substance Dependence from the DSM-IV TR.

- Unlike DSM-IV TR, tolerance and withdrawal due solely to prescribed medication taken as directed do not count towards a DSM-5 Substance Use Disorder diagnosis.

Data from American Psychiatric Association. Diagnostic and statistical manual of mental disorders. Fifth edition (DSM-5). Arlington (VA): American Psychiatric Association; 2013.

---

safe, and observational studies have associated low-level drinking with reduced cardiovascular risk, although causality is not clearly established. Brief intervention has been found to reduce weekly alcohol consumption rates, increase adherence to recommended drinking limits, and reduce health care utilization.[12–14] In a meta-analysis of 7 trials it was found that participants had 3.6 fewer drinks per week, and 12% of participants had fewer heavy drinking episodes at 12 months.[15] For patients with moderate to severe alcohol use disorders (corresponding to alcohol dependence in DSM-IV), brief interventions on their own have not been found effective.[16] However, brief interventions can be used to help promote successful engagement in evidence-based treatment of this subgroup of patients, including adherence to alcohol use disorder pharmacotherapy, mutual help group attendance, or participation in specialty treatment programs.

Brief interventions can vary greatly in their components and time, but typically include multiple short encounters providing feedback, discussing safe amounts, assessing readiness for change, discussing goals, and arranging follow-up (**Fig. 2**, **Box 6**). There are a variety of evidence-based psychosocial approaches that are effective in alcohol use disorders. Although it is not typically feasible in a primary care setting to provide regular and extended therapy using these approaches, they can be used to tailor responses to harmful drinking, develop rapport, and support

---

Box 5
Medical and psychiatric cooccurring disorders

Medical

- *Dermatologic*: skin abscesses

- *Cardiovascular*: essential hypertension, angina, myocardial infarction, heart failure, arrhythmias, infective endocarditis, cardiomyopathies

- *Respiratory*: nasal septal perforation, COPD, asthma

- *Gastrointestinal*: viral hepatitis, hepatic carcinoma, peptic ulcer disease, IBD, pancreatitis, gastritis, cirrhosis, cirrhotic varices

- *Hematologic*: anemia, thrombocytopenia, coagulopathies

- *Neurologic*: stroke, encephalopathy, traumatic brain injury, epilepsy, epidural abscess, peripheral neuropathy, Wernicke/Korsakoff syndrome

- *Endocrine*: hypo/hyperthyroidism, type 2 diabetes mellitus, hypogonadism

- *Immunologic*: HIV, immune suppression leading to opportunistic infections (eg, TB, pneumonia), necrotizing vasculitis

- *Metabolic*: electrolyte abnormalities, hypoxia, dehydration

Psychiatric

It is important to note whether the psychiatric disorder preceded the substance-use disorder, to distinguish whether it is a substance-induced disorder.

- *Alcohol*: Depressive disorders, anxiety disorders, psychotic disorders, bipolar disorders, antisocial personality disorder, and PTSD

- *Opioids*: Depressive disorders, sleep disorders, sexual dysfunctions, delirium, anxiety disorders, other substance-use disorders (especially tobacco, alcohol, cannabis, stimulants, benzodiazepines to moderate/modulate opioid withdrawal and intoxication), antisocial personality disorder, posttraumatic stress disorder

- *Stimulants*: Psychotic disorders, bipolar disorders, depressive disorders, anxiety disorders, obsessive compulsive disorders, sleep disorders, sexual dysfunction disorders, delirium, posttraumatic stress disorder, antisocial personality disorder, attention–deficit/hyperactivity disorder, gambling disorder.

---

self-efficacy (**Box 7**). No studies have assessed brief intervention in adolescents, but it has been found efficacious in pregnant populations.[17]

Pharmacotherapy for Alcohol Use Disorders

Ambulatory medically supervised withdrawal

Many patients with moderate to severe alcohol use disorders will have physical dependence. Symptoms of alcohol withdrawal can start within 6 hours of the last drink and can proceed through the early withdrawal to delirium tremens and seizures if untreated. Mild symptoms include tremors, anxiety, insomnia, headaches, loss of appetite, nausea, emesis, and diarrhea. Moderate symptoms can include elevated blood pressure and pulse, sweating, and confusion. Patients who are 5 days out from their last drink and who have no withdrawal symptoms will not need pharmacotherapy for their withdrawal. Alcohol withdrawal symptoms severity can be assessed with the CIWA-Ar (Clinical Institute Withdrawal Assessment for Alcohol, Revised).[18] In addition to reviewing a patient's medical and psychiatric stability, the CIWA-Ar can be used to help assess the most appropriate treatment setting, because scores greater than 15 are best handled in inpatient facilities. Patients eligible for ambulatory

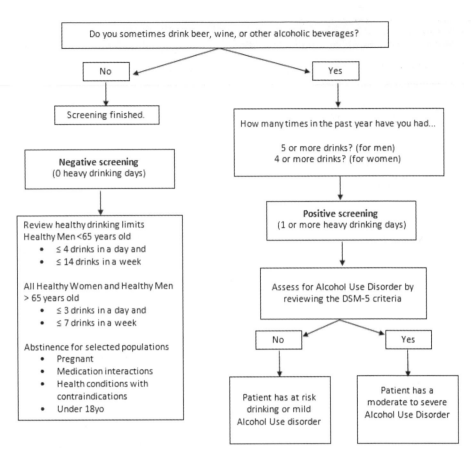

Fig. 1. Approach to initial alcohol screening in primary care. (*From* National Institute on Alcohol Abuse and Alcoholism. Helping patients who drink too much: a practitioner's guide. 2005. Available at: http://pubs.niaaa.nih.gov/publications/Practitioner/CliniciansGuide2005/clinicians_guide.htm. Accessed June 27, 2014.)

detoxification should also be medically and psychiatrically stable, have no other current substance problems, have no history of alcohol withdrawal seizures, be able to take oral medications, have family support that can monitor the patient, and be able to commit to daily medical visits.[19] Patients should be monitored daily until their symptoms have decreased. Symptoms typically resolve after 7 days. Thiamine 100 mg daily for prevention of Wernicke syndrome, and 1 mg of folic acid daily for nutritional replacement, should be started at the beginning of their supervised withdrawal.

Medications for alcohol withdrawal with the best evidence are benzodiazepines and anticonvulsants. Benzodiazepines reduce withdrawal symptoms and are the only medications found to prevent withdrawal seizures[20]; thus, they remain first-line treatment. There is no evidence that one benzodiazepine is better than another, although long-acting benzodiazepines like chlordiazepoxide and diazepam are thought to provide a smoother withdrawal experience. These medications can be administered in either a fixed dose schedule or a symptom-triggered schedule. Symptom-triggered approaches have been found to reduce medication use and have shorter inpatient stays.[21]

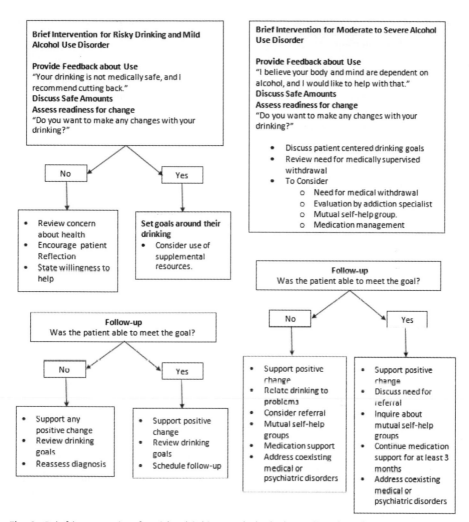

Fig. 2. Brief intervention for risky drinking and alcohol use disorders. (*From* National Institute on Alcohol Abuse and Alcoholism. Helping patients who drink too much: a practitioner's guide. 2005. Available at: http://pubs.niaaa.nih.gov/publications/Practitioner/CliniciansGuide2005/clinicians_guide.htm. Accessed June 27, 2014.)

Anticonvulsants have also been studied for ambulatory medically supervised alcohol withdrawal. For instance, gabapentin has been found to be as effective in treating alcohol withdrawal symptoms as both lorazepam and chlordiazepoxide.[22,23] In addition, the gabapentin groups had less craving and less sedation by the end of treatment. For both of these studies, a fixed dose schedule was set, with maximum doses of 1200 mg daily for 3 days and tapered over 4 days.

Medication management for relapse prevention
Prescribing medications for moderate to severe alcohol use disorder is useful to help patients stop drinking and in relapse prevention. Medication management for alcohol use disorders is an approach to provide both medication treatment follow-up and brief

---

Box 6
Aspects of brief intervention

Basics

- Multiple contacts: Project TrEAT (Trial for Early Alcohol Treatment) included 4 total contacts, 2 in person with a primary care provider 1 month apart, and two 5-minute calls with a nurse 2 weeks after each visit.[71]

- Brief: 6- to 15-minute encounters have been the most effective.[72]

- Counseling approaches can vary (see **Box 6**).

- Identify and reflect positive and negative aspects of drinking.

Components

  Providing feedback about harmful use

    Feedback on their use should be specific to the patient and may incorporate current psychosocial or medical issues related to their use.

    "You're drinking more than is medically safe and it is likely contributing to your [current problem]."

  Discussing safe amounts and explicit recommendations

    Describing what a standard drink is can be helpful for patients to understand how much they are actually drinking.

    "Drinking less than 14 drinks (7 for women) in a week will help you avoid some of the bad things associated with alcohol."

  Assessing readiness for change

    Patients may or may not be ready to change anything about their drinking. Some patients may not be aware they have risky drinking.

    "With what I have reviewed with you, is there anything you would like to change about your drinking?"

  Discussing goals and explicit recommendations

    Goals will vary depending on the patient's interest in making change. It is helpful to take a patient-centered approach to establishing drinking goals. Goals may include everything from reducing the amount of alcohol consumed to sobriety. Goals can also include steps the patient is currently taking to make change. Identifying specific strategies to achieve those goals is helpful. This may include tracking their drinks, eating better, alternating alcoholic and nonalcoholic beverages, managing triggering situations, utilizing friends or family.

  Arranging for follow-up

    Follow-up has been clearly shown to be superior to a one-time intervention.[72] This will provide opportunities for further assessment, and supporting and reviewing goals.

---

behavioral support to promote recovery by increasing medication adherence, education, and referrals to support groups (**Box 8**).[24]

When prescribing relapse prevention medications, such as naltrexone, XR-naltrexone IM, acamprosate, and disulfiram, close weekly follow-up is helpful initially. Naltrexone, an opioid antagonist that reduces cravings and peak drinking amounts, is a reasonable first choice for patients desiring to cut back or stop drinking and not taking opioids. This medication can be started while the patient is drinking or at the end of their medically supervised withdrawal.[25,26] Acamprosate, working on the glutamate and GABA neurotransmitter systems, has been shown to help prevent

---

Box 7
Psychosocial counseling approaches for alcohol use disorders

Motivational Interviewing

Motivational interviewing is a patient-centered conversation style whereby the provider's role is to guide the conversation to develop discrepancy between the patient's use and their goals and to work toward resolving that discrepancy.[73] It avoids confrontation, or the "righting reflex," whereby the provider wants to correct unhealthy behaviors, and instead, works to have the patient identify their own reasons for changing. It works through using an interviewing style that uses open-ended questions, affirming something positive in the patient, reflective listening in an effort to clarify what the patient is saying, and summarizing what the patient has said, which can demonstrate understanding and promote engagement. An example version of motivational interviewing called motivational enhancement therapy can be found at: http://pubs.niaaa.nih.gov/publications/ProjectMatch/match02.pdf.

Harm Reduction

Harm reduction approaches look at specific techniques a patient can take to reduce the harms they experience from their alcohol use, which often includes reducing drinking quantity. Strategies can include spacing out drinks, drinking with food in the stomach, alternating alcoholic and nonalcoholic beverages, tracking amount of alcohol drinking, and not drinking and driving. A harm reduction approach for adults can be found in Denning and Little's, *Practicing harm reduction psychotherapy: an alternative approach to addictions.*[74]

Cognitive Behavioral Therapy

Cognitive behavioral therapy (CBT) emphasizes developing skills to deal with high-risk situations, cravings, triggers, and lapses. This has been done individually and in group settings. This approach makes an effort to show the patient how their thoughts relate to their behaviors in a step-wise approach, to better understand what leads to relapses. In a meta-analysis of 53 studies of adults with alcohol or drug disorders, a modest positive effect was found compared with other interventions or controls.[75] An example can be found at: http://pubs.niaaa.nih.gov/publications/ProjectMatch/match03.pdf.

12-Step Facilitation and 12-Step Programs

Twelve-step facilitation emphasizes alcoholism as a disease and promotes and helps facilitate participation in 12-step groups like Alcoholic Anonymous (AA). Patients are encouraged to try different groups, find a sponsor, do service, and work the 12 steps. An example of this approach can be found at: http://pubs.niaaa.nih.gov/publications/ProjectMatch/match01.pdf.

AA

AA is a mutual support fellowship for people who want to stop drinking. Meetings are widely accessible, and in larger urban areas, there are meetings that will often cater to special groups, helping to reduce the anxiety around social situations. Believing in a "higher power" does not always mean believing in a deity and should not be a barrier to participation. Observational studies have shown effectiveness for this approach, with higher rates of abstinence at 12 months among military veterans participating in AA versus those in CBT (26% vs 19%).[76]

---

relapse and increase accumulated days of abstinence.[27] Acamprosate is useful in patients with contraindications to naltrexone, such as those taking opioids. Disulfiram blocks alcohol metabolism and leads to the buildup of acetaldehyde, which is responsible for flushing, sweating, nausea, and tachycardia. Disulfiram has been found effective in preventing relapse in alcohol dependence and in patients with cocaine and

> **Box 8**
> **Components of a medication management visit**
>
> *Initial visits*
>
> • Review of medical evaluation, including alcohol-affected comorbidities
>
> • Physical signs of substance use, including signs of withdrawal
>
> • Reviewing laboratory results
>
> • Reviewing any negative aspects of drinking
>
> • Discussion of their diagnosis
>
> • Interest in abstinence
>
> • Utility of medication, including its mechanism, adverse effects, and adherence strategies[58]
>
> • Encourage participation in a mutual support group
>
> *Follow-up visits*
>
> • Assess drinking amounts
>
> • Functional status
>
> • Medication adherence
>
> • Medication adverse effects
>
> *Data from* A detailed template of this is available at: http://pubs.niaaa.nih.gov/publications/ Practitioner/CliniciansGuide2005/guide.pdf. Accessed June 27, 2014.

alcohol dependence.[28] All of these oral medication formulations are most effective in motivated patients, or patients whose adherence can be monitored. Gabapentin has also been found effective in treating alcohol dependence (especially at the 1800 mg total daily dosing) when compared with placebo by improving rates of abstinence, decreasing heavier drinking days, as well as improving sleep, cravings, and mood (**Box 9**).[29]

Primary care physicians with appropriate experience, training, and support can treat patients with more significant alcohol problems. Referral to a higher level of specialty addiction treatment can be indicated for several reasons, including the need for inpatient medically supervised withdrawal, poor response to primary care treatment, complicated comorbid mental health conditions, or need for case management services.

SUBSTANCE USE DISORDER ISSUES IN CHRONIC PAIN MANAGEMENT

One of the most common and problematic issues in primary care practice is the intersection between SUD and opioid prescribing, particularly for chronic pain problems. Because SUD may present differently in the context of chronic opioid prescribing, the recognition and management of SUD must be integrated into an overall clinical approach to chronic pain management.

Opioid Treatment Risks

In an effort to more effectively treat chronic pain, chronic opioid therapy has become increasingly prevalent in general practice over the last decades,[30,31] although evidence for long-term effectiveness is limited, with short-term trials providing evidence for reduction in pain intensity, but mixed result for functional improvement.[32] Accompanying the increase in opioid prescribing has been worrisome trends in prescription

---

Box 9
Alcohol use disorder medications

Naltrexone

Start 50 mg daily. Range 25–150 mg daily. Significant interaction with opioids. Avoid in active hepatitis. Well-tolerated. May be used for harm reduction as well as abstinence-based goals. Stop for 5 days before using opioids. Liver function tests should be checked at baseline and followed every few months after that. Potential adherence problems.

XR Naltrexone IM

380 mg every 4 weeks. Significant interaction with opioids. Avoid in active hepatitis. Nausea, fatigue, and injection site reactions common. Side effects often improve by 5 days and can be managed with over-the-counter medications. May be used for harm reduction as well as abstinence-based goals.

Acamprosate

Start 666 mg 3 times a day. Range: 333–666 mg 3 times a day. An alternative for patients taking opioids. Diarrhea most common side effect. Suicidal ideation rare but reported. Renal excretion, so reduce dose with CrCl 30–50 mL/min. No liver toxicity or drug interactions. Potential adherence problems.

Disulfiram

Start 250 mg daily. Range: 125–500 mg daily. Should have abstained from alcohol for at least 24 hours. Most effective for those committed to abstinence with good social support for observed ingestion. Avoid in severe cardiac disease and active hepatitis. Review alcohol disulfiram reaction and forgotten forms of alcohol (eg, cologne, deodorant, cough syrups, vinegars). Several significant drug-drug interactions, including anticoagulants, isoniazid, metronidazole, and phenytoin, among others. Monitor liver function throughout.

Topiramate

Start 50 mg daily. Range 50–300 mg daily, divided, 2 times a day. Titrate over several weeks. Side effects include cognitive impairment, paresthesias, weight loss, headache, fatigue, dizziness, and depression. Not US Food and Drug Administration (FDA) approved for alcohol use disorder, but multiple positive trials.[77]

Gabapentin

Start 900 to 1200 orally for 3 days, followed by a taper over the next 4 days for ambulatory supervised withdrawal. Range: 900–1200 mg/d (withdrawal) and 1800 mg/d (alcohol dependence), divided 3 times a day. Useful for ambulatory medically supervised withdrawal and protracted alcohol withdrawal symptoms: depression, anxiety, and insomnia. Not FDA approved for alcohol use disorder.

---

opioid abuse by youth and adults emergency department and addiction treatment admissions associated with prescription opioids, and opioid-related overdose deaths.[33–35] These trends have led to multiple efforts to reduce the risk of opioid prescribing for noncancer pain, including development of state level prescription monitoring programs that allow providers to access records of all dispensed controlled substances, tamper-resistant formulation of opioid medications, and clinical guideline recommendations for safer opioid prescribing for noncancer pain.[36]

The use of higher doses of opioids for chronic noncancer pain is particularly problematic. Although no clinical trials comparing opioid dose levels for chronic noncancer pain have been reported,[37] higher prescribed opioid doses have been associated with multiple complications (**Box 10**). Opioid dose escalation should be avoided, but mixed evidence exists about the dose limits for opioids prescribed for noncancer pain. Risks appear to increase when daily use exceeds 50 to 100 mg of morphine or the equivalent,[38] and multiple opioid prescribing guidelines recommend avoiding doses greater than 90 to 200 mg of morphine equivalents daily.[36]

Approaching Patients on High-Dose Opioids

Conversations with patients on high doses of prescribed opioids can be challenging. Patients, particularly those with a history of substance use disorder, often feel scrutinized and stigmatized as they attempt to access medical care and have their symptoms taken seriously. Providers struggle to provide pain management safely while maintaining the rapport that is the basis of primary care practice.[39] In addition, patients may be afraid that their pain will be poorly controlled with dose tapering, or that they may experience opioid withdrawal. It is important to validate pain complaints and work with patients to improve their nonopioid medication regimens and their nonmedication approaches to chronic pain while also educating them on the risks of higher-dose therapy. Assessment of patient-attributed problems related to opioid therapy[40] may highlight ways in which a patient might benefit from dose reduction. Patients with safety issues related to higher dose therapy, for instance, an opioid overdose or inability to take the medication as prescribed, may need more rapid tapering. However, for stable patients who are not using other drugs or taking their medication in risky ways, slower opioid tapering may be possible and can avoid opioid withdrawal. Those who have difficulty tapering due to emergent substance use disorder symptoms may require opioid use disorder treatment with methadone or buprenorphine.

Detection and Management of Problems During Opioid Prescribing

Safely prescribing chronic opioid therapy for noncancer pain requires procedures that integrate comprehensive pain management and detection of emergent problems,

---

Box 10
Complications associated with high-dose opioid prescribing[a]

- Overdose and overdose death[78–80]
- Fractures among the elderly[81]
- Opioid misuse[82]
- Opioid use disorder diagnoses[83]
- Alcohol and drug-related emergency department visits[84]
- Increased mental health and substance use problems[a,85–89]
- Problems that patients attribute to prescribed opioids
  - Psychosocial problems (eg, low mood, sluggishness, poor concentration)
  - Concerns about control over opioid use (eg, self or other thought they might be addicted, wanted to cut down, tolerance).[40,90]

[a] It is not known to what extent higher-dose opioids cause these problems or, conversely, whether they are prescribed more frequently to patients with these preexisting problems, a scenario described as "adverse selection."[91]

some of which may indicate a substance use disorder. A "universal precautions" approach whereby all patients are monitored, rather than only those seen as high risk or who have manifested problems, can aid in detection of problems and reduce conflicted interactions that threaten the primary care relationship (**Box 11**).[41]

Fig. 3 provides a general clinical approach to detection and management of problems in patients prescribed opioids for chronic noncancer pain. In addition to the "universal precautions" approach, the development of a comprehensive chronic pain treatment plan can form the basis for monitoring adherence and identifying problems, including SUD, which may require additional treatment. Treatment plans generally require both active strategies that patients must engage in regularly on their own (eg, exercise, physical therapy, sleep hygiene) as well as medications and more passive nonmedication approaches, such as acupuncture, massage, or Tanscutaneous Electrical Nerve Stimulation units. Identifying functional goals and a patient-centered plan allow more objective assessment of the benefits of opioid prescribing over time.[42]

Problems that commonly arise during opioid prescribing include unexpected prescription-monitoring program or urine toxicology results, requests for early refills, lost or stolen prescriptions, behavioral problems in the clinic setting, and poor adherence to the chronic pain treatment plan. These problems may arise from a simple error or misunderstanding of the treatment agreement, or be caused by a new or worsening mental health problem, social instability, diversion of opioid medication, unsafe use, or a substance use disorder, all of which require assessment. Potential responses to sample problem behaviors are shown in **Fig. 3**. Appropriate responses to such problems include prompt conversations with patients and considering asking them to return between opioid dispensing visits for unscheduled urine toxicology testing and pill counts to assess for diversion. Some problems will be simple to assess, but others may require more prolonged assessment through intensification of treatment and more frequent monitoring visits. Because urine toxicology tests are potentially prone to error or misinterpretation (**Box 12**), it is recommended that opioid-prescribing decisions not be made solely on the basis of a single test, but instead considered in light of behavioral patterns and the overall clinical scenario. Some more dangerous problems, such as overdose events, may require prompt action to lower or discontinue opioids. Patients whose behavioral problems do not respond to the initial approach described above and have recurrent problems will often need their opioids discontinued for safety reasons. The Collaborative Opioid Prescribing Education program provides

---

Box 11
"Universal precautions" for opioid prescribing

All patients are monitored with the following components,[36] not just those considered high risk:

- Frequency of monitoring based on risk of problems, especially past substance use disorder
- Use of opioid risk tools[92,93]
- Treatment agreements describing patient and provider responsibilities during opioid therapy
- Routine urine toxicology testing
- Review of state prescription monitoring program for overlapping scheduled prescriptions

Data from Gourlay DL, Heit HA, Almahrezl A. Universal precautions in pain medicine: a rational approach to the treatment of chronic pain. Pain Med 2005;6(2):107–12.

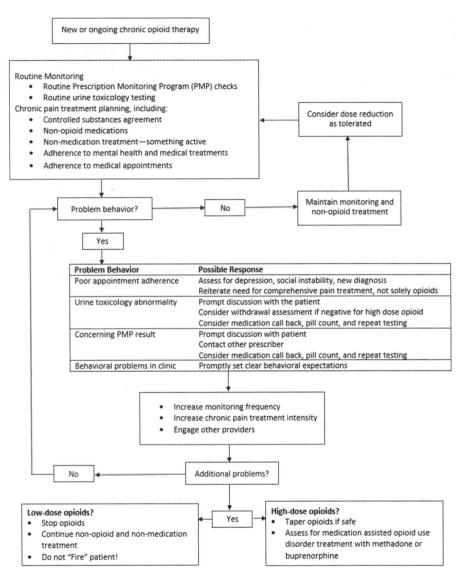

Fig. 3. Clinical approach to detection and management of problems during opioid prescribing.

examples of language clinicians can use to effectively communicate prescribing decisions and handle difficult situations.[43,44] Those with a clear diagnosis of opioid use disorder should be treated with methadone in an Opioid Treatment Program or with buprenorphine by a physician qualified to treat opioid use disorders. Methadone for the treatment of opioid use disorder is not permitted in a primary care setting and can only be provided in specially licensed and accredited Opioid Treatment Programs. Patients on high doses of opioids for pain who cannot safely be treated in primary care settings, and who cannot tolerate opioid tapering, may also need medication-assisted treatment of opioid use disorder.

Box 12
Urine toxicology testing issues and pitfalls

General Considerations

Urine toxicology testing can aid in identification of SUD, monitor patients with known disorders, and monitor patients receiving opioid therapy in primary care. Tests vary greatly in sensitivity and cost, with screening assays (enzymatic immunoassay or enzyme-multiplied immunoassay technique) and point-of-care tests generally less reliable but cheaper, and confirmatory tests (gas chromatography, GC/mass spectrometry, MS) more specific and expensive. Must understand characteristics of each test to correctly interpret results, which requires good communication with laboratory medicine expertise. Never make an important clinical decision based on a single test in isolation, but instead use results in the clinical context to guide further clinical and laboratory assessment.

Opioids

Screening assay for methadone is sensitive and specific. Opioid screening tests not sensitive for oxycodone or oxymorphone unless the dose is high, so negative tests in patients taking low doses can occur; consider including a specific oxycodone assay. Fentanyl poorly detected by opioid screening assays. Confirmatory testing (GC/MS) can be complex, because opioid metabolites may be present and confusing to interpret. For instance, hydromorphone is a common metabolite, but not of oxycodone. Poppy seeds can cause a positive test. Detection window 2–4 days.

Stimulants

Cocaine screening tests are sensitive and highly specific with minimal false positive tests. Many common medications (pseudoephedrine, bupropion, trazodone, others) cross-react with amphetamine/methamphetamine screening assays, so caution is warranted in interpreting positive tests. Consider using a reflex confirmation test for all positive amphetamine/methamphetamine screening tests. Methylphenidate (ritalin) is not an amphetamine and is thus not detected on standard drug screens. Detection window 2 days for amphetamine/methamphetamine, 2–4 days for cocaine.

Cannabis

Cannabis tests may remain positive for weeks in patients who were heavy users. Some methadone programs choose not to test for cannabis because, like nicotine, no important treatment decisions will be made based on the result. Detection window 3 days (single use) to greater than 30 days (heavy daily use).

Benzodiazepines

Some more potent benzodiazepines, such as clonazepam, are present in the urine at such low concentrations that they are poorly detected in most urine drug screening assays. Diazepam and alprazolam are well detected. Sertaline can cause a false positive result. Detection window 3 days (short acting) to 3 weeks (long acting).

Alcohol

Usual screening test detection window 7–12 hours. Urine ethyl glucuronide testing is highly specific and detectable for longer, but may be too sensitive (mouthwash, hand sanitizer can cause a positive test).

Other Drugs

Many synthetic drugs, or "designer drugs," do not have urine toxicology tests available.

> **Sample Test Panel for Patients on Long-term Opioids for Chronic Pain**
>
> Screening test for opioids, methadone, cocaine, benzodiazepine, barbiturate, amphetamine/methamphetamine. Suggest reflex confirmation of positive amphetamine/methamphetamine screen and a specific test for oxycodone.
>
> *Data from* Moeller KE, Lee KC, Kissack JC. Urine drug screening: practical guide for clinicians. Mayo Clin Proc 2008;83(1):66–76.

TREATMENT OF OPIOID USE DISORDERS

Patients with opioid use disorders require specific medication-assisted treatment for optimal outcomes, and these disorders can be identified in primary care settings.[45] Although there are complexities in making a clear substance use disorder diagnosis in patients prescribed opioids for chronic pain,[46] if patients are unable to safely manage their opioid medications in the context of a comprehensive pain management plan and are unable to be weaned from their prescriptions, opioid use disorder treatment should be considered. Detoxification treatment in the setting of opioid use disorders is unlikely to be successful, although it may be a reasonable approach for patients with a mild disorder or short duration of opioid use. Rapid and ultrarapid opioid detoxification has not been shown effective.[47] Medications for the treatment of opioid use disorders are presented in **Box 13** and include the opioid antagonist naloxone, which, along with overdose education, can be prescribed to patients at risk for opioid overdose and their families and friends.

Methadone Maintenance Treatment

Methadone maintenance treatment of opioid use disorders has more than 40 years of clinical research supporting its effectiveness in reducing drug use, criminal behavior, infectious disease transmission, overdose, and death.[48] It is superior to even richly supported detoxification programs in randomized trials,[49] and the poor outcomes after discontinuation of methadone maintenance support recommendations for its long-term use. In contrast to opioids prescribed in the medical setting for chronic non-cancer pain, higher doses of methadone provided in Opioid Treatment Programs have been shown to improve outcomes, as has a longer duration of treatment and inclusion of moderate amounts of psychosocial treatment.[50] Access to methadone maintenance, which is heavily regulated and frequently threatened with defunding, is largely limited to larger metropolitan areas, and its status as separate from medical settings limits physician understanding and coordination of care. Methadone maintenance programs have limited clinical flexibility, often do not have integrated medical or mental health services, and require specific signed authorization from patients to discuss their care unless it is a medical emergency.

Patients in methadone maintenance are required to attend treatment 6 days per week at the start of treatment so that medication ingestion can be observed, although patients who do well in treatment over a period of at least 3 months can become eligible for additional take-home doses, up to a full month of medication after years of successful treatment. Primary care providers can assess the stability of methadone maintenance patients by asking them how often they are required to attend treatment, as well as asking them the results of their recent urine toxicology tests. The patient should be advised to remain in treatment until their substance use has ceased and their medical, psychiatric, legal, family, and employment problems have stabilized. If methadone is tapered, it should be done slowly to avoid relapse.

Box 13
Treatments for opioid use disorders

Methadone

Full opioid agonist that may be used for opioid use disorder treatment only through specially licensed and accredited Opioid Treatment Programs, not through a physician prescription. Physicians may prescribe methadone for pain, although additional training specific to methadone is recommended because of increased risk of overdose when prescribed for pain. Starting doses for opioid use disorder are 10–40 mg daily and titrated every few days. Usual maintenance doses 80–120 mg daily. Requires daily observed dosing initially, but take-home doses are permitted after demonstration of stable recovery.

Buprenorphine/Naloxone

Partial opioid agonist that may be prescribed for opioid use disorder treatment by physicians who have completed a specific 8-hour course and obtained a federal waiver. Naloxone included to reduce intravenous abuse of buprenorphine, but is not absorbed if taken sublingually as directed. Dose range generally 8–24 mg daily. Induction requires tolerant patients to enter mild to moderate opioid withdrawal before the first dose. Similar drug use outcomes as methadone, but less effective at retaining patients in treatment. Primary care provision of buprenorphine in primary care involves development of protocols for screening, assessment, induction, monitoring, psychosocial treatment, termination, and referral.

Buprenorphine (mono)

Generally reserved for pregnant women, who have a higher risk if exposed to naloxone. Similar rates of neonatal abstinence syndrome in babies born to mothers on buprenorphine and methadone, but severity and duration of neonatal abstinence syndrome is lower with buprenorphine.[94]

Naltrexone

For opioid-use disorder, start 50 mg daily. Range 25–150 mg daily. Limited data of effectiveness in the United States, as adherence is low.[95] Will cause withdrawal in opioid-tolerant patients, so must be preceded by successful detoxification and a naloxone challenge test. Avoid in active hepatitis. Liver function tests should be checked at baseline and followed every few months after that. There is poor evidence supporting rapid opioid detoxification with naltrexone or naltrexone combined with anesthesia or heavy sedation.[47]

XR Naltrexone IM

380 mg every 4 weeks. Limited data support effectiveness for opioid use disorders, but adherence is improved. Similar issues as oral naltrexone. Nausea, fatigue, and injection site reactions common.

α-2 Adrenergic Agonists

Clonidine or other α-2 adrenergic agonists can relieve some opioid withdrawal symptoms, but are far less effective than agonist or partial agonist medications.

Naloxone with Overdose Education

Emerging harm reduction strategy to promote emergency lay administration of the opioid antagonist naloxone.[96,97] Provided to those at risk of opioid overdose and their families and friends. Education includes identification of opioid overdose and the appropriate responses, including rescue breathing, calling 911, and administration of naloxone (see stopoverdose.org).

Opioid Treatment programs can provide methadone only for the treatment of opioid use disorders and are not permitted to provide methadone for the treatment of pain. If a patient prescribed opioids for chronic pain is found to require treatment for opioid use disorder, he or she must seek treatment specifically for their substance use problem rather than requesting pain management from a methadone program. If a patient prescribed opioids for chronic pain is found to have a cocaine or methamphetamine problem, for instance, he or she may require admission to opioid use disorder treatment with methadone or buprenorphine if they cannot tolerate withdrawal of their opioids. Substance use disorder treatment programs that do not use methadone or buprenorphine will generally not admit patients with ongoing opioid or other controlled substance prescriptions.

Buprenorphine Treatment of Opioid Use Disorders

Buprenorphine is a partial opioid agonist that is effective for opioid use disorder treatment and can be prescribed in the medical setting by physicians who have completed a specific 8-hour training program and received a waiver from the federal government.[51] Federal legislation, the Drug Addiction Treatment Act of 2000, was required to allow integration of opioid use disorder treatment into medical settings for the first time, as well as outlining training and record keeping requirements, and limiting the number of patients a physician may treat at one time. Gaining knowledge and experience in opioid use disorder treatment with buprenorphine can greatly assist physicians in their management of opioid prescribing for chronic pain, and it is a gratifying form of treatment. Few treatments in primary care practice can have as much positive impact on patients' lives as buprenorphine for opioid use disorder.

Buprenorphine binds opioid receptors and activates them, but as the dose is raised, there is a ceiling effect, unlike full opioid agonists. This ceiling effect makes buprenorphine less prone to opioid overdose and thus safer than full agonists, but its activity at the opioid receptor is adequate to relieve opioid withdrawal even in highly tolerant patients. Buprenorphine also has very high affinity for opioid receptors, so that once it is on the receptor, other opioids are blocked. These features make buprenorphine an excellent choice for opioid use disorder treatment. The most commonly used form of buprenorphine in the United States also contains naloxone, which is included solely as an abuse deterrent, because it is not absorbed if the medication is taken as directed under the tongue. If a tolerant patient crushes and injects the combined buprenorphine/naloxone, the naloxone can precipitate opioid withdrawal. The high affinity of buprenorphine has implications for initiation of treatment, as patients must be in mild to moderate withdrawal before taking the first dose or risk precipitated withdrawal as buprenorphine displaces other opioids from the receptor and potentially reduces receptor activity. Scales assessing opioid withdrawal severity are available for use when inducing patients onto buprenorphine.[52]

Multiple comparative trials have tested the relative efficacy of buprenorphine and methadone and found comparable rates of drug use during treatment. However, meta-analyses of these trials found that methadone is more effective in retaining patients in treatment, a key outcome in addiction treatment.[53,54] No clear patient predictors of response to buprenorphine or methadone have been established, although patients needing more structure may benefit from a methadone program. For most patients seeking pharmacotherapy for the first time, the less restrictive structure of treatment in a physician office setting is preferred. Psychosocial services for patients on buprenorphine can consist of simple medication management and support, whereas higher levels of psychosocial treatment or cognitive behavioral therapy have not been shown more effective.[55–57]

The decision to undertake training to prescribe buprenorphine in a general medical setting requires understanding of the limitations of treatment as well as the profound benefits that can occur with successful treatment (see **Box 8**). Prescribers can choose to take on only patients within their practice who might benefit, due to a known opioid use disorder through having difficulty with opioid pain medications and being unable to successfully taper off. Providing effective treatment for opioid use disorders can be a lifesaving and positive clinical experience.

SUMMARY AND FUTURE DIRECTIONS

Addiction disorders are common in primary care settings and can have a major impact on treatment of medical problems, including chronic pain. Evidence-based screening, brief interventions, and pharmacotherapies are available for primary care providers and can improve patient outcomes. As physicians become experienced in prescribing pharmacotherapies for addiction disorders, integration of treatment of SUD into primary care settings will become more common and new models of providing medication and psychosocial services for these patients will need development. If successful, these models hold the promise of more integrated and effective treatment for patients with addiction disorders.

REFERENCES

1. Madras BK, Compton WM, Avula D, et al. Screening, brief interventions, referral to treatment (SBIRT) for illicit drug and alcohol use at multiple healthcare sites: comparison at intake and 6 months later. Drug Alcohol Depend 2009;99(1 3): 280–95.
2. Substance Abuse and Mental Helath Services Administration. Results from the 2011 National Survey on drug abuse and health: summary of national findings. Rockville (MD): 2012.
3. Merrill JO. Policy progress for physician treatment of opiate addiction. J Gen Intern Med 2002;17(5):361–8.
4. Miller PM, Thomas SE, Mallin R. Patient attitudes towards self-report and biomarker alcohol screening by primary care physicians. Alcohol Alcohol 2006;41(3):306–10.
5. Ray MK, Beach MC, Nicolaidis C, et al. Patient and provider comfort discussing substance use. Fam Med 2013;45(2):109–17.
6. Williams EC, Kivlahan DR, Saitz R, et al. Readiness to change in primary care patients who screened positive for alcohol misuse. Ann Fam Med 2006;4(3):213–20.
7. Moyer VA, Preventive Services Task Force. Screening and behavioral counseling interventions in primary care to reduce alcohol misuse: U.S. preventive services task force recommendation statement. Ann Intern Med 2013;159(3): 210–8.
8. Saitz R. Clinical practice. Unhealthy alcohol use. N Engl J Med 2005;352(6): 596–607.
9. Rubinsky AD, Kivlahan DR, Volk RJ, et al. Estimating risk of alcohol dependence using alcohol screening scores. Drug Alcohol Depend 2010;108(1–2):29–36.
10. Wilcox HC, Conner KR, Caine ED. Association of alcohol and drug use disorders and completed suicide: an empirical review of cohort studies. Drug Alcohol Depend 2004;76(Suppl):S11–9.
11. McLellan A, Lewis DC, O'Brien CP, et al. Drug dependence, a chronic medical illness: implications for treatment, insurance, and outcomes evaluation. JAMA 2000;284(13):1689–95.

12. Ballesteros J, Duffy JC, Querejeta I, et al. Efficacy of brief interventions for hazardous drinkers in primary care: systematic review and meta-analyses. Alcohol Clin Exp Res 2004;28(4):608–18.

13. Bertholet N, Daeppen JB, Wietlisbach V, et al. Reduction of alcohol consumption by brief alcohol intervention in primary care: systematic review and meta-analysis. Arch Intern Med 2005;165(9):986–95.

14. Fleming MF, Mundt MP, French MT, et al. Brief physician advice for problem drinkers: long-term efficacy and benefit-cost analysis. Alcohol Clin Exp Res 2002;26(1):36–43.

15. Jonas DE, Garbutt JC, Amick HR, et al. Behavioral counseling after screening for alcohol misuse in primary care: a systematic review and meta-analysis for the U.S. Preventive Services Task Force. Ann Intern Med 2012;157(9):645–54.

16. Saitz R. Alcohol screening and brief intervention in primary care: absence of evidence for efficacy in people with dependence or very heavy drinking. Drug Alcohol Rev 2010;29(6):631–40.

17. O'Connor MJ, Whaley SE. Brief intervention for alcohol use by pregnant women. Am J Public Health 2007;97(2):252–8.

18. Sullivan JT, Sykora K, Schneiderman J, et al. Assessment of alcohol withdrawal: the revised clinical institute withdrawal assessment for alcohol scale (CIWA-Ar). Br J Addict 1989;84(11):1353–7.

19. Blondell RD. Ambulatory detoxification of patients with alcohol dependence. Am Fam Physician 2005;71(3):495–502.

20. Mayo-Smith MF. Pharmacological management of alcohol withdrawal. A meta-analysis and evidence-based practice guideline. American Society of Addiction Medicine Working Group on pharmacological management of alcohol withdrawal. JAMA 1997;278(2):144–51.

21. Daeppen JB, Gache P, Landry U, et al. Symptom-triggered vs fixed-schedule doses of benzodiazepine for alcohol withdrawal: a randomized treatment trial. Arch Intern Med 2002;162(10):1117–21.

22. Myrick H, Malcolm R, Randall PK, et al. A double-blind trial of gabapentin versus lorazepam in the treatment of alcohol withdrawal. Alcohol Clin Exp Res 2009; 33(9):1582–8.

23. Stock CJ, Carpenter L, Ying J, et al. Gabapentin versus chlordiazepoxide for outpatient alcohol detoxification treatment. Ann Pharmacother 2013;47(7–8): 961–9.

24. Anton RF, O'Malley SS, Ciraulo DA, et al. Combined pharmacotherapies and behavioral interventions for alcohol dependence: the COMBINE study: a randomized controlled trial. JAMA 2006;295(17):2003–17.

25. Garbutt JC, Kranzler HR, O'Malley SS, et al. Efficacy and tolerability of long-acting injectable naltrexone for alcohol dependence: a randomized controlled trial. JAMA 2005;293(13):1617–25.

26. Rosner S, Hackl-Herrwerth A, Leucht S, et al. Opioid antagonists for alcohol dependence. Cochrane Database Syst Rev 2010;(12):CD001867.

27. Rosner S, Hackl-Herrwerth A, Leucht S, et al. Acamprosate for alcohol dependence. Cochrane Database Syst Rev 2010;(9):CD004332.

28. Skinner MD, Lahmek P, Pham H, et al. Disulfiram efficacy in the treatment of alcohol dependence: a meta-analysis. PLoS One 2014;9(2):e87366.

29. Mason BJ, Quello S, Goodell V, et al. Gabapentin treatment for alcohol dependence: a randomized clinical trial. JAMA Intern Med 2014;174(1):70–7.

30. Boudreau D, Von Korff M, Rutter CM, et al. Trends in long-term opioid therapy for chronic non-cancer pain. Pharmacoepidemiol Drug Saf 2009;18(12):1166–75.

31. Sullivan MD, Edlund MJ, Fan MY, et al. Trends in use of opioids for non-cancer pain conditions 2000-2005 in commercial and Medicaid insurance plans: the TROUP study. Pain 2008;138(2):440–9.
32. Ballantyne JC, Mao J. Opioid therapy for chronic pain. N Engl J Med 2003; 349(20):1943–53.
33. Hall AJ, Logan JE, Toblin RL, et al. Patterns of abuse among unintentional pharmaceutical overdose fatalities. JAMA 2008;300(22):2613–20.
34. McCabe SE, Cranford JA, West BT. Trends in prescription drug abuse and dependence, co-occurrence with other substance use disorders, and treatment utilization: results from two national surveys. Addict Behav 2008;33(10): 1297–305.
35. Paulozzi LJ, Xi Y. Recent changes in drug poisoning mortality in the United States by urban-rural status and by drug type. Pharmacoepidemiol Drug Saf 2008;17(10):997–1005.
36. Nuckols TK, Anderson L, Popescu I, et al. Opioid prescribing: a systematic review and critical appraisal of guidelines for chronic pain. Ann Intern Med 2014; 160:38–47.
37. Noble M, Treadwell JR, Tregear SJ, et al. Long-term opioid management for chronic noncancer pain. Cochrane Database Syst Rev 2010;(1):CD006605.
38. Washington State Agency Medical Directors' Group. Interagency Guideline on Opioid Dosing for Chronic Non-Cancer Pain: An Educational Aid to Improve Care and Safety With Opioid Therapy. Olympia, WA: Washington State Agency Medical Directors' Group; 2010. Available at: http://www.agencymeddirectors. wa.gov/opioiddosing.aspf. Accessed June 27, 2014.
39. Merrill JO, Rhodes LA, Deyo RA, et al. Mutual mistrust in the medical care of drug users: the keys to the "narc" cabinet. J Gen Intern Med 2002;17(5):327–33.
40. Banta-Green CJ, Von Korff M, Sullivan MD, et al. The prescribed opioids difficulties scale: a patient-centered assessment of problems and concerns. Clin J Pain 2010;26(6):489–97.
41. Gourlay DL, Heit HA, Almahrezi A. Universal precautions in pain medicine: a rational approach to the treatment of chronic pain. Pain Med 2005;6(2):107–12.
42. Sullivan MD. Collaborative Opioid Prescribing Education - Risk Evaluation and Mitigation Strategy (COPE-REMS). 2013. Available at: http://www.trainingxchange. org/our-programs/cope-rems. Accessed February 12, 2014.
43. Sullivan MD, Gaster B, Russo J, et al. Randomized trial of web-based training about opioid therapy for chronic pain. Clin J Pain 2010;26(6):512–7.
44. Sullivan MD, Leigh J, Gaster B. Brief report: training internists in shared decision making about chronic opioid treatment for noncancer pain. J Gen Intern Med 2006;21(4):360–2.
45. Smith PC, Schmidt SM, Allensworth-Davies D, et al. A single-question screening test for drug use in primary care. Arch Intern Med 2010;170(13):1155–60.
46. Banta-Green CJ, Merrill JO, Doyle SR, et al. Measurement of opioid problems among chronic pain patients in a general medical population. Drug Alcohol Depend 2009;104(1–2):43–9.
47. O'Connor PG, Kosten TR. Rapid and ultrarapid opioid detoxification techniques. JAMA 1998;279(3):229–34.
48. Fullerton CA, Kim M, Thomas CP, et al. Medication-assisted treatment with methadone: assessing the evidence. Psychiatr Serv 2014;65(2):146–57.
49. Sees KL, Delucchi KL, Masson C, et al. Methadone maintenance vs 180-day psychosocially enriched detoxification for treatment of opioid dependence: a randomized controlled trial. JAMA 2000;283(10):1303–10.

50. Saxon AJ, Wells EA, Fleming C, et al. Pre-treatment characteristics, program philosophy and level of ancillary services as predictors of methadone maintenance treatment outcome. Addiction 1996;91(8):1197–209.

51. Substance Abuse and Mental Health Services Administration. Buprenorphine. 2014. Available at: www.buprenorphine.samhsa.gov. Accessed April 10, 2014.

52. Wesson DR, Ling W. The clinical opiate withdrawal scale (COWS). J Psychoactive Drugs 2003;35(2):253–9.

53. Mattick RP, Kimber J, Breen C, et al. Buprenorphine maintenance versus placebo or methadone maintenance for opioid dependence. Cochrane Database Syst Rev 2003;(2):CD002207.

54. Thomas CP, Fullerton CA, Kim M, et al. Medication-assisted treatment with buprenorphine: assessing the evidence. Psychiatr Serv 2014;65(2):158–70.

55. Ling W, Hillhouse M, Ang A, et al. Comparison of behavioral treatment conditions in buprenorphine maintenance. Addiction 2013;108(10):1788–98.

56. Fiellin DA, Barry DT, Sullivan LE, et al. A randomized trial of cognitive behavioral therapy in primary care-based buprenorphine. Am J Med 2013;126(1): 74.e11–7.

57. Weiss RD, Potter JS, Fiellin DA, et al. Adjunctive counseling during brief and extended buprenorphine-naloxone treatment for prescription opioid dependence: a 2-phase randomized controlled trial. Arch Gen Psychiatry 2011; 68(12):1238–46.

58. National Institute on Alcohol Abuse and Alcoholism. Helping patients who drink too much: a practitioner's guide. 2005. Available at: http://pubs.niaaa.nih.gov/publications/Practitioner/CliniciansGuide2005/clinicians_guide.htm. Accessed June 27, 2014.

59. Smith PC, Schmidt SM, Allensworth-Davies D, et al. Primary care validation of a single-question alcohol screening test. J Gen Intern Med 2009;24(7):783–8.

60. Bush K, Kivlahan DR, McDonell MB, et al. The AUDIT alcohol consumption questions (AUDIT-C): an effective brief screening test for problem drinking. Ambulatory Care Quality Improvement Project (ACQUIP). Alcohol Use Disorders Identification Test. Arch Intern Med 1998;158(16):1789–95.

61. Bradley KA, DeBenedetti AF, Volk RJ, et al. AUDIT-C as a brief screen for alcohol misuse in primary care. Alcohol Clin Exp Res 2007;31(7):1208–17.

62. Fiellin DA, Reid MC, O'Connor PG. Screening for alcohol problems in primary care: a systematic review. Arch Intern Med 2000;160(13):1977–89.

63. Yudko E, Lozhkina O, Fouts A. A comprehensive review of the psychometric properties of the Drug Abuse Screening Test. J Subst Abuse Treat 2007;32(2):189–98.

64. Chang G, Wilkins-Haug L, Berman S, et al. Alcohol use and pregnancy: improving identification. Obstet Gynecol 1998;91(6):892–8.

65. Burns E, Gray R, Smith LA. Brief screening questionnaires to identify problem drinking during pregnancy: a systematic review. Addiction 2010;105(4):601–14.

66. Chiodo LM, Sokol RJ, Delaney-Black V, et al. Validity of the T-ACE in pregnancy in predicting child outcome and risk drinking. Alcohol 2010;44(7–8): 595–603.

67. American College of Obstetrtitions and Gynecologists, Committee on Health Care for Underserved Women. Committee opinion no. 496: at-risk drinking and alcohol dependence: obstetric and gynecologic implications. Obstet Gynecol 2011;118(2 Pt 1):383–8.

68. Chasnoff IJ, Wells AM, McGourty RF, et al. Validation of the 4P's Plus screen for substance use in pregnancy validation of the 4P's Plus. J Perinatol 2007;27(12): 744–8.

69. Chang G, Orav EJ, Jones JA, et al. Self-reported alcohol and drug use in pregnant young women: a pilot study of associated factors and identification. J Addict Med 2011;5(3):221–6.
70. National Institute on Alcohol Abuse and Alcoholism. Alcohol screening and brief intervention for youth: a practitioner's guide. Rockville (MD): National Institutes of Health; 2011.
71. Fleming MF, Barry KL, Manwell LB, et al. Brief physician advice for problem alcohol drinkers. A randomized controlled trial in community-based primary care practices. JAMA 1997;277(13):1039–45.
72. Jonas DE, Garbutt JC, Brown JM, et al. Screening, behavioral counseling, and referral in primary care to reduce alcohol misuse. Rockville (MD): Agency for Healthcare Research and Quality (US); 2012.
73. Miller WR, Rollnick S. Motivational interviewing: helping people change. 3rd edition. New York: Guilford Press; 2013.
74. Denning P, Little J. Practicing harm reduction psychotherapy: an alternative approach to addictions. 2nd edition. New York: Guilford Press; 2012.
75. Magill M, Ray LA. Cognitive-behavioral treatment with adult alcohol and illicit drug users: a meta-analysis of randomized controlled trials. J Stud Alcohol Drugs 2009;70(4):516–27.
76. Ouimette PC, Finney JW, Moos RH. Twelve-step and cognitive–behavioral treatment for substance abuse: a comparison of treatment effectiveness. J Consult Clin Psychol 1997;65(2):230–40.
77. Johnson BA, Rosenthal N, Capece JA, et al. Topiramate for treating alcohol dependence: a randomized controlled trial. JAMA 2007;298(14):1641–51.
78. Bohnert AS, Valenstein M, Bair MJ, et al. Association between opioid prescribing patterns and opioid overdose-related deaths. JAMA 2011;305(13):1315–21.
79. Dunn KM, Saunders KW, Rutter CM, et al. Opioid prescriptions for chronic pain and overdose: a cohort study. Ann Intern Med 2009;152(2):85–92.
80. Gomes T, Mamdani MM, Dhalla IA, et al. Opioid dose and drug-related mortality in patients with nonmalignant pain. Arch Intern Med 2011;171(7):686–91.
81. Saunders KW, Dunn KM, Merrill JO, et al. Relationship of opioid use and dosage levels to fractures in older chronic pain patients. J Gen Intern Med 2009;25(4):310–5.
82. Sullivan MD, Edlund MJ, Fan MY, et al. Risks for possible and probable opioid misuse among recipients of chronic opioid therapy in commercial and Medicaid insurance plans: The TROUP Study. Pain 2010;150(2):332–9.
83. Edlund MJ, Martin BC, Fan MY, et al. Risks for opioid abuse and dependence among recipients of chronic opioid therapy: results from the TROUP study. Drug Alcohol Depend 2010;112(1–2):90–8.
84. Braden JB, Russo JE, Fan MY, et al. Emergency department visits among recipients of chronic opioid therapy. Arch Intern Med 2010;170(16):1425–32.
85. Braden JB, Sullivan MD, Ray GT, et al. Trends in long-term opioid therapy for noncancer pain among persons with a history of depression. Gen Hosp Psychiatry 2009;31(6):564–70.
86. Edlund MJ, Martin BC, Devries A, et al. Trends in use of opioids for chronic noncancer pain among individuals with mental health and substance use disorders: the TROUP study. Clin J Pain 2010;26(1):1–8.
87. Edlund MJ, Martin BC, Fan MY, et al. An analysis of heavy utilizers of opioids for chronic noncancer pain in the TROUP study. J Pain Symptom Manage 2009;40(2):279–89.

88. Morasco BJ, Duckart JP, Carr TP, et al. Clinical characteristics of veterans pre-scribed high doses of opioid medications for chronic non-cancer pain. Pain 2010;151(3):625–32.
89. Weisner CM, Campbell CI, Ray GT, et al. Trends in prescribed opioid therapy for non-cancer pain for individuals with prior substance use disorders. Pain 2009; 145(3):287–93.
90. Merrill JO, Von Korff M, Banta-Green CJ, et al. Prescribed opioid difficulties, depression and opioid dose among chronic opioid therapy patients. Gen Hosp Psychiatry 2012;34(6):581–7.
91. Sullivan MD. Who gets high-dose opioid therapy for chronic non-cancer pain? Pain 2010;151(3):567–8.
92. Webster LR, Webster RM. Predicting aberrant behaviors in opioid-treated pa-tients: preliminary validation of the opioid risk tool. Pain Med 2005;6(6):432–42.
93. Turk DC, Swanson KS, Gatchel RJ. Predicting opioid misuse by chronic pain pa-tients: a systematic review and literature synthesis. Clin J Pain 2008;24(6): 497–508.
94. Jones HE, Kaltenbach K, Heil SH, et al. Neonatal abstinence syndrome after methadone or buprenorphine exposure. N Engl J Med 2010;363(24):2320–31.
95. Minozzi S, Amato L, Vecchi S, et al. Oral naltrexone maintenance treatment for opioid dependence. Cochrane Database Syst Rev 2006;(1):CD001333.
96. Beletsky L, Rich JD, Walley AY. Prevention of fatal opioid overdose. JAMA 2012; 308(18):1863–4.
97. Bowman S, Eiserman J, Beletsky L, et al. Reducing the health consequences of opioid addiction in primary care. Am J Med 2013;126(7):565–71.

Psychiatric Disorders and Sleep Issues

Eliza L. Sutton, MD

KEYWORDS

- Anxiety • Cognitive-behavioral therapy for insomnia • Depression • Insomnia
- Restless leg syndrome • Circadian rhythm disorders • Obstructive sleep apnea

KEY POINTS

- Sleep issues and psychiatric disorders commonly coexist and can influence each other (eg, insomnia and depression).
- Medications for psychiatric disorders can affect sleep and sleep disorders, particularly restless legs syndrome, positively or negatively.
- Medications for sleep disorders can cause or affect psychiatric symptoms (eg, dopamine agonists given for treatment of restless legs syndrome can cause gambling or other compulsive behaviors).
- Cognitive-behavioral therapy for insomnia in 4 to 8 sessions is the preferred treatment of chronic insomnia if acceptable to the patient and accessible.
- For depressed patients with insomnia, a sleep-promoting medication may be useful as adjunct therapy (zolpidem, eszopiclone, trazodone, or amitriptyline) or as monotherapy (mirtazapine, nefazodone, or trazodone).

INTRODUCTION

Psychiatric disorders and sleep problems are both common, with an estimated prevalence in 12 months of about 30% for any of the *Diagnostic and Statistical Manual of Mental Disorders, Fourth Edition* (DSM-IV) disorders[1] and about 30% for insomnia experienced at least a few days a week for at least a month (as part of a greater but less well-determined prevalence for all types of sleep issues).[2] Psychiatric and sleep problems overlap significantly and are related. Insomnia, for example, correlates with likelihood of having at least 1 psychiatric diagnosis with an odds ratio of 5.0 for severe insomnia, 2.6 for moderate insomnia, and 1.7 for mild insomnia.[3]

In this review article, the neurobiology of the sleep/wake states and mental health and observed associations between selected psychiatric disorders and sleep issues

Disclosure: No financial relationships to disclose.
Department of Medicine, University of Washington, 4245 Roosevelt Way Northeast, Box 354765, Seattle, WA 98105, USA
E-mail address: esutton@uw.edu

Med Clin N Am 98 (2014) 1123–1143
http://dx.doi.org/10.1016/j.mcna.2014.06.009

(**Table 1**) are described, and treatment considerations relevant to primary care (**Tables 2** and **3**) are presented.

NEUROBIOLOGY COMMON TO SLEEP, WAKEFULNESS, AND MENTAL HEALTH

Although the purposes and mechanisms of sleep are not truly known, sleep is clearly crucial to optimal functioning of the brain. Insufficient quantity or quality of sleep affects alertness, hormone regulation, memory formation, emotional regulation, executive function, and multiple facets of behavior. Multiple experiments subjecting small groups of healthy people to total sleep deprivation for a night or 2 have shown myriad specific impairments. In the area of emotional regulation, those findings include increase in symptoms of psychopathology (depression, anxiety, paranoia, and somatic complaints),[69] reduction in the physical expression of emotion,[70] and impairment in the ability to recognize emotion in others.[71]

In observational studies, psychiatric conditions are associated with alterations in sleep architecture,[72] although the direction of the effect and its importance are not known. However, there is increasing evidence that basic brain functions regulating sleep and wake play a role in psychiatric disorders. For example, alterations in the circadian pattern of release of the wake-promoting neurotransmitter orexin may contribute to hypersomnia and insomnia in depression.[73] Narcolepsy, well known as *the* condition of orexin deficiency, is associated with a roughly 2.5-fold higher risk of psychiatric disorder, including major depressive disorder (MDD) and social anxiety disorder.[12]

The association between sleep problems and affective disorders may be rooted at the genetic level. Circadian clock gene polymorphisms seem to be associated with mood regulation and affective disorders,[74,75] with blunting of the normal circadian pattern of gene expression in certain areas of the brain, including the limbic system, in people with MDD.[76] An orexin receptor antagonist is currently in phase 3 trials for treatment of insomnia, and other orexin receptor antagonists are being studied in animals for potential therapeutic effect in anxiety disorders and in compulsive behaviors, including eating and addiction.[77]

The remainder of this review focuses on observations in populations and in clinical studies, beginning with insomnia as the most common sleep issue and the one most commonly associated with psychiatric disorders, then considering specific types of psychiatric disorders in more depth.

INSOMNIA: STATE OF THE ART

Insomnia, the most common sleep problem, has been the target of research and reconsideration. In the most recent sleep medicine and psychiatric clinical diagnostic manuals, the distinction of persistent insomnia as primary versus secondary (eg, secondary to psychiatric or medical conditions) has largely been removed. DSM-5, released in 2013, gives "insomnia disorder" for persistent insomnia not completely explained by any coexisting mental disorders.[78] Similarly, the *International Classification of Sleep Disorders, Third Edition*,[79] released in 2014, introduced "chronic insomnia disorder" to replace the multiple subtypes of chronic insomnia described in previous classifications, including insomnia coexisting with psychiatric conditions. In each case, an important criterion is that another sleep disorder such as restless legs syndrome (RLS), sleep apnea, or a circadian rhythm disorder does not better explain the sleep impairment; those conditions, although often experienced as insomnia by the patient, are distinct sleep disorders, each with specific treatment approaches.[80]

For chronic insomnia not explained by another sleep disorder, cognitive-behavioral therapy for insomnia (CBTI) is considered to be the preferred treatment. CBTI has

Table 1
Observed associations between selected psychiatric disorders and sleep disorders

	Insomnia or Nonspecific Disrupted Sleep	Circadian Rhythm Disorder	Restless Leg Syndrome	Obstructive Sleep Apnea	Narcolepsy	Sleep Paralysis	Sleepwalking
Depressive disorders	A[4], B[5], S[6]	A[7]	A[8], B[9], PM[25]	A[10,11], M	A[12], S[12]	A[13]	A[14], PM[14]
Anxiety disorders	A[4,15–17], P[4], M	A (for OCD)[16,18]	M	A[10]	A[12]	A[19,20]	A (for OCD)[14], PM[14]
Posttraumatic stress disorder	A[21], B[22]				A[12]	A[23]	
Schizophrenia	A[24]	A[24]	PM[25,26]	PM[27]	S[28], M[29]		PM[30]
Suicidality	A[31–33]						
Attention-deficit/ hyperactivity disorder	PM	A[34]	A[35]	A in children[36] Not adults[37]			
Impulse control disorders			SM[33]				

Abbreviations: A, association observed; B, bidirectional association observed; M, sleep condition can mimic psychiatric condition; OCD, obsessive-compulsive disorder; P, psychiatric condition precedes sleep condition; PM, psychiatric medication causes or worsens sleep condition; S, sleep condition precedes psychiatric condition; SM, sleep medication causes or worsens psychiatric condition.

Table 2
Treatment approaches for insomnia in depression

Therapy	Effect on Sleep	Other Observations
CBT for depression without specific insomnia treatment	Improvement in sleep with improvement in depression, similar to pharmacologic antidepressant therapy[39]	
CBTI without specific depression treatment	Improvement in sleep is similar for people with high and low depression scores[40]	Beck Depression Index scores improve (with sleep item removed), including suicidality, vs control[40]
CBTI + SSRI	On escitalopram, insomnia remitted in 50% with CBTI vs 8% with sleep hygiene and other control therapy[41]	On escitalopram, depression remitted in 62% with CBTI vs 33% with sleep hygiene and other control therapy[41]
Exercise + SSRI	Mixed results: Sleep improved with exercise (16 kcal/kg/wk for 12 wk)[42] Sleep did not improve overall with exercise (45 min 3 times/wk × 16 wk, target heart rate 70%–85% of maximum for 30 min/session). Subset showed trend toward improvement early in study[43]	Depression improved more with exercise for those who had hypersomnia at baseline[42]
SSRI, SNRI	Insomnia occurs as an emergent symptom, can be moderately severe,[44] is more likely in those whose depression response is delayed beyond 6 wk[45]	
Bupropion	More improvement in fatigue and hypersomnolence on bupropion than on SSRI or placebo (no comment on effect on sleep)[46]	
SSRI + zolpidem	Improved sleep on SSRIs and zolpidem 10 mg.[47] Improved sleep and next-day functioning on escitalopram and zolpidem CR 12.5 mg[48]	No difference in depression outcome up to 24 wk[48]. FDA has advised starting dose should not exceed zolpidem 5 mg or zolpidem CR 6.25 mg for women and suggested these doses for men[49]

SSRI + eszopiclone	Improved sleep on eszopiclone 3 mg in titated with fluoxetine, maintained over 8 wk.[50] Improvement maintained over 2 wk after discontinuation of eszopiclone[51]	On fluoxetine, depression scores improved faster and more with eszopiclone than placebo[50] and did not relapse with discontinuation of eszopiclone after 2 wk[51]; FDA has advised eszopiclone starting dose should not exceed 1 mg in women and men[53]
SSRI + quetiapine	Improvement in insomnia seen early on quetiapine[54]	No difference in improvement in moods on quetiapine.[54] Can cause metabolic syndrome[55,56]
St John's wort + zolpidem	St John's wort reduces zolpidem levels to a variable degree, combined use not advised[52]	
Antidepressant + trazodone	Substantial improvement in antidepressant-associated insomnia[57,58] at trazodone 25–100 mg	
Trazodone monotherapy	Effective solo or as adjunct for depression[59]	Once-daily extended-release form may improve tolerability[59]
Mirtazapine monotherapy	Improves sleep more than paroxetine or venlafaxine; sedation is similar to amitriptyline; sleep effects may be better at mirtazapine doses ≤30 mg[60]	Effect may be more rapid than SSRIs, and is greater than venlafaxine.[61] Commonly causes weight gain
Nefazodone monotherapy	Sleep improved early on nefazodone vs worsening on paroxetine[62] and on fluoxetine[63]; differences minimal by 8 wk[62,63]	Can cause hepatotoxicity

Abbreviations: CBT, cognitive-behavioral therapy; CBTI, CBT for insomnia; FDA, US Food and Drug Administration; SNRI, serotonin-norepinephrine reuptake inhibitor; SSRI, serotonin reuptake inhibitor.

Table 3
Effect of psychiatric medications on selected common sleep disorders

	RLS	OSA	Sleepwalking or Sleep-Related Eating
Antidepressant: Bupropion	Does not worsen, and may improve, RLS[64]		
Antidepressant: Mirtazapine	Causes RLS in 28% of patients[65]		
Antidepressants: SSRIs	Associated with 3-fold increase in RLS risk[66]		
Antidepressants: SSRIs and SNRIs	Causes RLS in 9% of patients[65]		
Antidepressants: SSRIs and SNRIs			Associated with 3-fold increase in risk of sleepwalking[14]
First-generation antipsychotics (neuroleptics)	People with RLS may be at increased risk of developing akathisia from dopamine antagonists[67]		
Atypical antipsychotics: Aripiprazole	Possibly causes RLS[25] but several case reports suggest, instead, improvement in RLS		
Atypical antipsychotics: Clozapine Olanzapine Quetiapine Risperidone	Case reports of RLS, most with quetiapine (especially in conjunction with antidepressants)[26]		
Atypical antipsychotics		Nearly 2-fold increase risk of severe OSA after adjustment for factors, including body mass index[27]	
Atypical antipsychotics			Reported association with sleepwalking[30]
Atypical antipsychotics: Quetiapine			Reported to cause sleep-related eating disorder[68]

Abbreviations: OSA, obstructive sleep apnea; SNRI, serotonin-norepinephrine reuptake inhibitor; SSRI, serotonin reuptake inhibitor.

been shown to be more effective after 4 to 8 once-weekly sessions than sleep medication and to have subjective benefit persisting well after the intervention.[81,82] In addition, it is effective in patients with psychiatric disorders.[83] CBTI has similar efficacy for insomnia in people with low and high scores on the Beck Depression Inventory, although those who are more depressed may be less likely to follow some of the behavioral steps.[40] In people with insomnia, CBTI can improve the Beck Depression score, including the item on suicidal ideation, without antidepressant medication,[40] and in 1 study,[41] it significantly improved the response of MDD to escitalopram. CBTI may be effective for insomnia in depression in as few as 2 sessions.[84]

CBTI cannot be provided on an individual basis to everyone who might benefit, and therefore the sleep medicine community is exploring[85] and testing[86] stepped-care models, in which the first step would be accessed as general information or self-help by the patient (eg, via the tested approaches of a computer-based or printed resource). Individual therapy by psychologists would be reserved as the highest step, for the subset who need (or want) a more intensive or personalized approach.

Pharmacologic treatment of insomnia is also a reasonable approach and one used more commonly than CBTI, because of availability, familiarity, and patient or physician preference. Medication treatment of insomnia would ideally be reserved for relatively short-term use at the lowest dose effective for that patient, because medications pose potential risks, and the long-term efficacy and safety of hypnotic medications are not well known. Zolpidem and eszopiclone are the preferred medications for insomnia in the absence of a contraindication such as sleepwalking (a marker for increased risk of sleep-related activities on these medications, although other medications have also been linked with this effect [see **Table 3**]). Zolpidem and eszopiclone measurably (although not markedly) improve sleep subjectively and objectively and are not associated with respiratory depression, dose escalation, or withdrawal. The US Food and Drug Administration (FDA) has warned that "all drugs taken for insomnia can impair driving and activities that require alertness the morning after use,"[49] and it announced changes in labeling for zolpidem in 2013[49] and for eszopiclone in 2014,[53] with changes in labeling for other medications potentially to follow.[49,53] Based on findings that morning levels of these drugs may be increased and impair functions such as driving even if the person feels alert, the new labeling advises initial prescribing of the lowest strength for zolpidem, zolpidem CR, and eszopiclone, with allowance for consideration of higher doses of zolpidem in men, and of either medication in anyone who has had insufficient benefit on the lower dose.[49,53] Treatment of insomnia beyond these considerations is discussed specifically in the section on depression and in **Table 2**.

INSOMNIA AND PSYCHIATRIC ILLNESS

Several epidemiologic studies have reported a strong association between insomnia and any psychiatric disorder. In a large multinational European study,[4] 18% of the population reported insomnia of 6 months' duration or longer, and of those, 26% had a past psychiatric disorder and 48% had a current psychiatric disorder using DSM-IV criteria. In contrast, only 8% of people without insomnia had any history of past psychiatric disorder. Current severe insomnia, chronic insomnia not explained by a medical or psychiatric condition, and insomnia related to a medical condition each had an odds ratio just less than 6 for having a past psychiatric history. Insomnia was severe in 45% of people with comorbid MDD and anxiety disorder, in 34% in people meeting criteria for a single psychiatric disorder, and in 21% for those meeting criteria for insomnia disorder (without another mental health disorder). Among a subset of people surveyed for the National Institute of Mental Health (NIMH) Epidemiologic Catchment Area project,[87] 40% of people with insomnia and 47% of those with excessive sleepiness were found to have a psychiatric disorder using DSM-III criteria, as opposed to 16% of those with no sleep issues.

Insomnia may be a residual symptom of psychiatric illness, but may also precede it. The evidence for a temporal relationship is discussed in the sections on depressive disorders and anxiety disorders.

Insomnia and other sleep problems may be associated not only with the presence of a psychiatric disorder but with its severity or manifestations. In patients admitted to a forensic psychiatry hospital, chronic insomnia and other sleep problems were associated with greater aggression, hostility, and impulsiveness and reduced tolerance for frustrations.[88]

Sleep difficulties, particularly insomnia, have been well correlated with suicidality, including in adolescents. Even in the absence of a known psychiatric disorder, disturbances in sleep are associated with a significant increase in completed suicide.[31] In people with MDD and insomnia, the severity of insomnia correlates with severity of suicidal ideation.[32] Patients with depression, posttraumatic stress disorder (PTSD), or panic disorder who experience difficulties with sleep are at roughly 3-fold higher risk for suicidal behavior than patients with those conditions whose sleep is not impaired; for people with schizophrenia, the risk may be even higher.[33]

DEPRESSIVE DISORDERS AND BIPOLAR DISORDER

Derangement of sleep or wakefulness is a cardinal symptom of, and diagnostic criterion of, MDD and bipolar disorder. However, sleep problems are not only symptoms or sequelae of depression; the associations are more complex. Several sleep problems have been associated with increased risk of depression.

Sleep Deprivation

Sleep deprivation increases the risk for subsequent depression[89]; however, total sleep deprivation has also shown benefit as part of a therapeutic approach to depression in MDD[90] and bipolar disorder.[91] Regulation of rapid eye movement (REM) sleep may be particularly germane to the development and treatment of depression, although the role of the observed effect of REM suppression by many antidepressants is unclear.[92]

Insomnia

The best characterized association between sleep problems and psychiatric disorders is between insomnia and both depression and anxiety; anxiety is discussed later. Insomnia is not only a common symptom of depression but also predisposes to (or at least precedes) depression, is a common emergent symptom with treatment, and may perpetuate depression.[93]

Insomnia has a well-described bidirectional association with depression.[5] In the large multinational European study mentioned earlier,[4] among those with insomnia and a mood disorder, the insomnia was present before the mood disorder 41% of the time, appeared with onset of the mood disorder 29% of the time, and appeared after onset of the mood disorder 29% of the time. Chronic insomnia predicted an at least 2-fold increase in risk for subsequent depression occurring a year or more later in a meta-analysis of 21 longitudinal studies,[6] including 1 study that reported doubling of risk over the subsequent 3 to 4 decades.[94]

Insomnia and sleep disturbances persist after initiation of treatment of depression in about 50% of people[95] and can also emerge as a new symptom after initiation of antidepressant therapy.[44] Sleep disturbance predicts relapse in depression[43] and may contribute to treatment resistance. Insomnia commonly presages relapse or recurrence of depression.[96,97]

There are limited data to suggest that insomnia treatment improves the outcome of the depression, but moderate to severe insomnia should be treated in depression to reduce the patient's suffering.

Medications (FDA-approved hypnotics as well as sedating psychiatric medications used off-label for insomnia) are commonly prescribed to improve the sleep experience during treatment, particularly in the initial phase, and CBTI is also effective (see **Table 2**). Approaches for treating a patient with insomnia and depression include initiating:

- Antidepressant therapy with a selective serotonin reuptake inhibitor (SSRI) or serotonin-norepinephrine reuptake inhibitor (SNRI) or bupropion without additional therapy for insomnia, anticipating that sleep will improve when the depression improves (a reasonable approach when insomnia is mild and tolerable)
- Antidepressant therapy with an SSRI or SNRI or bupropion, plus also a sleep-promoting hypnotic or adjunct antidepressant medication for use until depression and insomnia improve
- Antidepressant therapy with an SSRI, SNRI, or bupropion, plus also nonmedication treatment of insomnia as CBTI over 4 to 8 weeks
- Antidepressant monotherapy with a sleep-promoting agent (mirtazapine, trazodone, nefazodone, or a sedating tricyclic antidepressant)

The sleep-promoting antidepressants have an antagonistic effect at $5-HT_2$ receptors or histamine receptors (trazodone, nefazodone, mirtazapine, amitriptyline, imipramine, and nortriptyline). These antidepressants can be effective for insomnia in depression, as can the benzodiazepine receptor agonists zolpidem and eszopiclone. Paroxetine, although sedating, results in more sleep disruption in the first 2 weeks of therapy than does nefazodone.[62]

Excessive daytime sedation is not uncommon as a side effect of any medium-acting to long-acting sedating medication taken at bedtime for sleep; besides being unpleasant for the patient, this sedation poses risk for injury. As discussed earlier, the FDA has warned that zolpidem levels can be sufficient to impair function such as driving the next morning even if the patient does not feel sleepy, particularly in women or at higher doses or with the extended-release form, and other medications taken for insomnia can also affect safe functioning of a motor vehicle.[49]

If acceptable to the patient and accessible, CBTI is the preferred approach for chronic insomnia, including insomnia associated with psychiatric disorders, given its relatively robust subjective effect after 4 to 8 sessions. CBTI has been shown to improve depression scores and even suicidal ideation in people with insomnia[40] but should not be first line for the treatment of a mood disorder.

Circadian Rhythm Disorders

Advanced sleep phase syndrome (ASPS), a circadian rhythm disorder in which affected people fall asleep early and wake early compared with social norms and light cycles, can be readily mistaken for depression, because early morning awakening is inherent to ASPS, and an early bedtime can restrict opportunities for social engagement. ASPS occurs uncommonly as a familial condition and also occurs with aging.

Delayed sleep phase syndrome (DSPS), a circadian rhythm disorder in which affected people fall asleep later and wake later compared with social norms and light cycles, is more common than ASPS. It can be genetic, or the same delayed sleep/wake pattern can occur as a result of habit or, perhaps, as a result of a psychiatric disorder. Delayed sleep phase is more common in adolescents with bipolar disorder with depressed mood and in MDD than in control individuals.[7]

Bright light therapy is a fundamental treatment of seasonal affective disorder and may have some benefit in other depressive disorders, although mania or hypomania is a risk in people with bipolar disorder.[98,99] Light therapy is also a cornerstone in the treatment of circadian rhythm disorders, for which the circadian timing of the exposure to light is key. Light exposure should be soon after awakening for DSPS and near the end of the day for ASPS.

RLS

RLS, experienced by 5% to 15% of the general population, also shows a bidirectional association with depression.[8] Prospective evaluation of women in the Nurses Health Study found that those who reported physician-diagnosed RLS but no depressive symptoms at baseline were at 1.5-fold greater risk for being diagnosed with depression in the subsequent 6 years than those without a diagnosis of RLS.[9] The same investigators performed a meta-analysis of all published studies of RLS and depression, calculating a pooled odds ratio of about 2.3 for the association.

RLS can be mistaken for agitation or for medication-induced akathisia, from which it can be distinguished by localization (most commonly experienced in the legs, rather than being described as a whole-body sensation or inner restlessness), its association with an urge to move and relief from movement, and its nocturnal timing.[100]

Treatment of moderate to severe RLS with a dopamine agonist can improve depressive symptoms,[101] and withdrawal of dopamine agonist therapy given for RLS has been reported to trigger major depression.[102] Adding complexity to this interrelationship, RLS can also be a common side effect of pharmacologic therapy for depressive disorders and bipolar disorder (see **Table 3**).

Obstructive Sleep Apnea

Increased scores on depression inventories are a common finding among people presenting for initial diagnosis with obstructive sleep apnea (OSA).[10] In those meeting criteria for MDD in a large cross-sectional survey using DSM-IV criteria, there was an odds ratio of 5.3 for also meeting criteria for OSA or related breathing disorder in sleep.[11]

Among people with OSA, depression is associated with reduced adherence to continuous positive airway pressure (CPAP) therapy.[103] Studies have found neutral to positive results from CPAP use in people with OSA and depression,[104] with persistence of excessive daytime sleepiness correlating with persistence of depressed moods.[105] Higher doses of hypnotic medications in people with depression are associated with higher risks of sleep apnea and of treatment-resistant depression,[106] but the factors may be interacting in a complex manner.

Sleepwalking

MDD is associated with a 3.5-fold increased risk of sleepwalking 2 times or more per month compared with people without psychiatric or sleep disorders.[14] SSRIs can also increase the risk (see **Table 3**). Although zolpidem can trigger complex sleep-related behaviors and thus should not be prescribed for someone already known to sleepwalk, published interventional studies of zolpidem for insomnia in people with MDD on SSRIs have not mentioned sleepwalking as an adverse effect.

Narcolepsy

MDD is common in people with narcolepsy. In a study of 320 people with narcolepsy,[12] nearly 20% were found to have MDD, a 2.7-fold increase in risk over the general population; in more than 85% of those with MDD, the narcolepsy developed first.

In an observational study of 517 people with narcolepsy or idiopathic hypersomno-lence,[107] 80% of whom were treated with stimulants and 26% with medications for cataplexy, 55% had depression of some degree. In that study, the presence and severity of depression correlated with multiple measures of the severity of the sleep/wake disorder: lower cerebrospinal fluid orexin levels, more cataplexy, more REM sleep manifestations such as sleep paralysis and hypnogogic hallucinations, more daytime sleepiness, and lower health-related quality of life.[107] The observed clin-ical correlation does not distinguish between (1) the 2 having a common neurochem-ical origin, and (2) narcolepsy causing functional impairment and subsequently causing depression.

Isolated Sleep Paralysis

Isolated sleep paralysis (ISP) (short episodes of paralysis with awareness occurring on awakening or falling asleep, sometimes accompanied by vivid hallucinations or fear) has been associated with bipolar disorders and to a lesser extent with depressive dis-orders. Almost 19% of people with frequent ISP meet DSM-IV criteria for bipolar dis-orders and just more than 6% meet DSM-IV criteria for MDD or dysthymia, compared with around 2.3% of people who had never experienced ISP.[13]

ANXIETY DISORDERS

Sleep disturbances are common in anxiety, with almost 75% of primary care patients with anxiety disorders reporting insomnia or restless sleep, particularly those with generalized anxiety disorder (GAD), PTSD, or comorbid MDD.[15]

Sleep disturbances including insomnia and short sleep time are common in obsessive-compulsive disorder (OCD); nocturnal rituals and coexisting depression may be contributing factors. Greater sleep difficulty correlates with increased OCD severity.[16]

Nightmares and disturbed sleep are, respectively, symptoms of intrusion and hyper-arousal that are included in the diagnostic criteria for PTSD.[78] In a population study in the Toronto area,[21] almost 76% of people with PTSD had at least 1 other psychiatric diagnosis and 70% of people with PTSD reported impaired sleep. In that study, those with PTSD were significantly more likely than those without PTSD to report sleep pa-ralysis, talking during sleep, violent behavior during sleep, difficulty initiating sleep or early awakening, or hypnogogic or hypnopompic hallucinations.[21] Nightmares and sleep disturbance before trauma seem to be a risk marker for future development of PTSD,[22] suggesting that, as with depression, there may be a bidirectional relationship between sleep issues and this psychiatric disorder.

Insomnia

Anxiety disorders are more likely than depression to precede the development of insomnia, but anxiety and insomnia may each be manifestations of the same underly-ing process or trait. In the large multinational European study mentioned earlier,[4] in people with an anxiety disorder and insomnia, the insomnia preceded the anxiety dis-order in 18%, appeared around the same time in 38%, and appeared after the anxiety disorder in 44%. In the NIMH study mentioned earlier,[87] people who reported insomnia at 2 interviews 1 year apart were 6 times more likely to have an anxiety dis-order than those without insomnia. In a large Norwegian study of people initially without anxiety or depression,[17] having insomnia at 2 survey points 11 years apart was associated with an almost 5-fold risk of having developed an anxiety disorder by the second survey, compared with not reporting insomnia in either survey. In comparison, the risk was 3.4-fold higher when insomnia was present at the first survey but not the second and was 1.6-fold higher when insomnia was present at the second survey but not the first.[17]

People with insomnia commonly experience heightened arousal of the mind or body with attempts to sleep. Persistent insomnia is more likely to develop in people who worry about their sleep, and people with persistent insomnia are more likely than those who sleep normally to monitor and focus on their attempts to sleep.[108] Such worry, heightened arousal, and focus on sleep (called psychophysiologic insomnia in prior nosologies) may be reported as anxiety at bedtime but can be differentiated from GAD by the absence of daytime worry.

For people with anxiety and insomnia, treatment with escitalopram has been studied in conjunction with extended-release zolpidem,[109] which improved sleep but not GAD, and with eszopiclone,[110] which improved sleep, daytime function, and GAD. CBTI has been less studied in GAD than in depression and PTSD, but cognitive-behavioral therapy for anxiety can improve sleep.[111]

Circadian Rhythm Disorders

Severe OCD has been associated with DSPS.[16,18]

RLS

RLS can mimic anxiety at bedtime, because feelings of restlessness and jitteriness prevent the patient from resting quietly in bed to fall asleep. The improvement of these symptoms with benzodiazepines can further mistakenly suggest anxiety. Other psychiatric medications used for anxiety can cause or worsen RLS (see **Table 3**).

OSA

People presenting for initial diagnosis with OSA have been reported to have increased scores on anxiety inventories as well as depression inventories.[10]

Uncontrolled studies suggest that CPAP for OSA in PTSD can reduce insomnia, nightmares, and PTSD symptoms[112]; however, adherence to CPAP is reduced in veterans with PTSD, particularly those reporting more frequent nightmares, with claustrophobia and air hunger being among the reasons given.[113]

Sleepwalking

People with OCD have a nearly 4-fold higher risk of sleepwalking, unrelated to medication use, compared with people without psychiatric or sleep disorders.[14]

Narcolepsy

Based on the study of 320 people with narcolepsy mentioned earlier,[12] anxiety disorders occur commonly in narcolepsy, including social anxiety disorder in 21% overall, and panic disorder and PTSD in 11% to 13% of women. The timing of onset varied in this study, with OCD and social phobia appearing before narcolepsy in about half of cases; PTSD, GAD, and agoraphobia occurred after narcolepsy in more than 75% of cases; and panic disorder and simple phobia were both apparent after narcolepsy in all cases.

ISP

ISP has been associated with panic disorder, PTSD, and other anxiety disorders. A review of 35 studies of lifetime prevalence of ISP[19] found that almost 32% of psychiatric patients, and 35% of psychiatric patients with panic disorder, reported experiencing sleep paralysis at least once in their lifetime, compared with less than 8% of the general population, and that nonwhites are more likely to experience sleep paralysis at least once than are whites. Among African Americans with ISP, more than 15% met diagnostic criteria for panic disorder.[20] Experiencing fear during paralysis episodes is more closely associated with PTSD than with other anxiety disorders.[23] No association has been found with antidepressant medications,[114] including specifically with SSRIs,[23] but the findings with regard to anxiolytics are mixed.[13,114]

SCHIZOPHRENIA

In a systematic review and meta-analysis,[33] patients with schizophrenia with sleep disturbances of all types were 12.66-fold more likely to have suicidal ideation, suicide attempts, and completed suicide than those without sleep disturbances, although the 95% confidence interval was wide: 1.40 to 114.44.

Insomnia and Circadian Rhythm Disorders

Insomnia is common in schizophrenia, with circadian abnormalities (phase advance, phase delay, or non-24-hour cycles) occurring in about half of people, and irregular, fragmented, or prolonged sleep occurring even in those with normal circadian cycles.[24] Physicians should be aware that worsening of insomnia can be the prodrome of a psychiatric exacerbation for a person with schizophrenia.

OSA

Atypical antipsychotic medications commonly cause weight gain but also increase the risk of severe OSA beyond that explained by weight (see **Table 3**).[27] The prevalence, presentation, and treatment of OSA have not been studied in schizophrenia in as much detail as in other groups, although there are case reports of schizophrenia symptoms improving (and in 1 case becoming exacerbated) with CPAP therapy.[115]

Narcolepsy

Narcolepsy can be confused for schizophrenia, because it can present with psychosis symptoms either from the narcolepsy itself or from stimulant use, and it can coexist with schizophrenia.[26] The psychosis of narcolepsy may be more common than realized. In 1 recent study,[116] 83% of people with narcolepsy reported having trouble distinguishing dreams from reality, and 95% reported experiencing such dream delusions at least once a month. When narcolepsy and schizophrenia are comorbid conditions, the schizophrenia may tend to present after the narcolepsy. A prospective study at the sole pediatric sleep clinic serving Taiwan[28] found that 10% of school-aged children diagnosed with narcolepsy-cataplexy developed schizophrenia in a mean of 2.6 ± 1.8 years, whereas retrospective review of records in the associated pediatric psychiatry division over the previous 10 years showed no teenagers with both conditions who had been diagnosed first with schizophrenia.

ATTENTION-DEFICIT/HYPERACTIVITY DISORDER

Sleep in attention-deficit/hyperactivity disorder (ADHD) has been investigated to a greater degree in children than in adults.

Insomnia

Stimulant medications (amphetamines and methylphenidate) and the nonstimulant medication atomoxetine cause insomnia,[117,118] particularly with long-acting or twice-daily dosing and with higher doses.[119] These medications can also improve sleep quality in adults with ADHD.[119,120]

Circadian Rhythm Disorders

In adults more than children, ADHD has been associated with delayed sleep phase; this association may trace back to the genetic level.[34]

RLS

In both children and adults, ADHD has been associated with RLS and periodic limb movements. Up to 44% of adults with ADHD have been found to have RLS, and up to 26% of those with RLS meet criteria for ADHD.[35] In children, treatment of RLS with L-DOPA does not improve ADHD,[121] and treatment of RLS has shown mixed results on ADHD.[122]

OSA

In children, ADHD is associated with breathing disorders of sleep (OSA and similar conditions) and improves after adenotonsillectomy.[36] However, in adults, this association has not been found.[37]

TREATMENT CONSIDERATIONS

Effects of sleep disorder treatments on psychiatric conditions have been noted in the discussion of that psychiatric condition. Treatment approaches for insomnia in depression are listed in **Table 2**. Effects of psychiatric medications on selected common sleep disorders are listed in **Table 3**.

Additional considerations regarding sleep disorder treatments relevant to psychiatric conditions of note for primary care physicians include the following:

- To avoid causing or exacerbating RLS (and perhaps even to improve existing RLS), the antidepressant of choice is bupropion, and the atypical antipsychotic of choice seems to be aripiprazole.
- Atypical antipsychotic medications commonly cause weight gain (especially olanzapine), extrapyramidal symptoms, akathisia (especially aripiprazole), fatigue, and sedation[123] as well as hyperlipidemia and hyperglycemia.[55]
- Quetiapine is particularly sedating and is prescribed off-label for insomnia,[56] despite its adverse effects, cost, and lack of studies directly comparing it with better studied hypnotic medications.[55]
- The psychiatrically relevant side effect of impulse control disorders can develop in patients taking even low-dose dopamine agonists for RLS; in 1 study, 7.6% of the patients on dopamine agonists for RLS developed 1 or more impulse control and compulsive behaviors, including gambling, shopping, and sexual behavior, sometimes with severe social consequences.[38]
- The wakefulness-promoting medications modafinil and armodafinil, currently FDA-approved only for narcolepsy, shift work sleep disorder, and residual excessive daytime sleepiness in OSA, have been studied off-label as treatments for psychiatric disorders and for side effects from psychiatric medications but have not shown significant benefits.
- In addition to its efficacy in chronic insomnia and insomnia associated with depression, CBTI is effective in insomnia in postpartum depression[124] and during abstinent recovery from alcohol dependence.[125] In conjunction with imagery rehearsal therapy to address nightmares,[112] CBTI has been shown to improve subjective sleep and daytime functioning in people with PTSD.[126]

SUMMARY/FUTURE CONSIDERATIONS

The associations described between psychiatric disorders and sleep issues include observations on the natural history of the overlap between sleep, wakefulness, and mental health. Awareness of these associations may help clinicians treating patients with psychiatric disorders or sleep disorders to recognize potential contributing factors from the other area, particularly when a treatment given for a psychiatric or sleep condition might be causing or exacerbating a problem in the other area. It is hoped that within the next few years, stepped care with CBTI will become a useful, accessible tool for the treatment of chronic insomnia, including that associated with psychiatric conditions. Sedating medications will continue to be part of our armamentarium as well as always requiring a balance between the desired promotion of sleepiness and the undesired side effects, including daytime sedation and functional impairment. Ongoing and future research to elucidate neurobiological mechanisms underlying both psychiatric disorders and sleep/wake disorders will likely provide a more solid basis for understanding the overlap areas as well as further means for diagnosis and effective treatment.

REFERENCES

1. Kessler RC, Demler O, Frank RG, et al. US prevalence and treatment of mental disorders, 1990 to 2003. N Engl J Med 2005;352(24):2515 23.
2. LeBlanc M, Mérette C, Savard J, et al. Incidence and risk factors of insomnia in a population-based sample. Sleep 2009;32(8):1027 37.
3. Sarsour K, Morin CM, Foley K, et al. Association of insomnia severity and comorbid medical and psychiatric disorders in a health plan-based sample: Insomnia severity and comorbidities. Sleep Med 2010;11(1):69–74.
4. Ohayon MM, Roth T. Place of chronic insomnia in the course of depressive and anxiety disorders. J Psychiatr Res 2003;37(1):9–15.
5. Sivertsen B, Salo P, Mykletun A, et al. The bidirectional association between depression and insomnia: the HUNT study. Psychosom Med 2012;74(7):758–65.
6. Baglioni C, Battagliese G, Feige B, et al. Insomnia as a predictor of depression: a meta-analytic evaluation of longitudinal epidemiological studies. J Affect Disord 2011;135(1–3):10–9.
7. Robillard R, Naismith SL, Rogers NL, et al. Delayed sleep phase in young people with unipolar or bipolar affective disorders. J Affect Disord 2013;145(2):260–3.
8. Szentkiralyi A, Völzke H, Hoffmann W, et al. The relationship between depressive symptoms and restless legs syndrome in two prospective cohort studies. Psychosom Med 2013;75(4):359–65.
9. Li Y, Mirzaei F, O'Reilly EJ, et al. Prospective study of restless legs syndrome and risk of depression in women. Am J Epidemiol 2012;176(4):279–88.
10. Macey PM, Woo MA, Kumar R, et al. Relationship between obstructive sleep apnea severity and sleep, depression and anxiety symptoms in newly-diagnosed patients. PLoS One 2010;5(4):e10211.
11. Ohayon MM. The effects of breathing-related sleep disorders on mood disturbances in the general population. J Clin Psychiatry 2003;64(10):1195–200.
12. Ohayon MM. Narcolepsy is complicated by high medical and psychiatric comorbidities: a comparison with the general population. Sleep Med 2013;14(6):488–92.
13. Ohayon MM, Zulley J, Guilleminault C, et al. Prevalence and pathologic associations of sleep paralysis in the general population. Neurology 1999;52(6):1194–200.

14. Ohayon MM, Mahowald MW, Dauvilliers Y, et al. Prevalence and comorbidity of nocturnal wandering in the U.S. adult general population. Neurology 2012; 78(20):1583–9.

15. Marcks BA, Weisberg RB, Edelen MO, et al. The relationship between sleep disturbance and the course of anxiety disorders in primary care patients. Psychiatry Res 2010;178(3):487–92.

16. Paterson JL, Reynolds AC, Ferguson SA, et al. Sleep and obsessive-compulsive disorder (OCD). Sleep Med Rev 2013;17(6):465–74.

17. Neckelmann D, Mykletun A, Dahl AA. Chronic insomnia as a risk factor for developing anxiety and depression. Sleep 2007;30(7):873–80.

18. Mukhopadhyay S, Fineberg NA, Drummond LM, et al. Delayed sleep phase in severe obsessive-compulsive disorder: a systematic case-report survey. CNS Spectr 2008;13(5):406–13.

19. Sharpless BA, Barber JP. Lifetime prevalence rates of sleep paralysis: a systematic review. Sleep Med Rev 2011;15(5):311–5.

20. Bell CC, Dixie-Bell DD, Thompson B. Further studies on the prevalence of isolated sleep paralysis in black subjects. J Natl Med Assoc 1986;78(7):649–59.

21. Ohayon MM, Shapiro CM. Sleep disturbances and psychiatric disorders associated with posttraumatic stress disorder in the general population. Compr Psychiatry 2000;41(6):469–78.

22. van Liempt S. Sleep disturbances and PTSD: a perpetual circle? Eur J Psychotraumatol 2012;3. http://dx.doi.org/10.3402/ejpt.v3i0.19142.

23. Sharpless BA, McCarthy KS, Chambless DL, et al. Isolated sleep paralysis and fearful isolated sleep paralysis in outpatients with panic attacks. J Clin Psychol 2010;66(12):1292–306.

24. Wulff K, Dijk DJ, Middleton B, et al. Sleep and circadian rhythm disruption in schizophrenia. Br J Psychiatry 2012;200(4):308–16.

25. Perez-Lloret S, Rey MV, Bondon-Guitton E, et al, French Association of Regional Pharmacovigilance Centers. Drugs associated with restless legs syndrome: a case/noncase study in the French Pharmacovigilance Database. J Clin Psychopharmacol 2012;32(6):824–7.

26. Rittmannsberger H, Werl R. Restless legs syndrome induced by quetiapine: report of seven cases and review of the literature. Int J Neuropsychopharmacol 2013;16(6):1427–31.

27. Rishi MA, Shetty M, Wolff A, et al. Atypical antipsychotic medications are independently associated with severe obstructive sleep apnea. Clin Neuropharmacol 2010;33(3):109–13.

28. Huang YS, Guilleminault C, Chen CH, et al. Narcolepsy-cataplexy and schizophrenia in adolescents. Sleep Med 2014;15(1):15–22.

29. Kishi Y, Konishi S, Koizumi S, et al. Schizophrenia and narcolepsy: a review with a case report. Psychiatry Clin Neurosci 2004;58(2):117–24.

30. Seeman MV. Sleepwalking, a possible side effect of antipsychotic medication. Psychiatr Q 2011;82(1):59–67.

31. Kodaka M, Matsumoto T, Katsumata Y, et al. Suicide risk among individuals with sleep disturbances in Japan: a case-control psychological autopsy study. Sleep Med 2014;15(4):430–5.

32. McCall WV, Blocker JN, D'Agostino R Jr, et al. Insomnia severity is an indicator of suicidal ideation during a depression clinical trial. Sleep Med 2010;11(9): 822–7.

33. Malik S, Kanwar A, Sim LA, et al. The association between sleep disturbances and suicidal behaviors in patients with psychiatric diagnoses: a systematic

review and meta-analysis. Syst Rev 2014;3:18. http://dx.doi.org/10.1186/2046-4053-3-18.

34. Baird AL, Coogan AN, Siddiqui A, et al. Adult attention-deficit hyperactivity disorder is associated with alterations in circadian rhythms at the behavioural, endocrine and molecular levels. Mol Psychiatry 2012;17(10):988–95.

35. Cortese S, Konofal E, Lecendreux M, et al. Restless legs syndrome and attention-deficit/hyperactivity disorder: a review of the literature. Sleep 2005; 28(8):1007–13.

36. Sedky K, Bennett DS, Carvalho KS. Attention deficit hyperactivity disorder and sleep disordered breathing in pediatric populations: a meta-analysis. Sleep Med Rev 2014;18(4):349–56. pii:S1087-0792(13) 00132-9.

37. Oğuztürk Ö, Ekici M, Çimen D, et al. Attention deficit/hyperactivity disorder in adults with sleep apnea. J Clin Psychol Med Settings 2013;20(2):234–9.

38. Voon V, Schoerling A, Wenzel S, et al. Frequency of impulse control behaviours associated with dopaminergic therapy in restless legs syndrome. BMC Neurol 2011;11:117.

39. Carney CE, Segal ZV, Edinger JD, et al. A comparison of rates of residual insomnia symptoms following pharmacotherapy or cognitive-behavioral therapy for major depressive disorder. J Clin Psychiatry 2007;68(2):254–60.

40. Manber R, Bernert RA, Suh S, et al. CBT for insomnia in patients with high and low depressive symptom severity: adherence and clinical outcomes. J Clin Sleep Med 2011;7(6):645–52.

41. Manber R, Edinger JD, Gress JL, et al. Cognitive behavioral therapy for insomnia enhances depression outcome in patients with comorbid major depressive disorder and insomnia. Sleep 2008;31(4):489–95.

42. Rethorst CD, Sunderajan P, Greer TL, et al. Does exercise improve self-reported sleep quality in non-remitted major depressive disorder? Psychol Med 2013; 43(4):699–709.

43. Combs K, Smith PJ, Sherwood A, et al. Impact of sleep complaints and depression outcomes among participants in the standard medical intervention and long-term exercise study of exercise and pharmacotherapy for depression. J Nerv Ment Dis 2014;202(2):167–71.

44. McClintock SM, Husain MM, Wisniewski SR, et al. Residual symptoms in depressed outpatients who respond by 50% but do not remit to antidepressant medication. J Clin Psychopharmacol 2011;31(2):180–6.

45. Fabbri C, Marsano A, Balestri M, et al. Clinical features and drug induced side effects in early versus late antidepressant responders. J Psychiatr Res 2013; 47(10):1309–18.

46. Papakostas GI, Nutt DJ, Hallett LA, et al. Resolution of sleepiness and fatigue in major depressive disorder: a comparison of bupropion and the selective serotonin reuptake inhibitors. Biol Psychiatry 2006;60(12):1350–5.

47. Asnis GM, Chakraburtty A, DuBoff EA, et al. Zolpidem for persistent insomnia in SSRI-treated depressed patients. J Clin Psychiatry 1999;60(10):668–76.

48. Fava M, Asnis GM, Shrivastava RK, et al. Improved insomnia symptoms and sleep-related next-day functioning in patients with comorbid major depressive disorder and insomnia following concomitant zolpidem extended-release 12.5 mg and escitalopram treatment: a randomized controlled trial. J Clin Psychiatry 2011;72(7):914–28.

49. US Food and Drug Administration. FDA Drug Safety Communication: risk of next-morning impairment after use of insomnia drugs; FDA requires lower recommended doses for certain drugs containing zolpidem (Ambien, Ambien

CR, Edluar, and Zolpimist). 2013. Available at: http://www.fda.gov/downloads/Drugs/DrugSafety/UCM335007.pdf. Accessed May 18, 2014.

50. Fava M, McCall WV, Krystal A, et al. Eszopiclone co-administered with fluoxetine in patients with insomnia coexisting with major depressive disorder. Biol Psychiatry 2006;59(11):1052–60.

51. Krystal A, Fava M, Rubens R, et al. Evaluation of eszopiclone discontinuation after cotherapy with fluoxetine for insomnia with coexisting depression. J Clin Sleep Med 2007;3(1):48–55.

52. Hojo Y, Echizenya M, Ohkubo T, et al. Drug interaction between St John's wort and zolpidem in healthy subjects. J Clin Pharm Ther 2011;36(6):711–5.

53. US Food and Drug Administration. FDA Drug Safety Communication: FDA warns of next-day impairment with sleep aid Lunesta (eszopiclone) and lowers recommended dose. 2014. Available at: http://www.fda.gov/downloads/Drugs/DrugSafety/UCM397277.pdf. Accessed May 18, 2014.

54. Garakani A, Martinez JM, Marcus S, et al. A randomized, double-blind, and placebo-controlled trial of quetiapine augmentation of fluoxetine in major depressive disorder. Int Clin Psychopharmacol 2008;23(5):269–75.

55. Anderson SL, Vande Griend JP. Quetiapine for insomnia: a review of the literature. Am J Health Syst Pharm 2014;71(5):394–402.

56. Hermes ED, Sernyak M, Rosenheck R. Use of second-generation antipsychotic agents for sleep and sedation: a provider survey. Sleep 2013;36(4):597–600.

57. Jacobsen FM. Low-dose trazodone as a hypnotic in patients treated with MAOIs and other psychotropics: a pilot study. J Clin Psychiatry 1990;51(7): 298–302.

58. Nierenberg AA, Adler LA, Peselow E, et al. Trazodone for antidepressant-associated insomnia. Am J Psychiatry 1994;151(7):1069–72.

59. Fagiolini A, Comandini A, Catena Dell'Osso M, et al. Rediscovering trazodone for the treatment of major depressive disorder. CNS Drugs 2012;26(12): 1033–49.

60. Dolder CR, Nelson MH, Iler CA. The effects of mirtazapine on sleep in patients with major depressive disorder. Ann Clin Psychiatry 2012;24(3):215–24.

61. Watanabe N, Omori IM, Nakagawa A, et al. Mirtazapine versus other antidepressive agents for depression. Cochrane Database Syst Rev 2011;(12):CD006528. http://dx.doi.org/10.1002/14651858.CD006528.pub2.

62. Hicks JA, Argyropoulos SV, Rich AS, et al. Randomised controlled study of sleep after nefazodone or paroxetine treatment in out-patients with depression. Br J Psychiatry 2002;180:528–35.

63. Rush AJ, Armitage R, Gillin JC, et al. Comparative effects of nefazodone and fluoxetine in outpatients with major depressive disorder. Biol Psychiatry 1998; 44(1):3–14.

64. Bayard M, Bailey B, Acharya D, et al. Bupropion and restless legs syndrome: a randomized controlled trial. J Am Board Fam Med 2011;24(4):422–8.

65. Rottach KG, Schaner BM, Kirch MH, et al. Restless legs syndrome as side effect of second generation antidepressants. J Psychiatr Res 2008;43(1):70–5.

66. Ohayon MM, Roth T. Prevalence of restless legs syndrome and periodic limb movement disorder in the general population. J Psychosom Res 2002;53(1): 547–54.

67. Young WB, Piovesan EJ, Biglan KM. Restless legs syndrome and drug-induced akathisia in headache patients. CNS Spectr 2003;8(6):450–6.

68. Tamanna S, Ullah MI, Pope CR, et al. Quetiapine-induced sleep-related eating disorder-like behavior: a case series. J Med Case Rep 2012;6(1):380.

69. Kahn-Greene ET, Killgore DB, Kamimori GH, et al. The effects of sleep deprivation on symptoms of psychopathology in healthy adults. Sleep Med 2007;8(3): 215–21.
70. Minkel J, Htaik O, Banks S, et al. Emotional expressiveness in sleep-deprived healthy adults. Behav Sleep Med 2011;9(1):5–14.
71. van der Helm E, Gujar N, Walker MP. Sleep deprivation impairs the accurate recognition of human emotions. Sleep 2010;33(3):335–42.
72. Benca RM, Obermeyer WH, Thisted RA, et al. Sleep and psychiatric disorders. A meta-analysis. Arch Gen Psychiatry 1992;49(8):651–68 [discussion: 669–70].
73. Nollet M, Leman S. Role of orexin in the pathophysiology of depression: potential for pharmacological intervention. CNS Drugs 2013;27(6):411–22.
74. Partonen T. Clock gene variants in mood and anxiety disorders. J Neural Transm 2012;119(10):1133–45.
75. McClung CA. Role for the Clock gene in bipolar disorder. Cold Spring Harb Symp Quant Biol 2007;72:637–44.
76. Li JZ, Bunney BG, Meng F, et al. Circadian patterns of gene expression in the human brain and disruption in major depressive disorder. Proc Natl Acad Sci U S A 2013;110(24):9950–5.
77. Merlo Pich E, Melotto S. Orexin 1 receptor antagonists in compulsive behavior and anxiety: possible therapeutic use. Front Neurosci 2014;8:26. http://dx.doi.org/10.3389/fnins.2014.00026. eCollection 2014.
78. American Psychiatric Association. Diagnostic and statistical manual of mental disorders. 5th edition. Arlington (VA): American Psychiatric Publishing; 2013.
79. American Academy of Sleep Medicine. International classification of sleep disorders. 3rd edition. Darien (IL): American Academy of Sleep Medicine; 2014.
80. Sutton EL. Insomnia. Med Clin North Am 2014;98(3):565–81.
81. Morin CM, Bootzin RR, Buysse DJ, et al. Psychological and behavioral treatment of insomnia: update of the recent evidence (1998-2004). Sleep 2006;29(11):1398–414.
82. Mitchell MD, Gehrman P, Perlis M, et al. Comparative effectiveness of cognitive behavioral therapy for insomnia: a systematic review. BMC Fam Pract 2012;13: 40. http://dx.doi.org/10.1186/1471-2296-13-40.
83. Sánchez-Ortuño MM, Edinger JD. Cognitive-behavioral therapy for the management of insomnia comorbid with mental disorders. Curr Psychiatry Rep 2012; 14(5):519–28.
84. Wagley JN, Rybarczyk B, Nay WT, et al. Effectiveness of abbreviated CBT for insomnia in psychiatric outpatients: sleep and depression outcomes. J Clin Psychol 2013;69(10):1043–55.
85. Mack LJ, Rybarczyk BD. Behavioral treatment of insomnia: a proposal for a stepped-care approach to promote public health. Nat Sci Sleep 2011;3:87–99.
86. Vincent N, Walsh K. Stepped care for insomnia: an evaluation of implementation in routine practice. J Clin Sleep Med 2013;9(3):227–34.
87. Ford DE, Kamerow DB. Epidemiologic study of sleep disturbances and psychiatric disorders. An opportunity for prevention? JAMA 1989;262(11):1479–84.
88. Kamphuis J, Dijk DJ, Spreen M, et al. The relation between poor sleep, impulsivity and aggression in forensic psychiatric patients. Physiol Behav 2014;123: 168–73.
89. Roberts RE, Duong HT. The prospective association between sleep deprivation and depression among adolescents. Sleep 2014;37(2):239–44.
90. Wu JC, Bunney WE. The biological basis of an antidepressant response to sleep deprivation and relapse: review and hypothesis. Am J Psychiatry 1990;147(1): 14–21.

91. Wu JC, Kelsoe JR, Schachat C, et al. Rapid and sustained antidepressant response with sleep deprivation and chronotherapy in bipolar disorder. Biol Psychiatry 2009;66(3):298–301.

92. Palagini L, Baglioni C, Ciapparelli A, et al. REM sleep dysregulation in depression: state of the art. Sleep Med Rev 2013;17(5):377–90.

93. Pigeon WR, Hegel M, Unützer J, et al. Is insomnia a perpetuating factor for late-life depression in the IMPACT cohort? Sleep 2008;31(4):481–8.

94. Chang PP, Ford DE, Mead LA, et al. Insomnia in young men and subsequent depression. The Johns Hopkins Precursors Study. Am J Epidemiol 1997; 146(2):105–14.

95. Nierenberg AA, Husain MM, Trivedi MH, et al. Residual symptoms after remission of major depressive disorder with citalopram and risk of relapse: a STAR*D report. Psychol Med 2010;40(1):41–50.

96. Perlis ML, Giles DE, Buysse DJ, et al. Self-reported sleep disturbance as a prodromal symptom in recurrent depression. J Affect Disord 1997;42(2–3): 209–12.

97. Gulec M, Selvi Y, Boysan M, et al. Ongoing or re-emerging subjective insomnia symptoms after full/partial remission or recovery of major depressive disorder mainly with the selective serotonin reuptake inhibitors and risk of relapse or recurrence: a 52-week follow-up study. J Affect Disord 2011; 134(1–3):257–65.

98. Tuunainen A, Kripke DF, Endo T. Light therapy for non-seasonal depression. Cochrane Database Syst Rev 2004;(2):CD004050.

99. Pail G, Huf W, Pjrek E, et al. Bright-light therapy in the treatment of mood disorders. Neuropsychobiology 2011;64(3):152–62.

100. Benes H, Walters AS, Allen RP, et al. Definition of restless legs syndrome, how to diagnose it, and how to differentiate it from RLS mimics. Mov Disord 2007; 22(Suppl 18):S401–8.

101. Benes H, Mattern W, Peglau I, et al. Ropinirole improves depressive symptoms and restless legs syndrome severity in RLS patients: a multicentre, randomized, placebo-controlled study. J Neurol 2011;258(6):1046–54.

102. Launois C, Leu-Semenescu S, Brion A, et al. Major depression after withdrawing dopamine agonists in two patients with restless legs syndrome and impulse control disorders. Sleep Med 2013;14(7):696.

103. Law M, Naughton M, Ho S, et al. Depression may reduce adherence during CPAP titration trial. J Clin Sleep Med 2014;10(2):163–9.

104. Giles TL, Lasserson TJ, Smith BJ, et al. Continuous positive airways pressure for obstructive sleep apnoea in adults. Cochrane Database Syst Rev 2006;(1):CD001106.

105. Gagnadoux F, Le Vaillant M, Goupil F, et al. Depressive symptoms before and after long term continuous positive airway pressure therapy in sleep apnea patients. Chest 2014. http://dx.doi.org/10.1378/chest.13-2373.

106. Li CT, Bai YM, Lee YC, et al. High dosage of hypnotics predicts subsequent sleep-related breathing disorders and is associated with worse outcomes for depression. Sleep 2014;37(4):803–9.

107. Dauvilliers Y, Paquereau J, Bastuji H, et al. Psychological health in central hypersomnias: the French Harmony study. J Neurol Neurosurg Psychiatry 2009;80(6): 636–41.

108. Norell-Clarke A, Jansson-Fröjmark M, Tillfors M, et al. Cognitive processes and their association with persistence and remission of insomnia: findings from a longitudinal study in the general population. Behav Res Ther 2014;54:38–48.

109. Fava M, Asnis GM, Shrivastava R, et al. Zolpidem extended-release improves sleep and next-day symptoms in comorbid insomnia and generalized anxiety disorder. J Clin Psychopharmacol 2009;29(3):222–30.

110. Pollack M, Kinrys G, Krystal A, et al. Eszopiclone coadministered with escitalopram in patients with insomnia and comorbid generalized anxiety disorder. Arch Gen Psychiatry 2008;65(5):551–62.

111. Bélanger L, Morin CM, Langlois F, et al. Insomnia and generalized anxiety disorder: effects of cognitive behavior therapy for GAD on insomnia symptoms. J Anxiety Disord 2004;18(4):561–71.

112. Maher MJ, Rego SA, Asnis GM. Sleep disturbances in patients with posttraumatic stress disorder: epidemiology, impact and approaches to management. CNS Drugs 2006;20(7):567–90.

113. El-Solh AA, Ayyar L, Akinnusi M, et al. Positive airway pressure adherence in veterans with posttraumatic stress disorder. Sleep 2010;33(11):1495–500.

114. Otto MW, Simon NM, Powers M, et al. Rates of isolated sleep paralysis in outpatients with anxiety disorders. J Anxiety Disord 2006;20(5):687–93.

115. Kalucy MJ, Grunstein R, Lambert T, et al. Obstructive sleep apnoea and schizophrenia–a research agenda. Sleep Med Rev 2013;17(5):357–65.

116. Wamsley E, Donjacour CE, Scammell TE, et al. Delusional confusion of dreaming and reality in narcolepsy. Sleep 2014;37(2):419–22.

117. Adler LA, Goodman D, Weisler R, et al. Effect of lisdexamfetamine dimesylate on sleep in adults with attention-deficit/hyperactivity disorder. Behav Brain Funct 2009;5:34.

118. Wietecha LA, Ruff DD, Allen AJ, et al. Atomoxetine tolerability in pediatric and adult patients receiving different dosing strategies. J Clin Psychiatry 2013; 74(12):1217–23.

119. Surman CB, Roth T. Impact of stimulant pharmacotherapy on sleep quality: post hoc analyses of 2 large, double-blind, randomized, placebo-controlled trials. J Clin Psychiatry 2011;72(7):903–8.

120. Boonstra AM, Kooij JJ, Oosterlaan J, et al. Hyperactive night and day? Actigraphy studies in adult ADHD: a baseline comparison and the effect of methylphenidate. Sleep 2007;30(4):433–42.

121. England SJ, Picchietti DL, Couvadelli BV, et al. L-Dopa improves restless legs syndrome and periodic limb movements in sleep but not attention-deficit-hyperactivity disorder in a double-blind trial in children. Sleep Med 2011; 12(5):471–7.

122. Cortese S, Angriman M, Lecendreux M, et al. Iron and attention deficit/hyperactivity disorder: what is the empirical evidence so far? A systematic review of the literature. Expert Rev Neurother 2012;12(10):1227–40.

123. Maher AR, Maglione M, Bagley S, et al. Efficacy and comparative effectiveness of atypical antipsychotic medications for off-label uses in adults: a systematic review and meta-analysis. JAMA 2011;306(12):1359–69.

124. Swanson LM, Flynn H, Adams-Mundy JD, et al. An open pilot of cognitive-behavioral therapy for insomnia in women with postpartum depression. Behav Sleep Med 2013;11(4):297–307.

125. Arnedt JT, Conroy DA, Armitage R, et al. Cognitive-behavioral therapy for insomnia in alcohol dependent patients: a randomized controlled pilot trial. Behav Res Ther 2011;49(4):227–33.

126. Talbot LS, Maguen S, Metzler TJ, et al. Cognitive behavioral therapy for insomnia in posttraumatic stress disorder: a randomized controlled trial. Sleep 2014; 37(2):327–41.

Psychiatric Care of the Older Adult
An Overview for Primary Care

Shaune DeMers, MD*, Kyl Dinsio, MD, Whitney Carlson, MD

KEYWORDS

- Geriatric patients • Primary care • Delirium • Dementia • Depression
- Substance abuse • Alcohol misuse • Caregivers

KEY POINTS

- Suspect delirium in any acute mental status change. Polypharmacy, medications, metabolic derangements, and infections are common causes for delirium.
- Dementia is a common and increasingly frequent diagnosis made in primary care settings. A structured approach combining history from patients, a collateral source, and bedside cognitive testing will usually establish a diagnosis.
- Depression is a common comorbidity that has negative impacts on health status and quality of life. Depression treatment should be tailored to the individual patient and treatment continued until remission is achieved.
- Although alcohol and substance misuse is less common among older adults, the prevalence is increasing. Older patients with changes in mood or cognition should be screened for alcohol and drug problems, particularly prescription medication overuse.
- Caregivers for older patients are usually a spouse or adult children and suffer significant morbidity. The primary care provider is often in the best position to assist caregivers with their own stress and to provide direction for more assistance.

INTRODUCTION: APPROACH TO OLDER ADULT PATIENTS

Primary care providers (PCPs) in the United States will be devoting increasing time to the management of geriatric patients. Between 2012 and 2050, the number of persons older than 65 years is expected to increase dramatically, from 43.1 million to 88.5 million.[1] This increase is a motivator for recent calls for an expansion of the primary care workforce by 52,000 physicians, with recognition that the numbers of geriatric specialists will not be sufficient to meet the demand.[2] In fact, the number of geriatric

The authors have no conflicts of interest to disclose.
Division of Geriatric Psychiatry, Harborview Medical Center and University of Washington, Box 359760, 325 Ninth Avenue, Seattle, WA 98104-2499, USA
* Corresponding author.
E-mail address: sdemers@uw.edu

Med Clin N Am 98 (2014) 1145–1168
http://dx.doi.org/10.1016/j.mcna.2014.06.010
medical.theclinics.com

internists and psychiatrists is expected to remain stable or even decline in the next decades.[3]

Older adults are in many ways similar to their younger counterparts, but important differences are highlighted in this overview as we consider the case of Mr Q (**Box 1**). Differential diagnoses for his presentation will allow us to review the most common psychiatric problems encountered in the primary care setting (delirium, dementia, depression, and substance misuse) and to discuss another critical issue, caregiver health and well-being.

DELIRIUM

Mr Q could be suffering from delirium. Most delirious patients are located in hospitalized or intensive care unit (ICU) settings, making it less common in primary care offices. However, although the base rate for delirium in outpatient settings is low (1%–2%), it increases dramatically with increasing age, increasing to 14% among individuals older than 85 years living in the community.[4,5] Primary care doctors are additionally likely to encounter an acute delirium in nursing home or end-of-life patients where prevalence increases to 60% and more than 80%, respectively.[5]

Delirium is an acute confusional state, characterized by deficits in attention, level of consciousness, orientation, memory, language, and ability to communicate and visual hallucinations or paranoia (**Box 2**). It is an abrupt change in mental status that is always driven by an underlying medical cause. The Confusion Assessment Method is an easy-to-use screening tool that has been validated for the detection of delirium.[6,7] The evolution of a delirium arises from some underlying vulnerability in patients combined with an acute medical insult or medication effect (**Box 3**). Older patients with dementia are particularly at risk for the development of a delirium, and the clinical picture of a delirium superimposed on top of dementia is quite common.[8] In elderly patients, even relatively minor medical disturbances, such as a urinary tract infection, mild dehydration, or even constipation, can cause a delirium. Other common causes are medications (particularly polypharmacy or postanesthesia), infections, and cardiac or cerebrovascular events.

Delirium is differentiated from dementia in that its onset is an *acute* change from the person's baseline. The time course of development of a delirium is hours to days, whereas in dementia it is months to years. The presence of a delirium necessitates an investigation into the underlying medical problems that are causing the change in mental status; often there are multiple contributing causes. In all cases, the

---

Box 1
The case of Mr Q

Mr Q is a 75-year-old retired anthropology professor with no psychiatric history whom you have been following for many years for the management of type II diabetes, hypertension, and occasional falls. He comes to the clinic for a 6-month check-up with his wife of 42 years and for the first time seems confused about his medications.

Questions

1. Is he delirious?

2. Has he developed cognitive impairment?

3. Could he be depressed?

4. What about alcohol or other drug intoxication or withdrawal?

5. How is his wife doing?

Box 2
Clinical features of delirium

Disturbance in attention and awareness

- Reduced ability to direct, focus, sustain, or shift attention
- Reduced awareness and orientation to the environment

Abrupt onset

- Disturbance develops abruptly, over the course of hours or days
- Disturbance represents a change from baseline attention, awareness, and cognitive abilities

Cognitive deficits

- Additional impairments in functions of memory, orientation, language
- Disorganized and incomprehensible speech or rambling and incoherent conversation

Alterations in levels of consciousness

- Difficulty maintaining normal alertness for even brief interactions, falls asleep during conversation
- Clouding of consciousness, with reduced clarity of awareness of the surrounding environment

Fluctuating course throughout the day

- Symptoms come and go or increase/decrease in severity over course of a day
- Lucid intervals sometimes present

Alterations in sleep-wake cycles

- Daytime sleepiness, nighttime agitation, difficulty falling asleep, excessive sleepiness throughout the day, or wakefulness throughout the night
- Complete reversal of the day-night, sleep-wake cycle

Psychomotor disturbances

- Hyperactivity marked by agitation, vigilance, and even violence
- Hypoactive marked by lethargy with markedly decrease level of motor activity
- Combination of hyperactive and hypoactive

Psychotic disturbances

- Illusions or hallucinations (typically visual)
- Paranoid ideation, fear, or concern for safety

Emotional disturbances

- Frequent and frequently shifting expressions of extreme emotions, including anxiety, fear, depression, irritability, anger, apathy, or euphoria
- May manifest behaviorally as calling out, screaming, cursing, muttering, moaning, or making other noises

Adapted from Inouye SK. Delirium in older persons. N Engl J Med 2006;354(11):1157–65.

treatment of a delirium begins with treatment of the underlying disorder or disturbance. This treatment will typically involve correction of the metabolic or electrolyte disturbance, antibiotics for an infection, discontinuing problematic medications, maintaining adequate nutrition and hydration status, and decreasing functional deconditioning through early mobilization and physical therapy. Even with adequate

---

Box 3
Predisposing and precipitating factors for delirium

Predisposing factors

Older age

Dementia diagnosis and severity

Polypharmacy

Alcoholism

Immobility

Hip fracture

Dehydration and poor nutritional status

Functional dependence

Severity of physical illness

Stroke

Metabolic abnormalities

Visual and hearing impairments

Anemia

Precipitating factors

Infections (eg, pneumonia, urinary tract infection, cellulitis)

Electrolyte disturbances (dehydration, hyponatremia/hypernatremia, or uremia)

Medication (particularly drugs with anticholinergic, sedative, or psychoactive effects)

Neurologic insult (stroke, seizure, hemorrhage)

Hypoxia

Alcohol withdrawal

Surgery and exposure to anesthesia

ICU admission

Sleep deprivation

Adapted from Burns A, Gallagley A, Byrne J. Delirium. J Neurol Neurosurg Psychiatry 2004;75(3):362–7; and Young J, Inouye SK. Delirium in older people. BMJ 2007;334(7598):842–6.

---

treatment, delirium may persist for weeks in many patients; some patients will not return to their prior cognitive baseline.[9–12]

DEMENTIA

The diagnosis and management of dementia in elderly persons is a common task and growing concern for PCPs. Recent epidemiologic data estimate that 13.9% of American adults older than 70 years have some form of dementia, most commonly caused by Alzheimer disease (AD).[13] This number continues to increase with age, composing 30% of 85 year olds.[14] In raw numbers, more than 5 million people in the United States currently have AD, and that number is expected to increase to more than 7 million by 2025.[15,16] Despite the striking prevalence of dementia in the community, PCPs continue to struggle with recognition, diagnosis, and documentation of cognitive impairment.[17]

If Mr Q's confusion does not have the acute onset or inattention consistent with delirium, then an investigation into dementia would be warranted. The chief feature suggestive of dementia is acquired cognitive impairment, usually in the domains of new learning and memory, severe enough to cause a decline in independent functioning. In dementia, memory impairment is observed in conjunction with deficits in at least one other cognitive domain. These deficits can include aphasia (difficulty understanding or producing speech), apraxia (difficulty performing tasks despite intact motor function), agnosia (difficulty with recognizing or naming familiar items), and executive dysfunction (inability to plan or organize complex tasks or make logical decisions). In the evaluation, it is critical to determine that the difficulties are related to actual cognitive loss rather than attributable to motor or sensory deficits or to an acute delirium. Unlike the acute nature of delirium, the development of a dementia is generally a subacute (months–years) process and represents a clear decline from a prior level of functioning in life.

Evaluation for dementia begins with a detailed history from both patients and at least one other informant. Individuals with suspected dementia do not often self-present for medical evaluation; concern by caregivers or family members usually brings individuals to attention. Lee and colleagues[10] describe a useful, structured approach for evaluating memory difficulties in primary care (**Fig. 1**).

History taking should focus on the time course of symptoms and their evolution. Patients should be observed and asked about changes in language, such as repetitive questioning, persistent word-finding difficulties, vague speech, or the frequent use of stereotyped phrases. Inquiry should elucidate evidence for functional impairment, particularly in the areas of activities of daily living (ADLs) and instrumental ADLs (IADLs). Asking explicitly about evidence for executive impairments, such as being taken in by telephone scams, choosing inappropriate clothing for the weather, or difficulty planning a shopping list or making meals, is also often useful.

In addition to a detailed history, routine evaluation should include some form of cognitive testing; several scales have been validated for the primary care population (**Table 1**).[19–21] One practice is to use the Mini-Cog as a screen, followed by the Montreal Cognitive Assessment (MoCA) or the Mini-Mental State Examination (MMSE) to further characterize the person's current deficits and to track the course of impairment over time.

The recommended laboratory and imaging workup for dementia is listed in **Box 4**. The primary purpose of the laboratory evaluation is to rule out any potential reversible cause for cognitive impairment and also to investigate for any comorbid medical illness that may be causing a mild delirium and temporarily worsening cognition. The routine use of neuroimaging in the evaluation of dementia is controversial because of concerns about cost-effectiveness and variable utility.[22–24] However, the American Academy of Neurology does recommend the use of structural neuroimaging (either computed tomography or magnetic resonance imaging) in the initial evaluation for dementia.[25] Potential reversible causes of dementia that could be found on neuroimaging include subdural hematomas, neoplasms, or significant hydrocephalus. In practice, many geriatric psychiatrists pursue imaging in cases when there are unexpected neurologic findings on examination, an atypical or unusual presentation, rapid decline, in young patients (aged <60 years), or when the imaging findings may be useful for families and caregivers to see. An observational study of patients evaluated in a memory clinic found that neuroimaging made some contribution to the diagnostic assessment more than 80% of the time.[26] **Box 5** lists suggestions for when to consider referring for specialty dementia evaluation.

Canadian Centre for Family Medicine Memory Clinic Clinical Reasoning Model
1. Is it delirium?
> Use the Confusion Assessment Method (Inouye 1990):
>> Acute onset and fluctuating course
>> +
>> Inattention
>> +
>> Disorganized thinking OR altered level of consciousness

2. Is it depression?
> Consider atypical presentations: anxiety, irritability, unexplained physical complaints, worsening cognition

3. Is there a reversible cause?
> Measure CBC, TSH, creatinine, electrolytes, calcium, glucose and vitamin B12; consider cranial imaging.

4. Is it dementia, MCI or normal aging?
- Dementia: objective findings of cognitive loss with impairment of ADLs
- MCI: objective findings of cognitive loss without impairment of ADLs
- Normal cognitive aging: no objective findings of cognitive loss

5. If it is dementia, what type or types?
- AD: initial short-term memory loss
- VaD: vascular risk factors; neuroimaging evidence of cerebrovascular involvement
- FTD: younger age, behavioral symptoms, or language impairment
- DLB: bradykinesia or features of parkinsonism, fluctuating cognition, visual hallucinations
- PDD: dementia occurring > 1 year after onset of Parkinson disease motor symptoms

6. How will you manage this?

7. Is driving a concern?

Fig. 1. Canadian Center for Family Medicine Memory Clinic Clinical Reasoning Model.[100–103] ADLs, activities of daily living; CBC, complete blood count; DLB, dementia with Lewy bodies; FTD, frontotemporal dementia; MCI, mild cognitive impairment; PDD, Parkinson disease dementia; TSH, thyroid-stimulating hormone; VaD, vascular dementia. (*From* Lee L, Weston WW, Heckman G, et al. Structured approach to patients with memory difficulties in family practice. Can Fam Physician 2013;59(3):249–54.)

Once there is established evidence of cognitive impairment, characterization of which dementia syndrome is present is helpful for patient and family education, treatment planning, and prognostic purposes. The 4 most common types of dementia are listed in **Table 2**. Importantly, syndromic overlap is quite common in dementia; it is not always possible to characterize a particular patient as having a singular cause for their cognitive impairment.[27]

Mild Cognitive Impairment

In recent decades, research into cognitive impairment has revealed an intermediate group of individuals with evidence of cognitive impairment not yet meeting the criteria for full dementia, now defined as mild cognitive impairment (MCI). MCI is a

Table 1
Cognitive testing

Test	Purpose	Sensitivity (%)	Specificity (%)
Mini-Cog (Borson et al,[104] 2003)	Screen for dementia	76	89
MMSE (cutoff of 24) (Folstein et al,[105] 1975, Crum et al,[106] 1993)	Diagnosis of dementia; track dementia progression over time	87	82
MoCA (Nasreddine et al,[20] 2005)	Diagnosis of MCI and dementia	90 100	87 87

Abbreviations: MCI, mild cognitive impairment; MMSE, Mini-Mental State Examination; MoCA, Montreal Cognitive Assessment.

heterogeneous concept, but individuals in this group are generally recognized to have deficits in at least one cognitive domain but otherwise continue to function independently. The presence of MCI greatly increases the risk for later development of dementia at a rate 3 times higher than individuals without MCI.[28,29] However, it has also been observed that 16% to 40% of patients have resolution of MCI and can revert back to normal cognition at follow-up assessments.[30,31] There is no current treatment of MCI that will prevent progression to dementia. Patients diagnosed with MCI should be monitored at least twice yearly for progression of cognitive impairment or deterioration of functioning.

PCPs will encounter an increasing number of middle-aged and older adults who are worried about the possibility of developing dementia and will wonder if their current memory problems are the start of this process. Normal aging can cause a subtle degradation in the speed and efficiency of information processing.[32] Older patients may notice that they are not able to multitask as easily, have some difficulty acquiring

Box 4
Evaluation of cognitive impairment

- History from patient and collateral informant (relative, friend, or caregiver)
- Mental status examination, including formal cognitive testing via MMSE or MoCA
- Physical examination, including neurologic examination
- Medication review
- Complete blood count
- Urinalysis
- Basic metabolic panel 10
- Liver function tests
- B_{12}, folate
- Thyroid-stimulating hormone, free T4
- Rapid plasma reagin test, Venereal disease research lab
- Head computed tomography or brain magnetic resonance imaging

Raskind MA, Bonner LT, Peskind ER. Cognitive Disorders. In: Blazer DG, Steffens DC, Busse EW. editors. Essentials of Geriatric Psychiatry. Washington, DC: American Psychiatric Publishing, Inc; 2007. p. 99–130.

Box 5
When to refer patients for specialty dementia evaluation
• Less than 65 years of age without family history of early onset dementia
• Atypical or rapid course
• Significant neurologic findings not accounted for by known prior cerebrovascular accident
• If considering a diagnosis of dementia with Lewy bodies or frontotemporal dementia
• Significant psychiatric comorbidity complicating presentation
• Patient or family request

Table 2
Four common causes of dementia

Dementia Type	Prevalence (%)	Age of Onset (y)	Cognitive Syndrome	Clinical Features
AD	50–60	>65	Insidious onset and progressive impairment Prominent memory impairment (impaired memory consolidation with rapid forgetting)	Aphasia Apraxia Agnosia Executive dysfunction Poor insight, apathy
Dementia with Lewy bodies	10–20	>65	Fluctuations in alertness Memory impairment Visuospatial deficits	Parkinsonian signs Visual hallucinations Neuroleptic sensitivity Falls (orthostatic hypotension) REM sleep behavior disorder
Vascular dementia	10–20	>65	Variable syndrome based on location of lesions Language/memory retrieval difficulties common	Focal neurologic deficits on examination Abrupt onset Executive dysfunction Vascular risk factors (hypertension, diabetes, AFib, hyperlipidemia) Pseudobulbar affect
Frontotemporal dementia	1–5	51–63 Rare after 75	Prominent personality/behavioral change Cognitive inflexibility Less obvious memory impairments in early years	Pronounced executive impairments Disinhibition or apathy Hyperorality, carbohydrate craving Hypersexuality Obsessive collecting/gathering behaviors

Abbreviations: AFib, atrial fibrillation; REM, rapid eye movement.
Adapted from Raskind MA, Bonner LT, Peskind ER. Cognitive Disorders. In Blazer DG, Steffens DC, Busse EW. editors. Essentials of Geriatric Psychiatry. Washington, DC: American Psychiatric Publishing, Inc; 2007. p. 99–130.

new information as fast as they once did, or have problems correctly remembering a newly learned list of items. However, unlike patients with MCI or dementia, cognitively normal individuals can acquire new information if given enough time and will recall a list if given cues or prompts. Most patients can be reassured that occasionally misplacing items or forgetting which word to use are not necessarily signs that they are becoming demented.[33]

AD

AD is the most common cause of dementia in older adults, accounting for 50% to 60% in autopsy samples.[27] The characteristic presentation for AD is insidious onset of memory impairment with a gradually progressive course starting after 65 years of age. The prognosis of AD is grim, with almost all patients requiring full care in the late stages. Survival varies by age at diagnosis, with most patients living an additional 7 to 10 years when diagnosed in the late 60s and early 70s.[34] **Table 3** describes the features of AD at mild, moderate, and severe stages and makes suggestions for possible interventions to help patients and families.

Food and Drug Administration–approved treatments for mild-moderate AD currently include 4 cholinesterase inhibitors (AChEIs) (donepezil, galantamine, rivastigmine, and tacrine) and one N-methyl-d-aspartate (NMDA) receptor antagonist (memantine) (**Table 4**: "Cognitive enhancers"). All AChEIs have similar side-effect profiles and tolerability, although tacrine is rarely used because of the risk of hepatotoxicity. There is ongoing disagreement regarding the effectiveness of AChEIs and memantine.[35–37] Controversy surrounds whether statistical significance found in research studies truly translates to clinically significant improvement. Common clinical practice is to choose one or more specific symptoms to target (such as word finding, language disturbance, or anxiety) when initiating a trial of an AChEI and/or memantine. If there is noticeable improvement or stabilization of the symptom after a few months, the medication is continued. Frequent reevaluation for efficacy and tolerability is needed, as patients' cognitive, behavioral, and medical symptom profiles change over time.

Dementia with Lewy Bodies

Once thought to be rare, dementia with Lewy bodies (DLB) has emerged in recent years as a significant cause of late-life dementia.[27] DLB is characterized by evidence of progressive cognitive decline consistent with dementia, combined with fluctuations in level of cognition and variable levels of alertness and attention, recurrent visual hallucinations that are well formed (typically of animals or small people), and spontaneous motor symptoms of parkinsonism.[38] The spontaneous parkinsonism typical of DLB is observed as bradykinesia and rigidity that affects the axial muscles more than peripheral, often resulting in a gait disorder and recurrent falls. The cognitive decline in DLB is similar to AD; but overall, the survival is shorter.[39,40]

Treatment of DLB involves symptomatic management for the most problematic aspects of the disease, such as with AChEIs or memantine for cognitive disruption, antiparkinsonian agents for significant gait and balance difficulties, low-potency atypical antipsychotics for disturbing visual hallucinations, or benzodiazepines for rapid-eye-movement sleep behaviors. Evidence for the cognitive enhancers is limited, but AChEIs and memantine may have modest benefits in DLB.[41–45] Antiparkinsonian agents, such as levodopa, can be considered for treatment of motor symptoms, although caution is advised to monitor for worsening of psychiatric symptoms.[38] Providers may consider treatment of the visual hallucinations if they are particularly disturbing or distressing to patients. Extreme neuroleptic sensitivity makes treatment particularly problematic in DLB, as extrapyramidal symptoms from antipsychotics

Table 3
Patient and caregiver experiences in dementia and possible interventions

Patient Characteristics	Caregiver Experiences	Possible PCP Interventions
Mild dementia (MMSE ~30–20)		
• Mild forgetfulness & word-finding trouble • Difficulty remembering appointments • Trouble with complex planning or multistep instructions • May have social withdrawal • May develop depression or anxiety related to cognitive decline	• Having to help more with planning, remembering, finances • Fearfulness about diagnosis & the future	• Diagnose & stage dementia in patient • Diagnose & treat any mood problems in patient • Counsel patient & family about legal issues, driving, advance care planning • Refer to memory clinic for diagnostic dilemmas or complex behavioral problems
Moderate dementia (MMSE ~20–10)		
• More language impairment • Difficulty with short-term memory, sequences, chronologies • More trouble with IADLS • Some trouble with ADLS • No longer able to drive or perform complex tasks • Beginnings of paranoia or fearfulness • May wander or get lost, leave stove on, succumb to scams	• Increasing burden of care • Frustration at memory trouble, language • Having to decrease working/activities to provide care • Increased vigilance as may not be able to leave patient alone • Poor sleep • Depression, anxiety, resentment, anger, grief	• Refer to caregiver support groups • Counsel regarding getting more help in the home • Refer patient for driving evaluation • Monitor caregiver for emergence of depression, fatigue • Involve family and friends to provide material & emotional support • Begin discussion about next steps in care: hiring help in the home, move to supported-living situation
Severe dementia (MMSE <10)		
• Physical manifestations begin: weakness, gait impairment, falls, swallowing trouble • Difficulty recognizing familiar people • Unable to perform any IADLs • Marked difficulty with ADLs • Apraxia • May have paranoia, delusions, agitation, aggression	• Fatigue may be severe • Medical complications emerge (eg, hypertension) • May feel guilt for placing patient in supervised care setting	• Refer to palliative medicine for goals of care discussion • Encourage caregiver to have close follow-up with their own PCP • Encourage respite, scheduled time away, exercise, self-care • Encourage support group and/or personal therapy
End stage		
• May be mute, bed bound • Requires complete care for ADLs	• Significant burden of daily care • Grief and/or relief at time of death	• Transition to hospice, either at home or in facility • Refer to bereavement support groups

Adapted from Merel S, DeMers S, Vig L. Palliative care in advanced dementia. Clin Geriatr Med, in press.

Table 4
Cognitive enhancers

Medication	Mechanism	Starting Dosage and Titration	Target Dosage	Take with Food	Major Side Effects
Donepezil pill or orally disintegrating tablet	AChEI	5 mg daily at bedtime Increase 5 mg in 4–6 wk	10 mg daily	No	Nausea, diarrhea, insomnia
Galantamine immediate-release tablet or solution	AChEI	4 mg BID increase 4 mg BID every 4–6 wk	12 mg BID	Yes	Nausea, vomiting, diarrhea
Galantamine extended-release tablet		8 mg daily Increase 8 mg every 4–6 wk	24 mg daily	Yes	
Rivastigmine pill or solution	AChEI	1.5 mg BID Increase 1.5 mg BID every 2–4 wk	6 mg BID	Yes	Dizziness, headache, nausea, diarrhea
Rivastigmine patch		4.6 mg/24 h Increase after 4 wk	9.5–13.3 mg/24 h		
Memantine	NMDA antagonist	5 mg daily Increase 5 mg every week in divided doses	10 mg BID	No	Dizziness, headache, confusion
Memantine extended-release tablet		7 mg daily Increase 7 mg daily every week	20 mg daily		

can increase agitation, worsen the movement disorder, and cause falls. If an antipsychotic medication is needed, use of a very-low-potency atypical, such as quetiapine, is a reasonable approach. Doses should be started low and titrated slowly. Patients and caregivers should be educated about the potential risks for worsening motor and behavioral symptoms and an increased risk of death with the use of antipsychotic agents in this population. Sleep disorders may improve with melatonin as a first trial, followed by low-dose clonazepam if necessary.[46] Consultation or comanagement with a neurologist or geriatric psychiatrist is usually indicated for these patients.

Vascular Dementia

Vascular dementia (VaD) represents an important cause for cognitive impairment in older adults, but the construct remains problematic.[47] Pure VaD is likely much less common than a mixed type, whereby cerebrovascular disease overlaps with other pathologies (particularly AD). In clinical practice, VaD is best conceptualized as dementia with an onset or dramatic worsening in the setting of a stroke or when evidence of significant cerebrovascular burden is found on imaging. Because the location and extent of vascular injury is highly variable, the clinical presentation of VaD can vary widely, from presentations similar to AD with primarily marked memory impairment to presentations with greater impairment in executive function and attention.

Treatment of VaD is focused on targeting risk factors for further cerebrovascular disease progression, including hypertension, diabetes, smoking, obesity, high cholesterol, high homocysteine, and atrial fibrillation.[48] The AChEIs and memantine are not currently approved for use in VaD but have some utility in clinical practice likely because there is so often overlap with AD.

Frontotemporal Dementia

Frontotemporal dementia (FTD; also called behavioral variant of frontotemporal lobar degeneration) is distinguished from the other dementias by a young age of onset and prominent changes in personality and behavior. Because it is most likely to present in younger individuals, FTD is often mistaken or misdiagnosed for a substance abuse, bipolar, or personality disorder. Neuroimaging can be helpful in the diagnosis of FTD, as a characteristic pattern of degeneration of the frontal and/or temporal lobes can be seen.

Treatment of FTD is largely symptomatic. AChEIs or memantine have not shown a clear symptomatic benefit in open-label studies and may even make behavioral disturbances worse.[49] Selective serotonin reuptake inhibitors (SSRIs) and trazodone may be useful for targeting impulsivity, sexually inappropriate behavior, and compulsive behaviors in some patients; but evidence is still preliminary.[49–51] Although antipsychotic medications are often used to treat behavioral symptoms in FTD, there have been no randomized controlled trials to examine this practice. As with patients with DLB, consultation with a specialist is helpful.

Neuropsychiatric Complications of Dementia

Although many different neurodegenerative diseases and medical conditions lead to dementia, the later stages of cognitive deterioration tend to look quite similar. Although depression and anxiety may emerge in earlier stages, significant behavioral problems, such as agitation, aggression, wandering, and resistance to care, tend to appear later in the course of disease.[52,53] Behavioral and environmental interventions are sometimes effective, but PCPs are often called on to prescribe medications to treat problem behaviors in their patients with dementia. The Clinical Antipsychotic Trials of Intervention Effectiveness-Alzheimer Disease study found that symptoms of anger, aggression, and paranoia did improve with active treatment with antipsychotics.[54] Caution needs to be used when prescribing these agents because of the risk of significant adverse effects, including orthostatic hypotension, sedation, falls, and an increase in cerebrovascular events and death.[55,56] Sink and colleagues[57] published a useful algorithm for evaluating and treating problematic behaviors in patients with dementia (summarized in **Box 6**).

DEPRESSION

Older adults receive most of their mental health treatment in the primary care setting because of the stigma and lack of access to mental health specialty services. Depression continues to be undertreated even when recognized, especially in older men and several minority groups.[58–61] Older adults often present to their PCP with somatic complaints rather than with mood concerns, which can make identifying depression more challenging without a high index of suspicion and an awareness of the prevalence of this disorder (**Box 7**). Many older adults have symptoms that fall short of meeting the criteria for major depression; but symptoms of minor depression, sometimes termed *depression not otherwise specified*, are associated with similar functional impairment, morbidity, mortality, and suffering. Clues to identifying depression include a lack of engagement with the provider (such as poor eye contact), failed appointments, providing vague or nonspecific concerns during an appointment, or

---

Box 6
Approach to the treatment of behavioral disturbances in patients with dementia

- Evaluate for occult medical problems and pain, and treat if present.
- Simplify the patients' medication list if possible, reducing or stopping medications that may be deliriogenic.
- Use nonpharmacologic behavioral and environmental strategies, including caregiver education.
- Consider a trial of a cholinesterase inhibitor if patients are not already taking one.
- Consider a trial of antidepressant if patients show signs of depression or anxiety.
- Consider a trial of antipsychotics only if no other options remain, there is concern for patient or caregiver safety, or patients seem to be experiencing considerable distress from delusions and agitation.
  - Have a risk-benefit discussion with the patients' surrogate discussing the possible increased risk of stroke or death before starting antipsychotics.
  - Check a baseline electrocardiogram for prolonged QT interval.
  - Reevaluate at least monthly for efficacy and side effects, and consider weaning and discontinuation every 6 months.

Adapted from Sink K, Holden K, Yaffe K. Pharmacologic treatment of neuropsychiatric symptoms of dementia: a review of the evidence. JAMA 2005;293(5):596–608.

---

somatic symptoms out of proportion to a patient's presenting concern. For example, Mr Q might be confused about his medications because he is apathetic about his medical care because of a new depression. Men may be more likely to present with substance abuse, irritability, anger, or social withdrawal and less likely to endorse sadness or psychological distress.[62] Please see **Box 8** for risk factors for depression.

The use of standardized scales can be helpful in identifying those who need a more in-depth interview to assess for depression. Such scales can be self administered or administered by medical assistants or nurses and the results provided to the PCP. Some of the most commonly used depression instruments are outlined in **Table 5**.[63–69]

Box 7
Why it can be difficult to diagnose depression

- Medication side effects can mimic depressive symptoms.
- The symptoms of concurrent medical illness overlap with symptoms of depression.
- There are clinician time pressures.
- The communication style of patients can lead to a difficulty in diagnosis.
- Multiple somatic concerns lead to a focus on medical causes.
- Clinician's, patients', or family's erroneous belief that
  - Depression is a normal consequence of aging.
  - Depression cannot or should not be treated.
  - Depression cannot improve with treatment.

Box 8
Risk factors for depression in older adults

- Social isolation
- Being widowed, divorced, or separated
- Lower socioeconomic status
- Female sex
- Uncontrolled pain
- Comorbid medical conditions
- Insomnia
- Cognitive impairment
- Functional impairment

Comorbidity

Depression is often embedded in a group of other symptoms; can be associated with medications or untreated medical issues, such as thyroid disease or diabetes; and can result in medical complications. **Box 9** lists some areas of clinical focus in patients identified as having depression. Looking at the full picture of patients' medical situation is warranted in order to identify medical issues that may contribute to depression or complicate treatment.

Depression often co-occurs with other mental health conditions, including anxiety disorders, somatization, cognitive impairment, personality disorders, and substance abuse or dependence involving alcohol, illicit drugs, pain medications, or sedative-hypnotic agents.[70–72] It is important to recognize these overlapping mental health syndromes, as older adults will sometimes receive medications for the other symptoms without recognition that they are related to the larger syndrome of depression. This practice can lead to polypharmacy and poor response to treatment and contribute to falls, accidents, and an increased risk of suicide.

Suicide

In the United States, older white men aged 85 years and older are the demographic group at the highest risk for completed suicide (**Box 10**). Older adults presenting with insomnia, psychotic symptoms, and agitation in combination with hopelessness, depression, unremitting pain, or active alcohol use are at a particularly high risk for

---

Table 5
Depression screening instruments

Instrument	Sensitivity (%)	Specificity (%)
2-item screen	97	67
Geriatric depression scale	94	81
Patient Health Questionnaire-9	88	88
Cornell Scale for Depression in Dementia	90	75
Patient Health Questionnaire-2	100	77

Adapted from Refs.[63–69]

Box 9
Areas of clinical focus in older adults with depression

- Review for medications with depressive side effects.
- Evaluate for contributing medical issues.
- Evaluate for complications and consequences of depression (eg, dehydration, malnutrition).
- Evaluate and adequately treat pain.
- Evaluate suicidality (plan, intent, lethality, and access to means).
- Ask about psychosis (may need additional medication or hospitalization).
- Screen for substance abuse, dependence, or withdrawal.
- Screen for cognitive impairment.
- Ask about prior treatment and success for patients and family members.

---

suicide.[70,73,74] In the United States, older adults attempt suicide less often but use more lethal means, such as firearms. Because of their often-debilitated medical status and social isolation, they are less likely to be discovered or to recover from an attempt.

Treatment

Once medical professionals identify depression, they should recognize the need to start conservative doses of medications for depression because of the physiologic changes in the geriatric population and their inability to tolerate standard starting adult doses. Starting one-half of a usual adult starting dose of medication is recommended. Unfortunately, failing to titrate the dose medication to the usual adult starting dose and then failing to further increase the dose to target ongoing symptoms commonly contributes to lack of relief from symptoms, ongoing suffering, and poor outcomes. It is important to monitor depression as an independent medical problem with a need for focused follow-up. Patients must be educated that these medications are to be taken every day and that response to and relief from symptoms often takes from 4 to 6 weeks and up to 12 to 14 weeks for full response because of the tendency for older adults to respond less rapidly to medications.

Box 10
Risk factors for suicide in older adults

- Social isolation
- Widowhood
- Chronic and inadequately treated pain
- Terminal or worsening physical illness
- Personality disorder
- Prior attempt
- Family history of suicide
- Substance abuse or dependence
- Access to lethal means, particularly firearms

Box 11
Tailoring antidepressant treatment

- Symptom profile (insomnia vs hypersomnia, poor appetite, pain)
- Cost of medication
- Drug interactions
- Medical comorbidities
- Safety
- Prior response of patient
- Prior or current response of family

Common variables to consider when choosing an antidepressant medication are shown in **Box 11**. Because in clinical trials antidepressants have shown relatively similar efficacy between classes, choosing an agent should be informed by patients' presentation, comorbid medical conditions, cost, safety, and prior treatment if any. Choosing a medication that a family member has had success with is a useful approach.[75] **Table 6** lists medications and other treatment modalities and potential reasons for use.

Although medications are often the primary focus of treatment of depression, older adults often despair at the idea of yet another medication to be added to their often already-complicated regimen or do not like the idea of taking a medication for depression.[76] Although educating patients that antidepressants can be very helpful and discussing depression as a medical problem can help with patients considering treatment with medication, respecting their decision not to take one is important. Identifying social issues that may benefit from the attention of social work, problem-solving therapy, and having information on available community resources for counseling that can be provided to patients are crucial.

Table 6
Depression treatments and considerations for use

Treatment	Useful for Patients with (Notes)
SSRIs (eg, citalopram)	Comorbid anxiety (safe, well tolerated, cost-effective)
Mirtazapine	Insomnia, poor appetite, weight loss, comorbid nausea
Serotonin norepinephrine reuptake inhibitors (eg, venlafaxine)	Comorbid neuropathic pain
Bupropion	Overweight, smoker, low energy
Tricyclic antidepressants (eg, nortriptyline)	Treatment resistance, need for/desire for blood level (third line; consider specialty referral)
Monoamine oxidase inhibitors (eg, tranylcypromine)	Treatment resistance (third line; consider specialty referral)
Electroconvulsive therapy	Inability to tolerate medications, rapid response needed, psychosis; prior response
Psychotherapy	Patient preference/adjunct

Behavioral activation is another important component of depression care and has been shown to be particularly beneficial for older adults.[77,78] Behavioral activation may include recommendations to increase social contacts, increase community connections, increase pleasurable activities identified by patients, and exercise. Problem-solving therapy is another approach and can help patients set goals and follow through on behavioral activation strategies toward solving problems they identify by making small incremental changes over time.[79]

Successful treatment of depression in primary care with collaborative care models has been shown repeatedly. Treatment involves care managers with the role of following up with depressed patients to identify side effects, investigate compliance, educate patients about depression and the course of treatment response, and to recommend a need for titration or change in the antidepressant regimen.[80–82] Collaborative care models have shown improved response to and remission of depressive symptoms and a decrease in suicidal ideation over usual care. PCPs and their staff can emulate collaborative care models by providing education to patients and their families about depression, medication side effects, response timeline, and the need to alert PCPs about side effects or a lack of response rather than stopping medication. A focused contact with patients either by phone or in the office 2 weeks after initiating medication to discuss side effects, assess the need for medication titration, discuss compliance issues, and to evaluate for clinical worsening or need for an increased level of care or specialty referral are particularly important. This practice is crucial for those who may be expressing hopelessness, passive death wishes, or suicidal ideation.

Treatment of depression can be successful if it is properly identified, treated with adequate doses of antidepressants with an important focus on response and remission of symptoms, and when follow-up for depression as an independent medical issue is provided. Failure to treat depression may lead to needless suffering, increased medical resource use, increased medical mortality, and suicide.

ALCOHOL AND SUBSTANCE MISUSE

Persons older than 65 years misuse alcohol and drugs less often than younger people, but the prevalence is increasing and is expected to continue to increase.[83] In a recent study of more than 10,000 older adults, 21% reported at-risk drinking (more than 2 drinks on average per day) and 17% binge drinking (more than 5 drinks per day at least once a month).[84] Although there are instruments to aid in screening for alcohol use disorders (such as the CAGE questionnaire for dependence and the Alcohol Use Disorders Identification Test for harmful drinking), simply asking patients about their specific pattern of alcohol use is probably the best first step.[85–87] It may also be necessary to query accompanying family members. Advice to older patients about their alcohol use needs to find a balance between recognition that low amounts of alcohol have been shown in several studies to have neuroprotective effects in some patients, whereas larger amounts and drinking in a binge pattern are clearly damaging to the brain.[88–90]

The drugs most commonly abused by older patients are prescription narcotics and benzodiazepines.[91] Less than 1% of illicit drug use is by persons older than 65 years, but this proportion too has been increasing in recent years. **Box 12** outlines risk factors for alcohol and substance misuse among the elderly. Mr Q should be asked about alcohol, any use of prescription narcotics and benzodiazepines, and illicit drugs as a cause for his confusion. Older patients with addiction problems should be referred for evaluation and treatment to a specialty clinic or addiction psychiatrist if possible.

Box 12
Warning signs and risk factors for alcohol or drug misuse

- Single
- Male
- Low income
- History of alcohol or substance misuse
- Few or no social connections
- Chronic pain
- Comorbid depression or anxiety
- Involvement in crime

Data from Taylor MH, Grossberg GT. The growing problem of illicit substance abuse in the elderly. Prim Care Companion CNS Disord 2012;14(4); and Culberson JW, Ziska M. Prescription drug misuse/abuse in the elderly. Geriatrics 2008;63:22–31.

CAREGIVERS

Many studies over the last decade have highlighted the increased morbidity and mortality associated with being a caregiver to an older adult, with and without dementia.[92–96] Screens have been developed to identify depression and strain among caregivers, but their utility in the primary care setting may be limited by time factors.[97,98] Asking the caregivers of older adults about their level of stress can reveal important problems not only affecting the caregivers but also the quality of the care they are providing and the well-being of the patients.[99] Once caregivers with high levels of strain or depression are identified, they can be referred for help to social workers or to outside resources or their own PCP can be alerted, with their permission. Mr Q's wife of many years should be asked about her own coping in the setting of his possibly diminished level of independent functioning.

CASE SUMMARY

The cause of Mr Q's confusion about his medications could be delirium, a sign of early dementia, apathy from depression, or caused by intoxication or withdrawal from alcohol or another substance of misuse. The initial approach to distinguishing these entities can be managed in the primary care setting, with referral to specialists in certain cases. Mr Q's wife should also be asked about her own coping (**Box 13**).

Box 13
What to do with Mr Q?

1. Screen for delirium
2. Screen for cognitive impairment
3. Screen for depression
4. Screen for alcohol or drug misuse
5. Assess his wife's coping

SUMMARY

The management of possible psychiatric issues in older adult patients will increasingly be done by PCPs. This overview summarizes an initial approach to delirium, dementia, depression, alcohol and substance misuse, and caregiver stress.

REFERENCES

1. Bureau USC, US Census Bureau. The next four decades the older population in the United States: 2010 to 2050. Statistics (Ber) 2010;2011:3–14.
2. Petterson SM, Liaw WR, Phillips RL, et al. Projecting US primary care physician workforce needs: 2010-2025. Ann Fam Med 2012;10:503–9.
3. Bartels SJ. Improving the system of care for United States Freedom Commission on Mental Health. Am J Geriatr Psychiatry 2003;11:486–97.
4. Folstein MF, Bassett SS, Romanoski AJ, et al. The epidemiology of delirium in the community: the Eastern Baltimore Mental Health Survey. Int Psychogeriatr 1991; 3(2):169–76.
5. Inouye SK. Delirium in older persons. N Engl J Med 2006;354(11):1157–65.
6. Inouye SK, van Dyck CH, Alessi CA, et al. Clarifying confusion: the confusion assessment method. A new method for detection of delirium. Ann Intern Med 1990;113(12):941–8.
7. Shi Q, Warren L, Saposnik G, et al. Confusion assessment method: a systematic review and meta-analysis of diagnostic accuracy. Neuropsychiatr Dis Treat 2013;9:1359–70.
8. Fick DM, Agostini JV, Inouye SK. Delirium superimposed on dementia: a systematic review. J Am Geriatr Soc 2002;50(10):1723–32.
9. Cole MG, Ciampi A, Belzile E, et al. Persistent delirium in older hospital patients: a systematic review of frequency and prognosis. Age Ageing 2009;38:19–26.
10. Dasgupta M, Hillier LM. Factors associated with prolonged delirium: a systematic review. Int Psychogeriatr 2010;22:373–94.
11. Kiely DK, Marcantonio ER, Inouye SK, et al. Persistent delirium predicts greater mortality. J Am Geriatr Soc 2009;57:55–61.
12. Saczynski JS, Marcantonio ER, Quach L, et al. Cognitive trajectories after postoperative delirium. N Engl J Med 2012;367:30–9.
13. Plassman BL, Langa KM, Fisher GG, et al. Prevalence of dementia in the United States: the aging, demographics, and memory study. Neuroepidemiology 2007; 29(1–2):125–32.
14. World Health Organization. Dementia: A Public Health Priority. Available at: http://www.who.int/mental_health/publications/dementia_report_2012. Accessed December 1, 2013.
15. Hebert LE, Weuve J, Scherr PA, et al. Alzheimer disease in the United States (2010-2050) estimated using the 2010 census. Neurology 2013;80(19):1778–83.
16. Thies W, Bleiler L. 2013 Alzheimer's disease facts and figures. Alzheimers Dement 2013;9(2):208–45.
17. Mitchell AJ, Meader N, Pentzek M. Clinical recognition of dementia and cognitive impairment in primary care: a meta-analysis of physician accuracy. Acta Psychiatr Scand 2011;124(3):165–83.
18. Lee L, Weston WW, Heckman G, et al. Structured approach to patients with memory difficulties in family practice. Can Fam Physician 2013;59(3):249–54.
19. Holsinger T, Plassman BL, Stechuchak KM, et al. Screening for cognitive impairment: comparing the performance of four instruments in primary care. J Am Geriatr Soc 2012;60:1027–36.

20. Nasreddine ZS, Phillips NA, Bédirian V, et al. The Montreal Cognitive Assessment, MoCA: a brief screening tool for mild cognitive impairment. J Am Geriatr Soc 2005;53(4):695–9.
21. Milne A, Culverwell A, Guss R, et al. Screening for dementia in primary care: a review of the use, efficacy and quality of measures. Int Psychogeriatr 2008;20:911–26.
22. Foster GR, Scott DA, Payne S. The use of CT scanning in dementia. A systematic review. Int J Technol Assess Health Care 1999;15(2):406–23.
23. Simon DG, Lubin MF. Cost-effectiveness of computerized tomography and magnetic resonance imaging in dementia. Med Decis Making 1985;5(3):335–54.
24. McMahon PM, Araki SS, Neumann PJ, et al. Cost-effectiveness of functional imaging tests in the diagnosis of Alzheimer disease. Radiology 2000;217(1):58–68.
25. Knopman DS, DeKosky ST, Cummings JL, et al. Practice parameter: diagnosis of dementia (an evidence-based review). Report of the Quality Standards Subcommittee of the American Academy of Neurology. Neurology 2001;56(9):1143–53.
26. Borghesani PR, DeMers SM, Manchanda V, et al. Neuroimaging in the clinical diagnosis of dementia: observations from a memory disorders clinic. J Am Geriatr Soc 2010;58:1453–8.
27. Knopman DS, Boeve BF, Petersen RC. Essentials of the proper diagnoses of mild cognitive impairment, dementia, and major subtypes of dementia. Mayo Clin Proc 2003;78(10):1290–308.
28. Bennett DA, Wilson RS, Schneider JA, et al. Natural history of mild cognitive impairment in older persons. Neurology 2002;59(2):198–205.
29. Manly JJ, Tang MX, Schupf N, et al. Frequency and course of mild cognitive impairment in a multiethnic community. Ann Neurol 2008;63(4):494–506.
30. Koepsell TD, Monsell SE. Reversion from mild cognitive impairment to normal or near-normal cognition: risk factors and prognosis. Neurology 2012;79(15):1591–8.
31. Larrieu S, Letenneur L, Orgogozo JM, et al. Incidence and outcome of mild cognitive impairment in a population-based prospective cohort. Neurology 2002;59(10):1594–9.
32. Blazer D, Steffens D, Busse E. Essentials of geriatric psychiatry. Arlington (TX): American Psychiatric Publishing, Inc; 2007.
33. Alzheimer's Association. Know the 10 signs. 2009. Available at: http://www.alz.org/national/documents/checklist_10signs.pdf. Accessed December 1, 2013.
34. Zanetti O, Solerte SB, Cantoni F. Life expectancy in Alzheimer's disease (AD). Arch Gerontol Geriatr 2009;49(Suppl 1):237–43.
35. Raina P, Santaguida P, Ismaila A, et al. Effectiveness of cholinesterase inhibitors and memantine for treating dementia: evidence review for a clinical practice guideline. Ann Intern Med 2008;148(5):379–97.
36. Qaseem A, Snow V, Cross JT, et al. Current pharmacologic treatment of dementia: a clinical practice guideline from the American College of Physicians and the American Academy of Family Physicians. Ann Intern Med 2008;148(5):370–8.
37. Yang Z, Zhou X, Zhang Q. Effectiveness and safety of memantine treatment for Alzheimer's disease. J Alzheimers Dis 2013;36(3):445–58.
38. McKeith IG, Dickson DW, Lowe J, et al. Diagnosis and management of dementia with Lewy bodies: third report of the DLB Consortium. Neurology 2005;65(12):1863–72.
39. Williams MM, Xiong C, Morris JC, et al. Survival and mortality differences between dementia with Lewy bodies vs Alzheimer disease. Neurology 2006;67(11):1935–41.

40. Hanyu H, Sato T, Hirao K, et al. Differences in clinical course between dementia with Lewy bodies and Alzheimer's disease. Eur J Neurol 2009;16(2):212–7.
41. McKeith I, Del Ser T, Spano P, et al. Efficacy of rivastigmine in dementia with Lewy bodies: a randomised, double-blind, placebo-controlled international study. Lancet 2000;356(9247):2031–6.
42. Mori E, Ikeda M, Kosaka K. Donepezil for dementia with Lewy bodies: a randomized, placebo-controlled trial. Ann Neurol 2012;72(1):41–52.
43. Rolinski M, Fox C, Maidment I, et al. Cholinesterase inhibitors for dementia with Lewy bodies, Parkinson's disease dementia and cognitive impairment in Parkinson's disease. Cochrane Database Syst Rev 2012;(3):CD006504.
44. Aarsland D, Ballard C, Walker Z, et al. Memantine in patients with Parkinson's disease dementia or dementia with Lewy bodies: a double-blind, placebo-controlled, multicentre trial. Lancet Neurol 2009;8(7):613–8.
45. Emre M, Tsolaki M, Bonuccelli U, et al. Memantine for patients with Parkinson's disease dementia or dementia with Lewy bodies: a randomised, double-blind, placebo-controlled trial. Lancet Neurol 2010;9(10):969–77.
46. Aurora RN, Zak RS, Maganti RK, et al. Best practice guide for the treatment of REM sleep behavior disorder (RBD). J Clin Sleep Med 2010;6:85–95.
47. Pohjasvaara T, Mäntylä R, Ylikoski R, et al. Comparison of different clinical criteria (DSM-III, ADDTC, ICD-10, NINDS-AIREN, DSM-IV) for the diagnosis of vascular dementia. National Institute of Neurological Disorders and Stroke-Association Internationale pour la Recherche et l'Enseignement en Neuro. Stroke 2000;31(12):2952–7.
48. Gorelick PB, Scuteri A, Black SE, et al. Vascular contributions to cognitive impairment and dementia: a statement for healthcare professionals from the American Heart Association/American Stroke Association. Stroke 2011;42(9): 2672–713.
49. Warren JD, Rohrer JD, Rossor MN. Clinical review. Frontotemporal dementia. BMJ 2013;347:f4827.
50. Manoochehri M, Huey ED. Diagnosis and management of behavioral issues in frontotemporal dementia. Curr Neurol Neurosci Rep 2012;12(5):528–36.
51. Huey ED, Putnam KT, Grafman J. A systematic review of neurotransmitter deficits and treatments in frontotemporal dementia. Neurology 2006;66(1):17–22.
52. Srikanth S, Nagaraja AV, Ratnavalli E. Neuropsychiatric symptoms in dementia-frequency, relationship to dementia severity and comparison in Alzheimer's disease, vascular dementia and frontotemporal dementia. J Neurol Sci 2005;236:43–8.
53. Lyketsos CG, Lopez O, Jones B, et al. Prevalence of neuropsychiatric symptoms in dementia and mild cognitive impairment: results from the Cardiovascular Health Study. JAMA 2002;288(12):1475–83.
54. Schneider LS, Tariot PN, Dagerman KS, et al. Effectiveness of atypical antipsychotic drugs in patients with Alzheimer's disease. N Engl J Med 2006;355: 1525–38.
55. Herrmann N, Lanctôt KL. Do atypical antipsychotics cause stroke? CNS Drugs 2005;19(2):91–103.
56. Brodaty H, Ames D, Snowdon J, et al. A randomized placebo-controlled trial of risperidone for the treatment of aggression, agitation, and psychosis of dementia. J Clin Psychiatry 2003;64:134–43.
57. Sink K, Holden K, Yaffe K. Pharmacological treatment of neuropsychiatric symptoms of dementia: a review of the evidence. JAMA 2005;293(5):596–608.
58. Lebowitz BD, Pearson JL, Schneider LS, et al. Diagnosis and treatment of depression in late life. Consensus statement update. JAMA 1997;278(14):1186–90.

59. Hybels CF, Blazer DG. Epidemiology of late-life mental disorders. Clin Geriatr Med 2003;19(4):663–96, v.

60. Unützer J. Clinical practice. Late-life depression. N Engl J Med 2007;357(22): 2269–76.

61. Fyffe DC, Sirey JA, Heo M, et al. Late-life depression among black and white elderly homecare patients. Am J Geriatr Psychiatry 2004;12(5):531–5.

62. Gallo JJ, Rabins PV, Lyketsos CG, et al. Depression without sadness: functional outcomes of nondysphoric depression in later life. J Am Geriatr Soc 1997;45(5):570–8.

63. Whooley MA, Avins AL, Miranda J, et al. Case-finding instruments for depression. Two questions are as good as many. J Gen Intern Med 1997;12(7):439–45.

64. Arroll B, Khin N, Kerse N. Screening for depression in primary care with two verbally asked questions: cross sectional study. BMJ 2003;327(7424):1144–6.

65. Montorio I, Izal M. The Geriatric Depression Scale: a review of its development and utility. Int Psychogeriatr 1996;8(1):103–12.

66. Rinaldi P, Mecocci P, Benedetti C, et al. Validation of the five-item geriatric depression scale in elderly subjects in three different settings. J Am Geriatr Soc 2003; 51(5):694–8.

67. Kroenke K, Spitzer RL, Williams JB. The PHQ-9: validity of a brief depression severity measure. J Gen Intern Med 2001;16(9):606–13.

68. Alexopoulos GS, Abrams RC, Young RC, et al. Cornell scale for depression in dementia. Biol Psychiatry 1988;23(3):271–84.

69. Li C, Friedman B, Conwell Y, et al. Validity of the Patient Health Questionnaire 2 (PHQ-2) in identifying major depression in older people. J Am Geriatr Soc 2007; 55(4):596–602.

70. Centers for Disease Control and Prevention (CDC). Homicides and suicides–National Violent Death Reporting System, United States, 2003-2004. MMWR Morb Mortal Wkly Rep 2006;55(26):721–4.

71. Cole MG, Dendukuri N. Risk factors for depression among elderly community subjects: a systematic review and meta-analysis. Am J Psychiatry 2003;160(6):1147–56.

72. Blow FC, Brockmann LM, Barry KL. Role of alcohol in late-life suicide. Alcohol Clin Exp Res 2004;28(Suppl 5):48S–56S.

73. Waern M, Runeson BS, Allebeck P, et al. Mental disorder in elderly suicides: a case-control study. Am J Psychiatry 2002;159(3):450–5.

74. Szanto K, Mulsant BH, Houck P, et al. Occurrence and course of suicidality during short-term treatment of late-life depression. Arch Gen Psychiatry 2003;60(6): 610–7.

75. Gartlehner G, Thaler K, Hill S, et al. How should primary care doctors select which antidepressants to administer? Curr Psychiatry Rep 2012;14:360–9.

76. Gum AM, Areán PA, Hunkeler E, et al. Depression treatment preferences in older primary care patients. Gerontologist 2006;46:14–22.

77. Pinquart M, Duberstein PR, Lyness JM. Treatments for later-life depressive conditions: a meta-analytic comparison of pharmacotherapy and psychotherapy. Am J Psychiatry 2006;163:1493–501.

78. Scogin F, Welsh D, Hanson A, et al. Evidence-based psychotherapies for depression in older adults. Clin Psychol Sci Pract 2005;12:222–37.

79. Arean P, Hegel M, Vannoy S, et al. Effectiveness of problem-solving therapy for older, primary care patients with depression: results from the IMPACT project. Gerontologist 2008;48:311–23.

80. Unützer J, Katon W, Callahan CM, et al. Collaborative care management of late-life depression in the primary care setting: a randomized controlled trial. JAMA 2002;288(22):2836–45.

81. Unützer J, Tang L, Oishi S, et al. Reducing suicidal ideation in depressed older primary care patients. J Am Geriatr Soc 2006;54(10):1550–6.

82. Bruce ML, Ten Have TR, Reynolds CF, et al. Reducing suicidal ideation and depressive symptoms in depressed older primary care patients: a randomized controlled trial. JAMA 2004;291(9):1081–91.

83. Han B, Gfroerer JC, Colliver JD, et al. Substance use disorder among older adults in the United States in 2020. Addiction 2009;104:88–96.

84. Blazer DG, Wu LT. The epidemiology of at-risk and binge drinking among middle-aged and elderly community adults: National Survey on Drug Use and Health. Am J Psychiatry 2009;166:1162–9.

85. Berks J, McCormick R. Screening for alcohol misuse in elderly primary care patients: a systematic literature review. Int Psychogeriatr 2008;20(6):1090–103.

86. Moore AA, Seeman T, Morgenstern H, et al. Are there differences between older persons who screen positive on the CAGE questionnaire and the Short Michigan Alcoholism Screening Test-Geriatric Version? J Am Geriatr Soc 2002;50:858–62.

87. Ewing JA. Detecting alcoholism. The CAGE questionnaire. JAMA 1984;252:1905–7.

88. Zahr NM, Kaufman KL, Harper CG. Clinical and pathological features of alcohol-related brain damage. Nat Rev Neurol 2011;7:284–94.

89. Panza F, Frisardi V, Seripa D, et al. Alcohol consumption in mild cognitive impairment and dementia: harmful or neuroprotective? Int J Geriatr Psychiatry 2012;27:1218–38.

90. Kim JW, Lee DY, Lee BC, et al. Alcohol and cognition in the elderly: a review. Psychiatry Investig 2012;9:8.

91. Simoni-Wastila L, Yang HK. Psychoactive drug abuse in older adults. Am J Geriatr Pharmacother 2006;4:380–94.

92. Gallagher D, Rose J, Rivera P, et al. Prevalence of depression in family caregivers. Gerontologist 1989;29:449–56.

93. Mausbach B, Chattillion E, Roepke S, et al. A comparison of psychosocial outcomes in elderly Alzheimer caregivers and noncaregivers. Am J Geriatr Psychiatry 2013;21(1):5–13.

94. Schulz R, Beach SR, Lind B, et al. Caregiving as a risk factor for mortality: the Caregiver Health Effects Study. JAMA 1999;285(24):2215–9.

95. Shaw WS, Patterson TL, Ziegler MG, et al. Accelerated risk of hypertensive blood pressure recordings among Alzheimer caregivers. J Psychosom Res 1999;46:215–27.

96. Lee S, Colditz GA, Berkman LF, et al. Caregiving and risk of coronary heart disease in U.S. women. Am J Prev Med 2003;24:113–9.

97. Brannan AM, Athay MM, Andrade AR. Measurement quality of the caregiver strain questionnaire-short form 7 (CGSQ-SF7). Adm Policy Ment Health 2012;39:51–9.

98. Sullivan MT. Caregiver Strain Index (CSI). Urol Nurs 2007;27:251–2.

99. Borson S, Scanlan JM, Sadak T, et al. Dementia services mini-screen: a simple method to identify patients and caregivers in need of enhanced dementia care services. Am J Geriatr Psychiatry 2013. [Epub ahead of print].

100. Gauthier S, Patterson C, Chertkow H, et al. Recommendations of the 4th Canadian Consensus Conference on the Diagnosis and Treatment of Dementia (CCCDTD4). Can Geriatr J 2012;15(4):120–6.

101. Chertkow H, Bergman H, Schipper HM, et al. Assessment of suspected dementia. Can J Neurol Sci 2001;28(Suppl 1):S28–41.

102. Garcia A. Cobalamin and homocysteine in older adults: do we need to test for serum levels in the work-up of dementia? Alzheimers Dement 2007;3(4):318–24.
103. Chow T. Structural neuroimaging in the diagnosis of dementia. Alzheimers Dement 2007;3(4):333–5.
104. Borson S, Scanlan JM, Chen P, et al. The Mini-Cog as a screen for dementia: validation in a population-based sample. J Am Geriatr Soc 2003;51(10):1451–4.
105. Folstein MF, Folstein SE, McHugh PR. "Mini-mental state". A practical method for grading the cognitive state of patients for the clinician. J Psychiatr Res 1975;12: 189–98.
106. Crum RM, Anthony JC, Bassett SS, et al. Population-based norms for the Mini-Mental State Examination by age and educational level. JAMA 1993;269(18): 2386–91.

Primary Care for Adults on the Autism Spectrum

Christina Nicolaidis, MD, MPH[a,b,d],*, Clarissa Calliope Kripke, MD[c],
Dora Raymaker, MS[a,d]

KEYWORDS

- Autism spectrum disorders • Primary care • Adults • Developmental disabilities

KEY POINTS

- The autistic population is very heterogeneous; individuals' skills or challenges fall along spectra on multiple axes (spoken language, written communication, ability to perform activities of daily living, need for consistency, sensory sensitivity, emotional regulation, and so forth) and can change depending on environmental stimuli, supports, and stressors.
- Autistic adults have increased rates of chronic medical illnesses, including epilepsy, gastrointestinal disorders, feeding and nutritional problems, metabolic syndrome, anxiety, depression, and sleep disturbances, and greater exposure to violence and abuse.
- Clinicians may improve quality of life by recommending accommodations, assistive technologies, therapies to improve adaptive function or communication, and caregiver training, and by supporting acceptance, access, and inclusion.
- Access to health care can be improved by using alternative communication strategies, reducing sensory stimuli, providing additional structure to visits, allowing extra time, and using visual aids.
- Illness often presents as a change from baseline behavior or function. When patients present with behavioral concerns, clinicians should consider medical and psychosocial causes.

INTRODUCTION

Although autism was once considered rare, it is now estimated that 1% of adults meet current criteria for autism spectrum disorder (ASD) with no difference in prevalence by

Disclosures: None.
[a] Regional Research Institute, School of Social Work, Portland State University, 1600 SW 4th Avenue, Suite 900, Portland, OR 97201, USA; [b] Departments of Medicine and Public Health & Preventive Medicine, Oregon Health and Science University; Academic Autism Spectrum Partnership in Research and Education, 3181 SW Sam Jackson Park Road, L475, Portland, OR 97239, USA; [c] Family and Community Medicine, University of California, San Francisco, 500 Parnassus Avenue, MU3E, Box 0900, San Francisco, CA 94143-0900, USA; [d] Academic Autism Spectrum Partnership in Research and Education, 1600 SW 4th Avenue, Suite 900, Portland, OR 97201, USA
* Corresponding author. Regional Research Institute, School of Social Work, Portland State University, 1600 SW 4th Avenue, Suite 900, Portland, OR 97201, USA.
E-mail address: nicol22@pdx.edu

age.[1] Because of changes in diagnostic criteria and their application over time, fewer adults have been formally diagnosed, but the large cohort of children diagnosed with ASD in the past 2 decades is rapidly approaching adulthood.

Autism, like other disabilities, does not preclude one from being healthy. However, cognitive and communication differences can complicate identification and management of illnesses unrelated to the disability. Also, autism is associated with increased prevalence of several medical conditions. The clinician's role is to prevent and treat illness, while providing support and accommodations for the disability. This article focuses on the identification of ASD in adults, potential referrals for services, the recognition of associated conditions, strategies, and accommodations to facilitate effective primary care services for autistic adults, and ethical issues related to caring for autistic adults. (Of note, we use terms such as "autistic adults" in this paper to respect the Autistic self-advocacy community's preference for identify first language over person-first language.)

As the literature on ASD in adults is at times sparse, we supplement existing evidence with recommendations from our professional and personal experiences as primary care physicians (PCPs), researchers, parents, and patients. Many of our recommendations arise from our National Institute of Mental Health–funded project with the Academic Autism Spectrum Partnership in Research and Education (AASPIRE, www.aaspire.org)[2] to develop a health care tool kit for autistic adults, their supporters, and their PCPs (http://autismandhealth.org), as well as from our work with the Office of Developmental Primary Care (http://ODPC.ucsf.edu).

We also extrapolate information from the body of literature on intellectual disability, although this extrapolation poses limitations. Some autistic individuals have intellectual disabilities. Others do not. Clinical data and strategies for people with intellectual disability are sometimes, but not always, applicable to people on the autism spectrum. Some notable differences are that autistic adults are more likely to struggle with communication pragmatics (eg, interpreting ambiguity or nuance, understanding context), have a higher level of education, and be impacted by atypical sensory experiences, and they are less likely to have a support system through county or state disability services. In general, clinicians should tailor their approach to the individual's needs, regardless of the patient's diagnostic label.

ASD DIAGNOSIS IN ADULTS

In 2013, the *Diagnostic and Statistical Manual of Mental Disorders, Fifth Edition* (DSM-5) unified autistic disorder, Asperger's disorder, childhood disintegrative disorder, and Pervasive Disorder Not Otherwise Specified into one diagnosis called ASD.[3] Although the DSM-5 conceptualizes ASD primarily as a social-communication disorder, there is also a growing literature supporting the hypothesis that ASD may be primarily characterized by differences in information processing.[4]

A large number of today's autistic adults may not have been formally diagnosed and/or may have been misdiagnosed with other conditions. PCPs may recognize characteristics of ASD in undiagnosed patients or in patients with other diagnoses. Patients also may diagnose themselves and offer this information to facilitate care or seek formal diagnosis. Recognition of ASD in adults can be challenging. Like people without disabilities, autistic individuals change and mature with age, and may develop coping strategies and skills that make autistic traits less noticeable. Furthermore, diagnostic criteria can manifest in multiple ways (see **Table 1**). For example, the DSM-5 criterion of "impaired social communication" may be met by someone with no speech or by someone with fluent speech and difficulty interpreting nonverbal cues.

Although ASD is referred to as a "spectrum" disorder, individuals do not fall on one linear spectrum of "low" and "high" functioning.[5] Instead, skills or challenges fall along spectra on multiple axes (spoken language, written communication, activities of daily living, need for consistency, sensory sensitivity, emotional regulation, and so forth). A patient with no spoken language may be able to read and write at a graduate level and an individual who speaks fluently may have profound learning disabilities. Within each axis, skills and challenges can change depending on environmental stimuli, supports, and stressors.

When considering a diagnosis, it is important not to rely on stereotypes. Autistic traits can be both strengths and challenges. Some autistic individuals develop great expertise in their areas of special interests, or capitalize on their need for consistency to self-manage chronic conditions. On the other hand, not all autistic individuals have stereotypically positive traits, such as memorization or computation, or possess savant skills. Autistic people do not always shy from social interactions, and many maintain strong friendships or relationships. Although, on average, autistic individuals have lower scores on tests of "cognitive empathy" (understanding another person's perspective) than nonautistic individuals, many score in the normal range. Moreover, autism is likely not associated with limitations in "affective empathy" (an observer's emotional response to the affective state of others).[6]

Clinicians should discuss risks and benefits of referral for formal diagnosis (**Box 1**). Referral can be challenging, as many autism specialists lack experience with adults. Diagnostic evaluation should draw on a variety of sources, including standardized diagnostic instruments such as the Autism Diagnostic Observation Schedule (ADOS).[7]

REFERRALS FOR ASSISTIVE TECHNOLOGIES AND THERAPIES

Assistive technologies, therapies, and services for autistic adults are not meant to treat or cure autism. They may improve function or quality of life by increasing coping strategies, treating co-occurring conditions, or providing access to accommodations and supports. Patients should select therapeutic goals and choose whether they wish to participate in therapy.

Assistive and augmentative communication (AAC) technology can improve communication for adults with limited or variable speech. AAC includes tools such as letter or picture boards or devices that translate text into speech. Adults can benefit even if such technology was not introduced in childhood. Sometimes patients' intellectual capabilities were underestimated, or the technology was not available. In other cases, patients develop the skills to use these technologies later in life. Some patients with fluent speech may lose their ability to speak when stressed or overwhelmed and can benefit from using AAC intermittently. Others may simply communicate more effectively using AAC. Previous failed attempts to use AAC, or the presence of speech, should not preclude consideration of an AAC referral. See **Table 2** for examples of AAC technology. Other assistive technologies that may be useful include speech-to-text (eg, Dragon Naturally Speaking) or word-completion programs, electronic or paper organizers, or visual or electronic reminders and alarms to help with prompting or sequencing. Consider offering referrals to speech and language pathologists or occupational therapists to address communication challenges or difficulty managing activities of daily living.

Depression, anxiety, posttraumatic stress disorder, and other mental health conditions may be more prevalent in autistic individuals;[8,9] however, mental health conditions are not inherent to autism. Mental health therapy may be useful to develop strategies for communication, organization, or sensory sensitivities, or to learn ways

Table 1
ASD characteristics in adults

DSM5 Criteria[3] for ASD		Examples of How Criteria May Manifest in Adults
A. Persistent deficits in social communication and social interaction across multiple contexts. (Diagnosis requires person meets all three criteria.)	1. Deficits in social-emotional reciprocity	Difficulty initiating or sustaining back and forth conversation; tendency to monologue without attending to listener cues; unusual response to greetings or other social conventions.
	2. Deficits in nonverbal communicative behaviors used for social interaction	Lack of eye contact; difficulty understanding non-verbal communication; unusual tone of voice or body language.
	3. Deficits in developing, maintaining, and understanding relationships	Challenges adapting behavior to match different social settings such as when interacting with family, friends, authority figures, or strangers; difficulty developing or sustaining friendships; greater than usual need for time alone.
B. Restricted, repetitive patterns of behavior, interests, or activities. (Diagnosis requires person meets at least two of four criteria.)	1. Stereotyped or repetitive motor movements, use of objects, or speech	Repetitive movements or "stimming" (eg, rocking, flapping, pacing, or spinning for enjoyment or as a coping mechanism); arranging objects in a very precise manner; echolalia; continuously repeating sounds, words, or phrases.
	2. Insistence on sameness, inflexible adherence to routines, or ritualized patterns of verbal or nonverbal behavior	Greater than expected degree of distress with changes in routines or expectations; difficulty transitioning between activities; need to do the same thing in the same way each time; greater than usual reliance on rituals for accomplishing daily tasks.
	3. Highly restricted, fixated interests that are abnormal in intensity or focus	Intense special interests (eg, looking at spinning objects for hours, learning the detailed schedules of an entire public transportation system, or becoming an expert in seventeenth century art) while having significant difficulty attending to topics outside of one's areas of special interest.
	4. Hyper- or hyporeactivity to sensory input or unusual interest in sensory aspects of the environment	Being hyper- or hypo-sensitive to sounds, lights, smells, or textures; having an abnormally high or low pain threshold; difficulty processing more than one sense at a time (eg, not being able to understand spoken language while looking at someone's face); tendency to become confused or overwhelmed by sensory stimuli; challenges with body awareness or separating different types of sensations.

C. Symptoms must be present in the early developmental period (but may not become fully manifest until social demands exceed limited capacities, or may be masked by learned strategies in later life)	Though characteristics should have been present throughout one's lifetime, a change in circumstances can disrupt coping strategies and make characteristics more pronounced; alternatively, environmental facilitators, supports, and coping strategies may make characteristics less noticeable.
D. Symptoms cause clinically significant impairment in social, occupational, or other important areas of current functioning.	Characteristics lead to difficulty obtaining or sustaining employment, doing basic or instrumental activities of daily living, maintaining social life, or integrating with community. For example, there may be significant mismatch between educational attainment and occupational history.
E. These disturbances are not better explained by intellectual disability or global developmental delay. Intellectual disability and autism spectrum disorder frequently co-occur; to make comorbid diagnoses of autism spectrum disorder and intellectual disability, social communication should be below that expected for general developmental level.	N/A

Data from American Psychiatric Association. Diagnostic and statistical manual of mental disorders, Fifth edition (DSM-5). Washington, DC: American Psychiatric Association; 2013.

Box 1
Potential risks and benefits of obtaining autism spectrum disorder (ASD) diagnosis in adult patients

Potential benefits of a formal diagnosis are as follows.

- Would confer anti-discrimination and legal rights to accommodations in school, at work, in health care, or in other settings.
- May assist the individual in developing a better understanding of self.
- May provide peace of mind through the professional confirmation of life experiences.
- May provide means to experience better coping or quality of life by more directly recognizing strengths and accommodating challenges.
- May provide other means to understand and support the individual.
- May qualify the individual for benefits and services for people who have an ASD diagnosis.
- May qualify the individual for programs for people with disabilities, such as scholarships or incentives that are meant to increase workplace diversity.

Potential risks associated with seeking an ASD diagnosis are as follows.

- The process of seeking and being evaluated for the diagnosis may be stressful.
- The person may perceive the interaction with the diagnostician or provider as negative, disrespectful, or otherwise uncomfortable.
- The interpretation of ASD criteria and subsequent diagnosis varies by provider, particularly in the adult presentation.
- Information about an individual's ASD could potentially negatively impact child custody cases.
- Others in the individual's life may still not be supportive, even with the diagnosis.

Adapted from the Academic Autistic Spectrum Partnership Research and Education (AASPIRE) Healthcare Toolkit. Available at: http://autismandhealth.org/. Accessed June 23, 2014.

to understand and manage social situations and change. Therapy may be helpful to understanding and responding to negative emotions or preventing melt-downs. However, it may be necessary to find a therapist with experience working with autistic patients. Because of the socio-communication differences inherent in autism, assumptions about how to communicate with patients, understand patient behavior, or foster therapeutic relationships may not apply.

Local autism centers, autism organizations, developmental disability programs, or professional organizations may have names of therapists with expertise working with autistic adults, or may be able to offer supports and services directly. Vocational rehabilitation services may be able to help patients obtain or sustain employment, including by assisting with referrals to therapists. **Box 2** lists potential resources.

ASSOCIATED CONDITIONS

Both genetic and environmental factors play a role in health outcomes.[10] Current evidence suggests autistic adults have high rates of associated chronic medical illness, especially epilepsy, gastrointestinal disorders, feeding and nutritional problems, metabolic syndrome, anxiety, depression, and sleep disturbances. Iatrogenic problems, such as side effects of medications, are also common,[11,12] as is exposure to violence and abuse.[13]

Table 2 Examples of alternative and augmentative communication (AAC) assistive technology			
	Text	**Image**	**Symbols**	**Gesture**
Unaided (no device)				• American Sign Language • Body language
Low-tech	• Writing with pencil/paper • Letter board	• Drawing with pencil/paper • Picture board • Photographs • Manipulation of physical objects/ models	• Braille • Symbolic language like Bliss Symbolics or MinSpeak on a board	
High-tech	• Text-to-speech device (example: DynaVox DynaWrite) • Text to speech software (example: Proloquo2Go for iPhone)	• Picture-based device (example: DynaVox Maestro) • Picture based software (example: AssistiveWare's LayoutKitchen)	• Symbolic device (example: DynaVox with Bliss Symbolics package) • Symbolic software (example: WinBliss software)	

Many of these devices can also be equipped with alternative interfaces, such as pointers, switches, and eye gaze systems for individuals with limited motor control or coordination. Assistive Ware's Layout Kitchen (Assistive Ware, Amsterdam, The Netherlands); DynaVox DynaWrite (DynaVox Mayer Johnson, Pittsburgh, PA); DynaVox Maestro (DynaVox Mayer-Johnson, Pittsburgh, PA); DynaVox with Bliss Symbolics package (DynaVox Mayer-Johnson, Pittsburgh, PA); Proloquo2Go for iPhone (Assistive Ware, Amsterdam, The Netherlands); WinBliss software (AnyCom AB, Yngsjö, Sweden).

Mortality

There is some evidence that autism is associated with modestly reduced life expectancy. The expected number of deaths is approximately 2 to 3 times higher than age-matched and sex-matched peers in the general population.[14] Risk factors include moderate to severe intellectual disability, epilepsy, and female sex. Death from seizures, sudden unexpected death in epilepsy, and accidents, such as suffocation and drowning, are more common, but there is also increased risk of mortality from a wide variety of causes that also are found at similar rates in the general population. The excess mortality from these causes might reflect difficulties in recognizing and reporting signs and symptoms or in accessing health care.[14–17]

Epilepsy

Approximately 20% to 30% of autistic adults have co-occurring epilepsy. The first seizure often occurs during adolescence. Autistic adults with intellectual disability have higher rates of epilepsy than those with normal intelligence.[14,18] Epilepsy can be misdiagnosed due to misinterpreting events as behavioral tics, lack of attention, emotional outbursts, stereotyped movements, or other presentations.[19] On the other hand, calming repetitive movements, atypical facial expressions, or unusual behaviors can be confused with seizure spells. Seizures can be missed more easily in patients who have nontraditional ways of communicating or who have complex teams providing their support.[20] Caregiver education and capturing spells on video can aid accurate diagnosis. Clinicians also should monitor side effects of antiepileptic

Box 2
Resources for autistic patients, families, and health care providers

Resources for Primary Care Providers

- *Academic Autism Spectrum Partnership in Research and Education (AASPIRE) Healthcare Toolkit.* Targeted to autistic adults, supporters, and primary care providers. Includes the Autism Healthcare Accommodations Tool (AHAT), worksheets and checklists, and step-by-step guides: www.autismandhealth.org.

- *University of California San Francisco Office of Developmental Primary Care.* Resources about developmental disabilities for primary care providers, including forms for behavior assessment: http://odpc.ucsf.edu/

- *Health Care for Adults with Intellectual and Developmental Disabilities.* Toolkit for Primary Care Providers: http://vkc.mc.vanderbilt.edu/etoolkit/

Information on Autism-Related Services and Resources

- *Autism NOW Center.* National Autism Resource and Information Center, sponsored by the Administration on Intellectual and Developmental Disabilities (AIDD): www.autismnow.org

- US Department of Health and Human Services *Administration for Community Living* maintains a comprehensive list of relevant agencies and resources: http://www.acl.gov/Get_Help/Help_Indiv_Disabilities/

- *Autism Society of America*: http://www.autism-society.org/

The Americans with Disabilities Act (ADA) in health care

- Main ADA page: http://www.ada.gov

- For more information on the ADA and health care: http://www.pacer.org/publications/adaqa/health.asp

- For an in-depth legal analysis of the ADA in health care, see http://www.ncbi.nlm.nih.gov/books/NBK11429/

- ADA Centers see http://adata.org/Static/Home.html

- ADAdata.org has a frequently asked questions page where you can learn more about the ADA: http://adata.org/faq-page

- The Autistic Self Advocacy Network has a series of policy briefs on health care and intellectual and developmental disabilities: http://autisticadvocacy.org/

Autistic Community Links for Patients

Books and Guides for Autistic Individuals from the Autistic Self-Advocacy Network (available at http://autisticadvocacy.org/about-asan/books/) include the following:

- Welcome To The Autistic Community: http://autisticadvocacy.org/wp-content/uploads/2014/02/WTTAC-Adult-FINAL-2.pdf

- Navigating College: http://navigatingcollege.org/

- Loud Hands: Autistic People, Speaking (ISBN-10: 1938800028)

Autistic Advocacy Groups and Forums

- The Autistic Self-Advocacy Network: http://autisticadvocacy.org/

- Autism Women's Network (AWN): http://autismwomensnetwork.org/

- Wrong Planet: largest online autistic forum with more than 80,000 members. WrongPlanet.net

- The Thinking Person's Guide to Autism: http://www.thinkingautismguide.com/

- Autism National Committee: http://www.autcom.org/

medications and do regular pharmacy reviews for drug interactions. Antiepileptics are a risk factor for osteoporosis and vitamin D deficiency.[21] Consider side effects of anti-seizure medication in the differential diagnosis of a change in behavior.

Gastrointestinal Disorders

Gastrointestinal disorders, such as gastroesophageal reflux, constipation, and food intolerances are commonly reported by autistic people.[22] However, the prevalence, etiology, and treatments for these conditions are not well studied.[23] Physical distress from gastrointestinal problems can increase agitation. Identifying and treating gastro-intestinal problems may reduce what appear to be symptoms of psychiatric illness. Dysphagia and esophageal reflux are common in people who have difficulty producing clear speech. Consider a swallow study in patients who cough or become short of breath with meals.

Feeding and Nutrition

Feeding problems and poor nutrition can result from unrecognized reflux, constipation, bowel motility problems, dysphagia, or dental problems. Feeding and nutritional issues also can be related to sensory sensitivities to flavors, textures, or smells. Some autistic patients may have difficulty identifying the sensation of hunger, managing cooking or the grocery store, or initiating the actions required to prepare or consume meals; these individuals may require prompts and support. Sometimes autistic people have not been offered basic education about healthy lifestyles in a format they can understand. Our tool kit includes a variety of accessible patient materials about nutrition and exercise (http://autismandhealth.org). Clinicians can encourage supporters and programs to facilitate healthy eating and exercise habits, and to avoid using foods as rewards.[24]

Metabolic Syndrome

Based on retrospective chart reviews, autistic adults appear to have a higher-than-average prevalence of hypertension, hyperlipidemia, obesity, and diabetes.[11,12] Clinicians should perform age-appropriate screening of weight, blood pressure, cholesterol, and blood sugar, minimize the use of medications, such as antipsy-chotics, that are known to exacerbate metabolic syndrome, and provide accessible information about lifestyle modifications.

Mental Health

A systematic review of 40 studies found high rates of anxiety in autistic children and adolescents.[8] One study of anxiety across the life span in autistic individuals found that anxiety rises from toddlerhood to childhood, decreases from childhood to young adulthood, but again increases from young adulthood into older adulthood.[25] There is also growing evidence that autistic individuals experience high rates of depressive ill-nesses.[9] Behavioral and psychiatric disorders in people with developmental disabil-ities are often the result of social and physical stressors, trauma, discrimination, and lack of effective communication. Some of the excess frequency of psychiatric illness may be preventable.[26] Mainstream mental health and disability support services often have inadequate training to work with autistic adults.[27] Referral to regional subspe-cialty services may be required.[28]

Psychiatric diagnoses can be made in people with intellectual disabilities or who communicate in nontraditional ways. The National Association for the Dually Diag-nosed has published an adaptation of the *Diagnostic and Statistical Manual of Mental Disorders, Fourth Edition, Text Revision* for intellectual disability,[29] although one does not yet exist specific to autism. Once a diagnosis is made, careful therapeutic trials of standard medications and treatments are reasonable.

Sleep Disturbances

Sleep disturbances are commonly reported both in autistic children[30] and adults.[31] Longitudinal studies show sleep problems persist as children age.[32] Sleep problems are associated with challenging behavior, respiratory disease, visual impairment, psychiatric conditions, and may be exacerbated by medications, especially psychotropic, antiepileptic, and antidepressant medications.[33] Patients should be assessed for possible medical problems, such as esophagitis or unrecognized pain.

Melatonin has the best evidence to support its effectiveness in autistic people and has a favorable side-effect profile. Patients can try 1 to 10 mg orally 30 minutes before bedtime.[34,35] Nonpharmacological approaches, such as sleep hygiene, also may be effective.[36]

Violence and Abuse

There is strong evidence to suggest both men and women with disabilities are more likely to experience violence victimization than the general population.[13] People with disabilities are at risk for physical and sexual violence from intimate partners, caregivers, and peers. Abuse also can take the form of refusal to provide assistance with essential activities of daily life, economic abuse, and the withholding of an assistive device. Clinicians should regularly screen for violence and should always keep violence or abuse in the differential diagnosis for injuries, changes in behavior, worsened mental health issues, or unexplained medical problems.

FACILITATING EFFECTIVE HEALTH CARE INTERACTIONS

People with disabilities face significant disparities in health and health care.[37–39] We have found that autistic adults experience greater unmet health care needs, greater emergency room use, less use of recommended preventive care services, lower satisfaction with health care, lower health care self-efficacy, and a greater number of barriers to health care than nonautistic adults.[40]

Many ASD characteristics can directly impact health care. Effective physician-patient communication correlates with improved patient health outcomes, even in general populations.[41] In our qualitative study, autistic adults described examples of how failure to accommodate communication, sensory integration, and executive functioning resulted in poor outcomes. They also reported that their uneven skills[42,43] led providers to make false assumptions about their abilities to understand health care issues, communicate, or navigate the health care system.[44]

Table 3 lists ASD-related characteristics that can impact health care interactions, with recommendations for strategies or accommodations. **Box 3** offers additional strategies and accommodations for facilitating physical examinations, tests, procedures, phlebotomy, and dentistry. As each patient is unique, it is important to understand his or her individualized needs and preferences. AASPIRE has created the Autism Healthcare Accommodations Tool (AHAT), an interactive tool for patients and supporters to create a provider-friendly report of individualized strategies and accommodations to facilitate health care; it can be accessed at http://autismandhealth.org.

When caring for autistic adults, obtain information about their communication, including speaking and understanding spoken language, reading and writing, use of AAC, and effects of stress on communication. Attempt to use the most effective communication mode for the patient, even if it means altering your usual interview

Table 3
Potential strategies and accommodations to address autism spectrum disorder (ASD)-related factors that can affect health care

ASD-Related Factor	Potential Strategies or Accommodations
Heterogeneity of communication skills between and within autistic individuals	• Obtain information on patient's 　○ Ability to understand spoken language. 　○ Ability to speak. 　○ Ability to read and write. 　○ Use of alternative and augmentative communication (AAC). 　○ Preferred communication mode. 　○ Ability to use the telephone for between-visit communications (and alternatives if telephone is not effective). 　○ Communication variability based on environmental factors or stress. • Do not assume that a patient cannot understand health care information or communicate because they cannot speak fluently. • Do not assume that a patient with fluid speech or an advanced vocabulary does not have significant communication difficulties. • Attempt to use the most effective communication mode, even if it means altering your usual interview style.
Tendency to take language literally and need for precise language	• Be very concrete and specific. • Avoid expressions and figures of speech. • Avoid very broad questions. (Some patients may need only "yes" or "no" questions; others may be able to answer open-ended questions if provided with specific instructions or examples.) • Show lists of symptoms to choose from. • Give examples of the types of things people may experience and have the patient tell you if he or she also experiences them. • Remind that it is OK to not know the answers to questions or not to be 100% exact. • Give very blunt and concrete examples when discussing your assessment and plan. • Direct to detailed information about health conditions and treatment options.
Atypical nonverbal communication	• Patient may have difficulty understanding tone of voice, facial expressions, or body language. • Patients may inadvertently seem rude because of their atypical body language or facial expressions (potentially in addition to use of very direct language). • Do not force patient to make eye contact; it may be uncomfortable or hinder effective communication.

(continued on next page)

Table 3
(continued)

ASD-Related Factor	Potential Strategies or Accommodations
Slow processing speed	• Give time to process what has been said or to respond. Check if ready to move on. • Give extra time to process sensory input before they respond. • Schedule longer appointments. • Encourage patients to prepare notes in advance about what they want to discuss. Carefully read any notes that patients bring to the visit. A variety of templates are available to help patients prepare for visits at http://autismandhealth.org. • Write down important information or instructions. • Direct to detailed information or resources about health conditions for review outside of the appointment. • Allow patient to communicate decisions at a later time. It may be possible to see another patient and then return to finish a visit with the original patient, or it may be best to schedule a follow-up visit.
Increased or decreased sensory sensitivity; difficulty processing multiple stimuli at once.	• Use natural light, turn off fluorescent lights, make the lighting dim. • Try to see the patient in a quiet room. • Only have one person talk at a time and try not to talk to the patient while there are other noises. • Avoid unnecessarily touching the patient (for example, to express concern). • Warn the patient before you touch him or her. • Encourage patient or supporters to bring objects to reduce or increase sensory stimuli. Examples may include headphones to block noise or sensory toys or fidgets.
Repetitive ("stimming") behaviors	• Stimming may be an effective coping mechanism, especially during times of stress, such as medical visits. Do not try to dissuade stimming behaviors or assume that a patient is not paying attention because he or she is fidgeting, making repetitive movements, or not looking at you.
Atypical body awareness, pain, and sensory processing	• Consider the possibility that differences in body awareness may be affecting how a patient recognizes or describes a symptom, or how a patient responds to illness. • In some cases, you may need to do additional testing or imaging, as information from the history and physical may be limited.

Need for consistency	• Before a visit, ask staff to:
	  ○ Let the patient or his or her supporters know what is likely to happen.
	  ○ Avoid rescheduling appointments and notify as soon as possible of unexpected changes.
	  ○ Enable the patient to procure pictures of the office and/or staff.
	  ○ When checking in, let the patient know how long the wait is likely to be, and give plenty of warning about delays.
	• During a visit:
	  ○ Make a problem list with the patient, and collaboratively decide what to address.
	  ○ Explain, in detail, what is likely to happen during the visit.
	  ○ Write down a list of topics and point out when there is a change of topic.
	  ○ Show the patient equipment before using it. If possible, do a "trial run" of difficult examinations or procedures.

Limited time awareness	• Link questions about time to important events in the patient's life. • Work with the patient to best explain time-based recommendations; for example, help the patient set up an alarm for when to take a pill, or link the act of taking a pill to specific parts of their daily routine.
Visual thinking	• Offer to use diagrams, pictures, or models with patients who may benefit from them. • Create (or have your staff or the patient's supporters create) visual schedules for your recommendations. For example, make a visual schedule for when a patient should take his or her medications.
Difficulties planning, organization, and sequencing	• Write out detailed step-by-step instructions. • Show the patient what you want him or her to do while the patient is still in your office. • Have office staff help the patient schedule follow-up visits, referrals, or tests. • Show or have someone show the patient how to get to other places in your office or medical center. • Have office staff contact the patient or his or her supporters after the visit to make sure that the patient has been able to follow your instructions. • Provide worksheets or diaries to keep track of symptoms. • Provide detailed information about how to communicate with office staff between visits.

Adapted from the Academic Autistic Spectrum Partnership Research and Education (AASPIRE) Healthcare Toolkit. Available at: http://autismandhealth.org/. Accessed June 23, 2014.

Box 3
Strategies and accommodations for successful physical examinations, tests, procedures, phlebotomy, and dentistry

Physical examinations, tests, and procedures[a]

The following are examples of accommodations or strategies that may help some patients:

- Explain what is going to be done before doing it.
- Show the patient equipment (or pictures of the equipment) before using it.
- If possible, let the patent do a "trial run" of difficult examinations or procedures.
- Tell the patient how long an examination or procedure is likely to take.
- Warn the patient before touching or doing something to him or her.
- Limit the amount of time a patient has to be undressed or in a gown.
- Give patients extra time to process things they need to see, hear, or feel before they respond.
- Allow the patient to sit, lie down, or lean on something during procedures, when possible.
- Let patients use a signal to tell you they need a break.
- Ask the patient from time to time if he or she is able to handle the pain or discomfort.

In many cases, thoughtful planning and appropriate accommodations can enable patients to tolerate examinations and procedures that have previously been intolerable. Still, there may be times when patients need anesthesia to tolerate examinations or procedures.

Phlebotomy[a] may be particularly challenging for some (but not all) patients on the autism spectrum. If a patient has had a particularly hard time with blood draws, you may consider some of the following strategies and accommodations:

- Only order blood tests when absolutely necessary and group them together to minimize the number of draws.
- Allow the patient to lie down or lean back on something.
- Use a numbing spray or cream.
- Be very patient and use a calm voice.
- Give the patient a very detailed explanation of what will happen, including how many tubes of blood you will fill.
- Consider giving the patient an anti-anxiety medication before the blood draw.
- Give the patient a lot of advance warning so he or she can prepare himself or herself emotionally.
- Give the patient something to distract his or her attention.

Dentistry may require additional accommodations to reduce barriers to accessing care. The following strategies may be useful to some patients.

- To accommodate sensory issues
  - Noise-reducing ear phones
  - Dark glasses or an eye pillow
  - Use of a private room or scheduling as the last of the appointment of the day to reduce or eliminate noise from other patients
- To tolerate examinations, cleanings, or procedures
  - Use of nitrous oxide during the visit
  - Use of valium or other sedative before the visit
  - Anesthesia

- To accommodate other stressors
  - Providing clear indication of the order of events
  - Indicating how long each event is likely to take
  - Decreasing wait time
  - Minimizing small talk and other distractions
- To accommodate challenges with dental hygiene
  - Adaptive toothbrushes
  - Water pic and suction
  - Chlorhexidine oral rinse on a swab or brush
  - Use of xylitol sprays or chewing gum
  - Increasing time between meals
  - Use of mouth rinse or baking soda in water

a *Adapted from* the Academic Autistic Spectrum Partnership Research and Education (AASPIRE) Healthcare Toolkit. Available at: http://autismandhealth.org/. Accessed June 23, 2014.

style. Also note that many patients cannot effectively communicate via telephone, even if they speak fluently, and need to establish alternate ways to communicate between visits.

Figures of speech, vague statements, and broad questions can be problematic for individuals who take language literally or who require very precise language. Patients may experience anxiety if they cannot answer a question with 100% accuracy. It is best to be concrete and specific. Some patients may be able to respond to questions better if offered multiple-choice–style answers, examples of the types of things people may experience, or are reassured that they do not need to be 100% accurate.

Patients may have difficulty understanding nonverbal cues and may inadvertently seem rude because of their atypical body language or facial expressions. Do not force a patient to make eye contact, as it may cause discomfort or hamper his or her ability to communicate.

Autistic individuals may have difficulty processing information quickly enough to respond to questions or make health care decisions in real time. For example, patients report insufficient time to indicate that an area is tender before the provider begins palpating a different area. Give patients time to process information or stimuli, and check for understanding before moving on. Encourage patients to prepare information before the visit and try to write down key information so that they can review it later. It may be necessary to schedule longer appointments or a second visit.

Autistic individuals commonly have atypical sensory processing, including increased or decreased sensitivity to sounds, lights, smells, touch, or taste. They may have great difficulty filtering background noise, processing information in overstimulating environments, or processing more than one sensation at a time. Sensory issues can compromise a patient's ability to communicate or tolerate a health care visit. It is important to assess a patient's sensory needs and find ways to remove environmental barriers to care. Repetitive behaviors ("stimming") may be an effective coping mechanism, especially during times of stress. Do not dissuade stimming behaviors or assume that a patient is not paying attention because of fidgeting, repetitive movements, or lack of eye contact.

Autistic patients may experience challenges related to limited body awareness. Examples include difficulty discriminating abnormal from normal body sensations, difficulty pinpointing the location of a symptom, difficulty characterizing the quality of a sensation, experiencing particularly high or low pain thresholds, displaying atypical body language when in distress, and difficulty recognizing normal stimuli such as hunger or the need to micturate. It is important to ask the patient about differences in body awareness that may affect recognition or description of symptoms, or responses to pain or illness. In some cases, you may need to do additional testing or imaging.

Autistic individuals often require great consistency. Changes in routine can provoke confusion or anxiety, leading to melt-downs or an inability to function. They may need clear agendas and more detailed explanations than other patients to plan for a visit or to stay focused and comfortable, or may benefit from trial runs for difficult procedures. Other autism-related factors that can affect health care interactions include limited time awareness, or difficulties with planning, organization, and sequencing.

Some autistic adults have difficulty accessing dental care because of sensory challenges, financial barriers, and a lack of qualified clinicians. Strategies include providing information on what to expect for how long, decreasing wait times, and minimizing small talk and other distractions, as well as sensory accommodations, such as seeing the patient in a private room where the sounds of concurrent dental work are reduced. Creative collaboration with patients and supporters can help reduce the need for dental care under sedation or anesthesia. However, some patients require the use of agents such as nitrous oxide or referral to hospital dentistry.[23,45]

Barriers to care may be more or less prominent depending on environmental factors, illness, and the supports available to a patient. It is important to work with patients and their supporters to determine useful strategies and accommodations. If possible, discuss strategies during routine visits, as they are often most needed during times of crisis when it is hardest to develop them de novo.

UNDERSTANDING AND ADDRESSING BEHAVIOR CHANGE

In people with nontraditional communication or atypical cognition, common medical problems can present in unusual ways. Illness often presents as a change from baseline behavior or function. For example, pain can present as social withdrawal or self-injurious or agitated behavior. If the behavior or illness makes caregiving easier (eg, amenorrhea or decreased activity levels) caregivers often fail to report the change. Therefore it is important to record the patient's baseline in the areas of cognition, mental health/behavior, fine and gross motor function, sensory integration and function, and seizure threshold.

Patients may not reliably volunteer information or may describe their symptoms in atypical ways. Caregivers also may not volunteer information, may misinterpret behavior, or have competing interests. Clinicians should always attempt to obtain a history directly from their patient. However, when needed, with permission, caregivers and supporters can be important supplementary sources of information.

Challenging Behavior

Challenging behavior is usually not a presenting complaint from a patient. Caregivers seek consultation because they feel challenged. As a first step, it is important to determine if the stress is due to a change in the function or behavior of the patient, or from a change in the caregiver's resiliency or ability to provide support. The solution may include helping the caregiver with additional supports, training, or relief from caregiving responsibilities.

Typically, caregivers are focused on stopping the target behavior. Determining the cause can take time and additional work when a caregiver is already overwhelmed. But understanding the cause of the behavior is critical. Start by asking the patient, even if the patient does not communicate in traditional ways. Remind caregivers that all behavior is a form of communication and that all people communicate. Clinicians should consider a full differential diagnosis, including common medical and psychosocial causes (**Boxes 4** and **5**). Psychiatric illness is only one possible cause of aggression or challenging behavior. Patients who present to specialty psychiatry services frequently have undiagnosed or undertreated medical problems contributing to their condition.

Pharmacologic and Nonpharmacologic Approaches to Challenging Behavior

The primary treatment for challenging behavior is to diagnose and address the underlying cause. However, the cause may not be readily apparent. Both pharmacologic and nonpharmacological approaches may need to be explored.

Although short-term use of risperidone or aripiprazole has been shown to be effective in treating irritability, hyperactivity, and stereotypies in autistic children, the risks and side effects often outweigh the benefits.[46] There are no data regarding the benefit of long-term antipsychotic medication in autistic individuals.[47–49] People with intellectual and developmental disabilities have high rates of complications from long-term use of antipsychotic medication, such as movement disorders, obesity, hyperprolactinemia, and metabolic syndrome.[50,51] In children, increased risk of diabetes is apparent within the first year of treatment with antipsychotic drugs, including newer atypical medications, and the risk increases with total cumulative dose.[52,53] Even after long-term use, discontinuing antipsychotic medication improves metabolic parameters. For antipsychotics prescribed for challenging behavior in adults with intellectual disability, discontinuing them is associated with improved behavioral function.[54] Although autism-specific data are not available, studies suggest that the use of antipsychotic medication is not

---

Box 4
Common medical causes of a change in behavior or function

Constipation

Dental problems

Dysphagia

Esophageal reflux

Headaches

Hearing changes

Hypothyroidism

Kidney stones

Seizures

Side effects of medications

Trauma

Urinary obstruction or retention or new incontinence

Urinary tract infections

Vision changes

Box 5
Common psychosocial causes of a change in behavior or function

Abuse or neglect

Caregiver stress causing a change in support

Escape or avoidance of demands

Increase or decrease arousal

Means to access an activity or object

Mental illness

Need for attention

Pursuit of control and autonomy

Reduction of anxiety

Substance use or abuse

---

cost-effective for adults with intellectual disability. Despite weak evidence to support the practice, long-term antipsychotic medications are frequently prescribed for autistic individuals. Before selecting a treatment, patients and caregivers should know that aggressive behavior frequently remits over the short-to-medium term.[48,55]

There are some data to support the efficacy of nonpharmacological treatment approaches. Mindfulness interventions are effective to reduce behavioral and psychological problems in people with developmental disabilities, including autism.[56–58] Cognitive behavioral therapy for anxiety also is effective in autistic people.[59] Physical exercise has been shown to reduce stereotypy, aggression, off-task behavior, and elopement in autistic people.[60] Functional assessment and improved communication have also been shown to reduce challenging behaviors.[61,62]

LEGAL AND ETHICAL CONSIDERATIONS
Decision-Making Capacity; Surrogate Decision Makers

Issues of autonomy can be particularly significant for autistic individuals, many of whom have been denied opportunities for self-determination. The capacity of autistic people to consent to treatment or participate in shared decision-making is often overlooked. With appropriate accommodations, people with communication or intellectual disabilities can usually understand the options, weigh the risks and benefits, and communicate a choice. Some medical decisions are more abstract than others, so capacity to make an informed decision should be assessed separately for each decision.

People who lack capacity to make a specific decision independently often can decide who they trust to support them in decision-making and complete a Power of Attorney form. Others may be able to contribute information about their values and priorities for consideration.

Clinicians, caregivers, family members, and case managers all have competing interests that need to be managed. One technique for managing this is to list and distinguish what is important to and for each team member (**Box 6**).

Some autistic adults have a conservator or guardian. When surrogates support a patient, they should be encouraged to solicit the patient's values and priorities. If it is impossible, even with supports, to include the patient in any way, surrogates should be encouraged to base their decision on their best estimate of what the patient would choose if he or she was able to be involved, rather than on what the surrogates prefer.

Box 6
Example of strategy listing what is important to and for patient and team members as a way to manage competing interests

Important *to* the patient: Avoid the pain of a needle stick.

Important *for* the patient: Get laboratory tests drawn.

Important *to* the caregiver: That she be the one to provide support.

Important *for* caregiver: End clinic visit to get to work on time.

Solution: Provider writes prescription for numbing cream to be applied 1 hour before a laboratory appointment on a convenient date.

Access to Care

Access to health care is a civil right under the Americans with Disabilities Act (ADA). The ADA does not list specific recommendations but instead requires individualized strategies to address the specific barriers posed by an individual's impairments. It is the responsibility of clinicians and health plans to provide access to care for people with disabilities. Examples include large print, translators, plain language, or visual presentations; sensory accommodations such as quiet rooms and dimmed lights; and longer appointment times. The act of requesting accommodations can in and of itself be challenging for autistic individuals who struggle with social communication. Our AHAT can help patients create personalized accommodations reports for health care providers. Taking the time to respond to accommodation requests can ultimately save time, improve the therapeutic relationship, and facilitate effective care.

SUMMARY

Clinicians can work with patients on the autism spectrum and their supporters to find effective strategies and accommodations to reduce barriers to care. In people with nontraditional communication or atypical cognition, illness often presents as a change from baseline behavior or function. Clinicians should consider a full differential diagnosis, including common medical and psychosocial causes. Appropriate supports and accommodations can reduce illness and disability and maximize patient autonomy and quality of life.

ACKNOWLEDGMENTS

Many of the recommendations in this article arise from the AASPIRE Healthcare Toolkit Project. Funding for the project was provided by the National Institute of Mental Health (R34MH092503). We would like to thank the many AASPIRE team members and study participants who have contributed to the project.

REFERENCES

1. Brugha TS, McManus S, Bankart J, et al. Epidemiology of autism spectrum disorders in adults in the community in England. Archives of general psychiatry 2011;68(5):459–65.
2. Nicolaidis C, Raymaker D, McDonald K, et al. Collaboration Strategies in Nontraditional Community-Based Participatory Research Partnerships: lessons from an academic–community partnership with autistic self-advocates. Prog Community Health Partnersh 2011;5(2):143.

3. American Psychiatric Association. Diagnostic and statistical manual of mental disorders, fifth edition (DSM-5). Washington, DC: American Psychiatric Association; 2013.

4. Markram K, Markram H. The intense world theory—a unifying theory of the neurobiology of autism. Front Hum Neurosci 2010;4:224.

5. Nicolaidis C. What can physicians learn from the neurodiversity movement? Virtual Mentor 2012;14(6):503.

6. Rogers K, Dziobek I, Hassenstab J, et al. Who cares? Revisiting empathy in Asperger syndrome. J Autism Dev Disord 2007;37(4):709–15.

7. Lord C, Rutter M, DiLavore P, et al. Autism diagnostic observation schedule: ADOS-2. Torrance (CA): Western Psychological Services; 2012.

8. White SW, Oswald D, Ollendick T, et al. Anxiety in children and adolescents with autism spectrum disorders. Clin Psychol Rev 2009;29(3):216–29.

9. Stewart ME, Barnard L, Pearson J, et al. Presentation of depression in autism and Asperger syndrome. A review. Autism 2006;10(1):103–16.

10. Doshi-Velez F, Ge Y, Kohane I. Comorbidity clusters in autism spectrum disorders: an electronic health record time-series analysis. Pediatrics 2014;133(1):e54–63.

11. Tyler CV, Schramm SC, Karafa M, et al. Chronic disease risks in young adults with autism spectrum disorder: forewarned is forearmed. Am J Intellect Dev Disabil 2011;116(5):371–80.

12. Kohane IS, McMurry A, Weber G, et al. The co-morbidity burden of children and young adults with autism spectrum disorders. PLoS One 2012;7(4):e33224.

13. Hughes RB, Lund EM, Gabrielli J, et al. Prevalence of interpersonal violence against community-living adults with disabilities: a literature review. Rehabil Psychol 2011;56(4):302.

14. Woolfenden S, Sarkozy V, Ridley G, et al. A systematic review of two outcomes in autism spectrum disorder—epilepsy and mortality. Dev Med Child Neurol 2012; 54(4):306–12.

15. Shavelle RM, Strauss D. Comparative mortality of persons with autism in California, 1989-1996. J Insur Med 1998;30(4):220–5.

16. Shavelle RM, Strauss DJ, Pickett J. Causes of death in autism. J Autism Dev Disord 2001;31(6):569–76.

17. Perkins EA, Berkman KA. Into the unknown: aging with autism spectrum disorders. Am J Intellect Dev Disabil 2012;117(6):478–96.

18. Viscidi EW, Triche EW, Pescosolido MF, et al. Clinical characteristics of children with autism spectrum disorder and co-occurring epilepsy. PLoS One 2013;8(7): e67797.

19. Chapman M, Iddon P, Atkinson K, et al. The misdiagnosis of epilepsy in people with intellectual disabilities: a systematic review. Seizure 2011;20(2):101–6.

20. Kerr M, Scheepers M, Arvio M, et al. Consensus guidelines into the management of epilepsy in adults with an intellectual disability. J Intellect Disabil Res 2009;53(8):687–94.

21. Srikanth R, Cassidy G, Joiner C, et al. Osteoporosis in people with intellectual disabilities: a review and a brief study of risk factors for osteoporosis in a community sample of people with intellectual disabilities. J Intellect Disabil Res 2011;55(1):53–62.

22. Charlot L, Abend S, Ravin P, et al. Non-psychiatric health problems among psychiatric inpatients with intellectual disabilities. J Intellect Disabil Res 2011;55(2): 199–209.

23. Buie T, Campbell DB, Fuchs GJ, et al. Evaluation, diagnosis, and treatment of gastrointestinal disorders in individuals with ASDs: a consensus report. Pediatrics 2010;125(Suppl 1):S1–18.

24. Humphries K, Traci MA, Seekins T. Nutrition and adults with intellectual or developmental disabilities: systematic literature review results. Intellect Dev Disabil 2009;47(3):163–85.
25. Davis TE III, Hess JA, Moree BN, et al. Anxiety symptoms across the lifespan in people diagnosed with autistic disorder. Res Autism Spectr Disord 2011;5(1):112–8.
26. Allen D, Langthorne P, Tonge B, et al. Towards the prevention of behavioural and psychiatric disorders in people with intellectual disabilities. J Appl Res Intellect Disabil 2013;26(6):501–14.
27. Rose N, Rose J, Kent S. Staff training in intellectual disability services: a review of the literature and implications for mental health services provided to individuals with intellectual disability. Int J Dev Disabil 2012;58(1):24–39.
28. Lunsky Y, Lin E, Balogh R, et al. Are adults with developmental disabilities more likely to visit EDs? Am J Emerg Med 2011;29(4):463–5.
29. Fletcher R, Loschen E, Stavrakaki C, et al. DM-ID: diagnostic manual-intellectual disability: a textbook of diagnosis of mental disorders in persons with intellectual disability. Kingston (NY): NADD Press; 2007.
30. Polimeni M, Richdale A, Francis A. A survey of sleep problems in autism, Asperger's disorder and typically developing children. J Intellect Disabil Res 2005;49(4):260–8.
31. Matson JL, Ancona MN, Wilkins J. Sleep disturbances in adults with autism spectrum disorders and severe intellectual impairments. J Ment Health Res Intellect Disabil 2008;1(3):129–39.
32. Sivertsen B, Posserud MB, Gillberg C, et al. Sleep problems in children with autism spectrum problems: a longitudinal population based study. Autism 2012;16(2):139–50.
33. van de Wouw E, Evenhuis H, Echteld M. Prevalence, associated factors and treatment of sleep problems in adults with intellectual disability: a systematic review. Res Dev Disabil 2012;33(4):1310–32.
34. Rossignol DA, Frye RE. Melatonin in autism spectrum disorders: a systematic review and meta-analysis. Dev Med Child Neurol 2011;53(9):783–92.
35. Hollway JA, Aman MG. Pharmacological treatment of sleep disturbance in developmental disabilities: a review of the literature. Res Dev Disabil 2011;32(3):939–62.
36. Hylkema T, Vlaskamp C. Significant improvement in sleep in people with intellectual disabilities living in residential settings by non-pharmaceutical interventions. J Intellect Disabil Res 2009;53(8):695–703.
37. Krahn GL, Hammond L, Turner A. A cascade of disparities: health and health care access for people with intellectual disabilities. Ment Retard Dev Disabil Res Rev 2006;12(1):70–82.
38. Iezzoni LI, O'Day BL, Killeen M, et al. Communicating about health care: observations from persons who are deaf or hard of hearing. Ann Intern Med 2004;140(5):356–62.
39. Iezzoni LI, Davis RB, Soukup J, et al. Satisfaction with quality and access to health care among people with disabling conditions. Int J Qual Health Care 2002;14(5):369–81.
40. Nicolaidis C, Raymaker D, Dern S, et al. Comparison of healthcare experiences in autistic and non-autistic adults: a cross-sectional online survey facilitated by an academic-community partnership. J Gen Intern Med 2012;28(6):761–9.
41. Stewart MA. Effective physician-patient communication and health outcomes: a review. CMAJ 1995;152(9):1423–33.

42. Joseph RM, Tager-Flusberg H, Lord C. Cognitive profiles and social-communicative functioning in children with autism spectrum disorder. J Child Psychol Psychiatry 2002;43(6):807–21.
43. Mayes SD, Calhoun SL. WISC-IV and WIAT-II profiles in children with high-functioning autism. J Autism Dev Disord 2008;38(3):428–39.
44. Nicolaidis C, Raymaker D, McDonald K, et al. "Respect the way I need to communicate with you": healthcare experiences of adults on the autistic spectrum. Paper presented at: Annual Meeting of the Society of General Internal Medicine. Phoenix, May 4–7, 2011.
45. Rada RE. Treatment needs and adverse events related to dental treatment under general anesthesia for individuals with autism. Intellect Dev Disabil 2013; 51(4):246–52.
46. Siegel M, Beaulieu AA. Psychotropic medications in children with autism spectrum disorders: a systematic review and synthesis for evidence-based practice. J Autism Dev Disord 2012;42(8):1592–605.
47. Spencer D, Marshall J, Post B, et al. Psychotropic medication use and polypharmacy in children with autism spectrum disorders. Pediatrics 2013;132(5): 833–40.
48. Dove D, Warren Z, McPheeters ML, et al. Medications for adolescents and young adults with autism spectrum disorders: a systematic review. Pediatrics 2012;130(4):717–26.
49. Ching H, Pringsheim T. Aripiprazole for autism spectrum disorders (ASD). Cochrane Database Syst Rev 2012;(5):CD009043.
50. Hellings JA, Cardona AM, Schroeder SR. Long-term safety and adverse events of risperidone in children, adolescents, and adults with pervasive developmental disorders. J Ment Health Res Intellect Disabil 2010;3(3):132–44.
51. Frighi V, Stephenson MT, Morovat A, et al. Safety of antipsychotics in people with intellectual disability. Br J Psychiatry 2011;199(4):289–95.
52. de Kuijper G, Mulder H, Evenhuis H, et al. Determinants of physical health parameters in individuals with intellectual disability who use long-term antipsychotics. Res Dev Disabil 2013;34(9):2799–809.
53. Bobo WV, Cooper WO, Stein CM, et al. Antipsychotics and the risk of type 2 diabetes mellitus in children and youth. JAMA Psychiatry 2013;70(10):1067–75.
54. Kuijper G, Evenhuis H, Minderaa R, et al. Effects of controlled discontinuation of long-term used antipsychotics for behavioural symptoms in individuals with intellectual disability. J Intellect Disabil Res 2014;58(1):71–83.
55. Cooper SA, Smiley E, Jackson A, et al. Adults with intellectual disabilities: prevalence, incidence and remission of aggressive behaviour and related factors. J Intellect Disabil Res 2009;53(3):217–32.
56. Hwang YS, Kearney P. A systematic review of mindfulness intervention for individuals with developmental disabilities: long-term practice and long lasting effects. Res Dev Disabil 2013;34(1):314–26.
57. Harper SK, Webb TL, Rayner K. The effectiveness of mindfulness-based interventions for supporting people with intellectual disabilities: a narrative review. Behav Modif 2013;37(3):431–53.
58. Spek AA, van Ham NC, Nyklicek I. Mindfulness-based therapy in adults with an autism spectrum disorder: a randomized controlled trial. Res Dev Disabil 2012; 34:246–53.
59. Lang R, Regester A, Lauderdale S, et al. Treatment of anxiety in autism spectrum disorders using cognitive behaviour therapy: a systematic review. Dev Neurorehabil 2010;13(1):53–63.

60. Lang R, Koegel LK, Ashbaugh K, et al. Physical exercise and individuals with autism spectrum disorders: a systematic review. Res Autism Spectr Disord 2010;4(4):565–76.
61. Lang R, Rispoli M, Machalicek W, et al. Treatment of elopement in individuals with developmental disabilities: a systematic review. Res Dev Disabil 2009; 30(4):670–81.
62. Walker VL, Snell ME. Effects of augmentative and alternative communication on challenging behavior: a meta-analysis. Augment Altern Commun 2013;29(2): 117–31.

Medical Conditions with Neuropsychiatric Manifestations

Margaret L. Isaac, MD[a],*, Eric B. Larson, MD, MPH[b]

KEYWORDS

- Cognitive impairment • Mood disorders • Neuropsychiatric symptoms • Dementia
- Autoimmune/inflammatory disease • Central nervous system (CNS)
- Peripheral nervous system

KEY POINTS

- Many medical conditions can have neuropsychiatric manifestations and a high index of suspicion is necessary, particularly in patients with other unexplained systemic symptoms and signs.
- These neuropsychiatric symptoms are nonspecific so additional information (eg, detailed history and physical examination, laboratory and imaging studies) may be needed to determine whether medical disease is the true cause.
- The most commonly implicated pathophysiologic categories that produce neuropsychiatric symptoms and signs include infectious, autoimmune, endocrinologic, metabolic, and neoplastic diseases.
- Involvement of subspecialty colleagues can be important when these conditions are suspected.
- Treatment of these disorders usually includes symptom-directed therapies, and also therapies directed at treating the underlying systemic condition. These therapies are widely variable depending on the specific disease process.

INTRODUCTION

Many medical conditions have neurologic and psychiatric symptoms, and early identification of the underlying cause can be critical in directing further management (**Table 1**). Medical conditions known to cause neuropsychiatric symptoms can also be varied in presentation, making diagnosis challenging. The number of medical conditions that potentially cause neurologic and psychiatric symptoms is extensive. This

Financial Disclosures: None.
[a] Medicine, Harborview Medical Center, University of Washington School of Medicine, 325 9th Avenue, Box 359892, Seattle, WA 98104, USA; [b] Medicine, Group Health Research Institute, University of Washington School of Medicine, Seattle, WA, USA
* Corresponding author.
E-mail address: misaac@uw.edu

Table 1
Medical conditions with neuropsychiatric manifestations

System	Disease
Infectious	HIV/AIDS • Opportunistic infections/malignancies Syphilis Lyme disease Prion disease
Rheumatologic/autoimmune	Systemic lupus erythematosus Sarcoidosis Vasculitides Multiple sclerosis
Endocrinologic	Hypothyroidism/hyperthyroidism Hypoparathyroidism/hyperparathyroidism Cushing syndrome Adrenal insufficiency
Metabolic	Vitamin deficiencies • Thiamine (vitamin B_1) • Vitamin B_{12} Micronutrient abnormalities • Hypocalcemia/hypercalcemia Acute hepatic porphyrias Wilson disease Amyloidosis Hepatic encephalopathy Uremia
Neoplastic	Paraneoplastic syndromes CNS tumors (primary and metastatic) Carcinomatous meningitis
Hematologic	Sickle cell disease (cerebrovascular disease)
Heritable/genetic	Huntington disease Lysosomal storage diseases

Abbreviations: AIDS, acquired immunodeficiency syndrome; CNS, central nervous system; HIV, human immunodeficiency virus.

article highlights several broad categories of medical diseases (infectious, autoimmune, endocrinologic, metabolic, and neoplastic), with a focus on pragmatic considerations in evaluation, diagnosis, and management in the primary care setting. The focus of this article is on common medical conditions with neuropsychiatric manifestations, as well as specific diseases that have a characteristic neuropsychiatric presentation requiring early detection and evaluation.

INFECTIOUS
Human Immunodeficiency Virus

Human immunodeficiency virus (HIV) disease can cause neuropsychiatric manifestations as a result of primary HIV disease, opportunistic infections and malignancies, medication side effects, and the psychosocial consequences and stigma associated with HIV infection. Common neuropsychiatric disorders that are associated or comorbid with HIV disease include minor cognitive impairment and dementia[1]; delirium; peripheral nervous system disorders such as polyneuropathy; and psychiatric syndromes such as bipolar affective disorder, major depression, schizophrenia, and substance abuse.[2] Cognitive impairment in the setting of HIV infection can be caused by encephalopathy attributed to the virus; central nervous system (CNS) lymphoma; and primary CNS infections such as progressive multifocal leukoencephalopathy (PML), cryptococcal meningitis, toxoplasmosis, and cytomegalovirus (CMV) encephalitis.

HIV-associated neurocognitive disorders (HAND), can be classified as asymptomatic neurocognitive impairment, mild neurocognitive disorder, or HIV-associated dementia, with HIV-associated dementia being the most severe, characterized by profound abnormalities in neuropsychological testing and significant impairment in a patient's ability to perform activities of daily living.[3] Some degree of neurocognitive impairment has been found to be present in between a quarter and half of all patients infected with HIV in one large study,[4] although other studies have found the rate of cognitive impairment in patients with early stage HIV and high viral loads to be similar to that in HIV-negative individuals.[5] HAND is characterized by the triad of memory impairment, mood (depressive) symptoms, and movement disorders such as ataxia, tremor, weakness, and bradykinesia.[6] Screening for HAND in patients infected with HIV includes neuropsychological testing, and is a diagnosis of exclusion made after alternate causes have been ruled out. Treatment includes antiretroviral (ARV) medications, medications intended to manage symptoms, such as stimulants and antipsychotics,[7] and supportive care (including psychiatric care and attention to functional needs with rehabilitation services).

PML, a demyelinating disease that affects the CNS, is caused by the opportunistic reactivation of polyomavirus (JC virus) infection. PML occurs in immunosuppressed patients, and, before the advent of ARV therapy, affected up to 5% of patients with advanced HIV disease.[8] The disease is far less prevalent since the broader use of ARVs. PML has historically been thought of as a disease of the white matter (specifically affecting oligodendrocytes and astrocytes) but it can also affect structures such as the cortical gray matter, thalamus, and basal ganglia.[9] It rarely affects the spinal cord.[10] Classic symptoms include weakness, sensory changes, cognitive dysfunction, ataxia, visual symptoms such as hemianopsia and diplopia, aphasia, and seizures.[9] Definitive diagnosis can be made by brain biopsy, but can also be made by using polymerase chain reaction to show the presence of JC virus in the cerebrospinal fluid (CSF) and by the characteristic demyelinating lesions seen on neuroimaging. The prognosis for patients with PML is poor, with a median survival in patients affected by HIV of 1.8 years in the post-ARV era. Prognosis is improved in patients with higher CD4 counts.[11] Treatment is focused on optimizing ARV therapies and although several specific treatment agents have been studied, there are no large-scale, robust data to support the use of these agents, and there is no treatment currently available that is designed to treat JC virus specifically.[12,13]

Cryptococcal meningitis is a protozoan infection that affects immunocompromised patients, including patients with advanced HIV/acquired immunodeficiency syndrome. Symptoms typically present insidiously and subacutely, with headaches, mental status changes, lethargy, and memory loss developing over a period of weeks. Diagnosis is made using lumbar puncture, which highlights the importance of a high index of suspicion in susceptible patients given that the diagnosis cannot be made from serology alone. Patients with cryptococcal meningitis classically have a markedly high opening pressure. CSF examination can be significant for low glucose and high protein levels, and cell counts are typically low when the infection is HIV associated. Cryptococcal meningitis is treated with antifungals including amphotericin B, flucytosine, and fluconazole, and is fatal if untreated.[13]

Toxoplasmosis gondii is a protozoan disease that is usually a manifestation of reactivation of latent cysts in immunosuppressed patients (typically patients with HIV with CD4 counts <100) and is also an important pathogen in pregnant women.

Toxoplasmosis in HIV-positive patients classically presents with headache, fever, and mental status changes, although focal neurologic symptoms and seizures are also common. Extracerebral manifestations can include posterior uveitis and pneumonitis. Diagnosis is made from serologies (positive antitoxoplasma immunoglobulin G), imaging, and a clinical presentation suggesting toxoplasmosis. Definitive diagnosis can be made by biopsy of a suspected lesion. First-line treatment includes sulfadiazine, pyrimethamine, and leucovorin.[13]

Ventriculoencephalitis related to CMV infection has declined since the advent of effective ARV treatments. CMV can affect various parts of the neurologic system and, when the brain is involved, classically presents subacutely with altered mental status, and commonly with memory impairment.[14] Diagnosis is made by isolating CMV antigen or DNA from the CSF, and imaging is also used to rule out other potential pathogens/causes.[15,16] Treatment of CMV encephalitis includes ganciclovir and foscarnet,[17] although the data supporting this treatment are limited to case reports and small, nonrandomized prospective studies.[18] Prognosis is poor and CMV infection is rapidly fatal, regardless of treatment.[19]

Syphilis

Neurosyphilis was once common, occurring in up to 40% of patients with documented syphilis[20] in the era before the advent of antibiotics. It is now rare, with the reduction attributed not just to increased treatment of early syphilis but also to the widespread prevalence of antibiotics in society and in the environment, outside the setting of specific treatment of bacterial illness in humans. Neuropsychiatric symptoms caused by syphilis are usually late manifestations of the disease. Early neurosyphilis can be either asymptomatic (diagnosed based on CSF studies) or symptomatic, presenting with acute meningitis, sometimes with leptomeningeal spread and the development of focal areas of CNS inflammation (gummas), ophthalmologic symptoms (uveitis), otic symptoms (hearing loss), and meningovascular symptoms. Many patients clear syphilitic meningitis spontaneously, whereas others develop chronic asymptomatic CNS disease, and this latter group of patients is at the highest risk for late neurosyphilis. Late neurosyphilis can present with a variety of clinical CNS syndromes, including dementia, paresis, and locomotor ataxia (tabes dorsalis). Neurosyphilis is diagnosed based on clinical presentation (history and physical examination, which can reveal characteristic abnormalities such as the Argyll-Robertson pupil in the setting of tabes dorsalis) and CSF or serum evaluation. No single laboratory test can diagnose neurosyphilis. Laboratory evaluation in a patient without known syphilis begins with nontreponemal serum testing (such as rapid plasma reagin or venereal disease research laboratory [VDRL]), and confirmed by specific treponemal testing.[21] In patients with late neurosyphilis, nontreponemal serum testing can sometimes be falsely negative,[22] although typically specific treponemal testing remains positive, making it an important part of diagnosis in patients for whom providers have a high suspicion for neurosyphilis. In patients with known prior syphilis or positive serum treponemal testing, lumbar puncture should be:

- Considered in patients with an unknown syphilis history who have neurologic or ophthalmologic symptoms consistent with neurosyphilis, and HIV-positive patients with a known history of syphilis even without symptoms of neurologic or ophthalmologic involvement
- Performed in patients with neurologic or ophthalmologic symptoms or signs with a known history of syphilis
- Performed in patients with active tertiary syphilis affecting other organ systems
- Performed in patients with documented evidence of treatment failure[23]

CSF VDRL is very specific for neurosyphilis, but has a low sensitivity, meaning that a positive test is diagnostic, but a negative test may not rule out the disease. Other CSF parameters may be helpful in suggesting the diagnosis as well; an increased cell count and protein level. In HIV-positive patients, the CSF VDRL can be falsely negative, so there may be a role for a more sensitive but less specific test of the CSF (such as the fluorescent treponemal antibody absorption).[23] Treatment of neurosyphilis requires parenteral antibiotics capable of crossing the blood-brain barrier: either intravenous (IV) penicillin G for 10 to 15 days, or procaine penicillin G intramuscularly and oral probenecid for 10 to 14 days. Ceftriaxone and doxycycline may be reasonable alternatives in patients who are allergic to penicillin.

Lyme Disease

Another spirochete infection, Lyme disease, caused by *Borrelia burgdorferi* and spread through the bite of the *Ixodes* tick, can present with dermatologic, musculoskeletal (joint), and neurologic manifestations. Spirochetes seed the nervous system through hematogenous spread and can cause a variety of neurologic symptoms that can be classified either by anatomic location (central vs peripheral) or time of onset (early disease, occurring within weeks or months of the initial tick bite, or late/chronic disease, with onset months to years later).

Many patients, and most of those who present with erythema migrans, can have nonspecific symptoms that are seemingly neuropsychiatric in origin, including fatigue, headache, and cognitive impairment. These ill-defined symptoms are not thought to be manifestations of CNS Lyme disease[24] or nervous system damage and are common across patients with other inflammatory and infectious diseases (and in patients without known medical disease as well). Approximately 15% of patients develop meningitis, cranial neuropathies, or radiculopathy/radiculitis acutely, with these three sequelae constituting the classic triad for acute, early neuroborreliosis.[25] Peripheral neuropathies (including radiculopathy, symmetric polyneuropathies, and carpal tunnel syndrome) and encephalomyelitis can occur either early in the disease course or much later, even months or years after initial infection.[26] Diagnosis depends on a known exposure (through the bite of the *Ixodes* tick); objective clinical evidence of nervous system involvement; and laboratory data, specifically positive Lyme serologies and anti-*Borrelia* antibodies in the CSF, although anti-*Borrelia* antibodies are not required for diagnosis. Evaluation of the CSF in the setting of Lyme meningitis typically reveals a modest, lymphocyte-predominant pleocytosis, moderately increased protein, and normal glucose levels.[27] Electromyogram/nerve conduction studies can be helpful to characterize peripheral nervous systems disorders as well. Treatment regimen and course depend on the timing and location of disease and ranges as follows[28]:

- Early disseminated disease with cranial nerve symptoms: oral antibiotics (doxycycline) for 2 to 4 weeks
- Early disseminated disease with meningitis: IV antibiotics (ceftriaxone) for 4 weeks
- Late disseminated disease with neurologic symptoms: IV antibiotics (ceftriaxone, cefotaxime, penicillin G) for 4 weeks

RHEUMATOLOGIC

Several autoimmune/rheumatologic diseases can cause neuropsychiatric symptoms, including, but not limited to, systemic lupus erythematosus (SLE), sarcoidosis, CNS vasculitis, and multiple sclerosis. This article focuses specifically on SLE and sarcoidosis.

SLE

Most patients with SLE develop neuropsychiatric symptoms,[29] typically within the first year of diagnosis.[30] Neurologic sequelae are included as a potential criterion for SLE diagnosis in both the original American College of Rheumatology diagnostic criteria[31,32] and also the revised criteria proposed by the Systemic Lupus International Collaborating Clinics.[33] The American College of Rheumatology divides neuropsychiatric manifestations of SLE into central and peripheral syndromes (see **Table 2** for details)[34] and has case definitions for each syndrome. Central syndromes can range from mild to severe, including (from most to least common) cognitive dysfunction, headaches, mood disorders, cerebrovascular disease, seizure disorders, and psychosis.[35] Peripheral syndromes include, but are not limited to, Guillain-Barré syndrome, peripheral neuropathies, and myasthenia gravis, with polyneuropathies being the most common.[35] The specific pathophysiologies underlying these various syndromes are varied. Medications used to treat SLE, such as steroids, can commonly cause symptoms such as psychosis and cognitive dysfunction, so considering iatrogenic causes is also imperative. Cognitive dysfunction may occur in patients with SLE and underlying psychiatric disorders or without any psychiatric history and can also be associated with CNS emboli in the setting of antiphospholipid antibodies.

Some biomarkers seem to be increased in patients with neuropsychiatric SLE,[36] and associations have been found between increased levels of antineuronal antibodies and other antibodies and both neuropsychiatric symptoms generally, and cognitive defects specifically.[37,38] These tools remain nonspecific in diagnosis. In addition, imaging for structural brain changes can be a helpful adjunctive tool for evaluation. SLE as a cause for neuropsychiatric symptoms remains a diagnosis of exclusion made after other potential causes have been evaluated and ruled out.

Treatment of neuropsychiatric lupus varies depending on the specific symptoms. Steroids and immunosuppressants such as azathioprine and cyclophosphamide are mainstays of treatment of lupus psychosis, as are symptom-directed treatments such as antipsychotic medications. For other neuropsychiatric symptoms such as cognitive dysfunction that can have variable underlying causes even in the setting of SLE, treatments are directed at the underlying cause: reduction or discontinuation of steroid medications if indicated, and, conversely, treating with steroid medications if the cause is thought to be antibody mediated, and/or anticoagulation if associated

Table 2 Central and peripheral syndromes in neuropsychiatric SLE	
Peripheral	**Central**
Acute inflammatory demyelinating polyradiculoneuropathy (Guillain-Barré syndrome)	Acute confusional state
Autonomic dysfunction	Anxiety disorder
Cranial neuropathy	Aseptic meningitis
Mononeuropathy (single or multiplex)	Cerebrovascular disease
Myasthenia gravis	Chorea (movement disorder)
Plexopathy	Cognitive dysfunction
Polyneuropathy	Demyelinating syndrome
	Headache
	Mood disorder
	Myelopathy
	Psychosis
	Seizure disorder

Data from The American College of Rheumatology nomenclature and case definitions for neuropsychiatric lupus syndromes. Arthritis Rheum 1999;42(4):599–608.

with embolic phenomena in the setting of antiphospholipid antibody syndrome. One particularly challenging diagnostic dilemma is distinguishing steroid psychosis from acute psychotic symptoms caused by CNS lupus, a situation with a very different treatment approach. Soliciting help from psychiatric and rheumatologic colleagues is appropriate in any patient thought to have CNS lupus.

Sarcoidosis

Sarcoidosis can present with a large variety of both systemic and neuropsychiatric symptoms. It is estimated that 5% to 15% of patients with sarcoidosis develop related neurologic symptoms.[39,40] However, sarcoidosis is rare, with an estimated incidence of 10 to 40 new cases per 100,000 patients per year,[41] making neurosarcoidosis rarer still. Sarcoidosis can affect both the central and peripheral nervous systems, and most frequently causes cranial neuropathies.[42] Neurosarcoidosis can cause nearly any neurologic symptom, including aseptic meningitis, seizures, peripheral neuropathies, psychiatric symptoms, and small fiber neuropathies causing symptoms such as pain, restless legs, and autonomic neuropathies.[43] Hypothalamic inflammation can cause a variety of symptoms including polyuria (caused by central diabetes insipidus or primary polydipsia) and changes in sleep, appetite, and temperature regulation.[44] The diagnosis of neurosarcoidosis is made based on history, radiologic and laboratory evaluation, and histology showing granulomatous disease. Useful diagnostic tests include images of the CNS and chest (to detect the presence of hilar adenopathy), serum angiotensin-converting enzyme (ACE) levels (which are neither specific nor sensitive and can be increased in a variety of systemic diseases), and CSF evaluation in the setting of CNS symptoms.[42] CSF findings suggesting neurosarcoidosis include pleocytosis, increased protein, and low glucose, although these levels are normal in about one-third of patients with neurosarcoidosis.[45] CSF ACE levels are also nonspecific but can be useful in monitoring response to therapy.

Neurosarcoidosis carries an uncertain prognosis, mainly because of its low incidence and the absence of long-term follow-up studies. Treatment recommendations similarly are based on expert opinion and clinical experience rather than data from randomized controlled trials. Treatment of neurosarcoidosis includes systemic steroids and cytotoxic immunosuppressants, as are used in treatment of sarcoidosis elsewhere in the body. The efficacy of tumor necrosis factor alpha blockers has also been shown in certain refractory cases.[46]

ENDOCRINOLOGIC
Thyroid Disorders

Both hypothyroidism and hyperthyroidism can cause neuropsychiatric symptoms. This article focuses on neurologic manifestations in adult-onset, rather than congenital, hypothyroidism. Hypothyroidism can cause cognitive impairment and symptoms of depression, usually co-occurring with other systemic symptoms of hypothyroidism including fatigue, cold intolerance, dry skin, weight gain, and lethargy.[47] In addition, hypothyroidism caused by autoimmune thyroiditis (Hashimoto disease) is associated with encephalopathy, although this is thought to be mediated by an immunologic process rather than by low levels of circulating thyroid hormone. Cognitive impairment in the setting of hypothyroidism has an unknown mechanism, although some investigators have postulated that anxiety and depression, both highly prevalent, may be impairing memory and concentration, as they can in euthyroid patients.[48] Screening for hypothyroidism in patients with newly diagnosed cognitive impairment is widespread, because this is considered to be a reversible form of impairment. However, the yield of such screening is low,[49] and the evidence for reversibility of cognitive symptoms with thyroid supplementation is mixed, with the possibility of incomplete recovery,[50] particularly in the case of subclinical hypothyroidism and in the presence of other common comorbid conditions such as Alzheimer disease. Hypothyroidism is also associated with other neurologic symptoms and syndromes including ataxia,[51] peripheral neuropathies (including carpal tunnel syndrome and symmetric polyneuropathies), and myopathies, which present with proximal muscle weakness and pain. Most of these syndromes respond to thyroid replacement.

Hyperthyroidism can also cause both CNS and peripheral nervous system syndromes. CNS manifestations can include psychiatric symptoms such as irritability and anxiety,[52] and, in the elderly, depression and lethargy.[53] In addition, patients can present with cognitive deficits, include memory impairment, inattention, and decreased productivity.[52] Other CNS symptoms of hyperthyroidism include tremor[54] and seizures,[55] and, rarely, stroke and chorea. Peripheral nervous system manifestations can include peripheral neuropathies (classically a symmetric distal sensory polyneuropathy), myasthenia gravis, hypokalemic periodic paralysis, and myopathy.[56] Diagnosis of these various syndromes is made using serum measurement of thyroid function, as well as possible additional testing for each specific symptom constellation (not discussed in this article). Many of these syndromes respond to treatment and either resolve or improve with restoration of euthyroidism.

Cushing Syndrome

Hypercortisolism (Cushing syndrome) causes neuropsychiatric symptoms in more than half of affected patients.[57,58] Common psychiatric symptoms include dysphoria, irritability, appetite changes, anxiety and panic attacks, mania, psychosis, and insomnia.[59,60] Excess cortisol can also have profound effects on cognitive function,[61] with memory impairment being the most common manifestation. Attention, reasoning, comprehension, and information processing can also be affected.[61] Neuropsychiatric and other symptoms of hypercortisolism are nonspecific, and diagnosis is made by measuring salivary or urinary cortisol levels, and by administration of the dexamethasone suppression test.[62] The specific cause of Cushing syndrome is established by ruling out exogenous administration of glucocorticoids, then by localizing the defect along the hypothalamic-pituitary-adrenal axis. Thus, subsequent measurement of serum adrenocorticotropic hormone (ACTH) is performed, followed by further laboratory testing and imaging of the pituitary or adrenal glands, if indicated. Treatment varies depending on the underlying cause. Related neuropsychiatric symptoms typically improve with treatment, but often do not fully resolve, and patients with a history of treated Cushing syndrome are commonly left with residual psychiatric symptoms and cognitive impairment.[63,64]

Adrenal Insufficiency, Including Primary Adrenal Insufficiency (Addison Disease)

Adrenal insufficiency, which can include deficiencies in glucocorticoids, aldosterone, and androgens, can also cause nonspecific systemic symptoms that overlap with psychiatric symptoms, most commonly fatigue, lassitude, generalized weakness, and loss of appetite.[65] In addition, patients with chronic adrenal insufficiency can have neuropsychiatric symptoms including cognitive impairment, depression, and psychosis.[66] Diagnosis is made from serum ACTH and cortisol levels, and subsequent laboratory evaluation (metyrapone testing, corticotropin-releasing hormone stimulation testing) as indicated. After hypocortisolism has been established, ACTH levels are used to determine whether the cause is central or peripheral, and then the underlying cause is sought.[65] Treatment with replacement of glucocorticoids, mineralocorticoids, and androgens is complex and depends on the clinical scenario and context. As with many of the other medical conditions described earlier, patients who are treated may not have complete resolution of neuropsychiatric symptoms or subjective health status.[67]

METABOLIC
Vitamin Deficiencies

Vitamin deficiencies can also cause neuropsychiatric symptoms, particularly thiamine (vitamin B_1) and cobalamin (B_{12}) deficiencies. Thiamine deficiency classically causes Wernicke-Korsakoff syndrome, which can be further subdivided into 2 distinct clinical entities: Wernicke encephalopathy (WE) and Korsakoff syndrome. WE is an acute syndrome characterized by cognitive impairment, ataxia, and oculomotor dysfunction, with most patients having some, but not all, of the classic symptom triad.[68] The cognitive impairment of WE typically includes inattention and disorientation. Korsakoff syndrome is a chronic condition characterized primarily by anterograde and retrograde memory impairment with conservation of long-term memory. Both syndromes are most commonly associated with excessive alcohol use and inadequate nutrition. Diagnosis is made by documentation of serum thiamine deficiency with a compatible clinical presentation. Imaging of the CNS can help suggest the diagnosis and rule out alternative causes. Although WE is treatable, significant deficits may persist even after adequate thiamine repletion.[68] Patients with Korsakoff syndrome typically respond poorly to treatment and require long-term supportive care.

Cobalamin (vitamin B_{12}) deficiency is usually caused by impaired absorption in the setting of pernicious anemia or gastric/small bowel disorders. Cobalamin deficiency can cause a wide range of neuropsychiatric symptoms, including mood disorders; psychosis; cognitive impairment; and disorders of the sensory, motor, and autonomic nervous systems (**Table 3** provides a list of possible neuropsychiatric symptoms).[69] These neuropsychiatric complications can occur in the absence of any hematologic evidence of megaloblastic anemia or other conditions associated with B_{12} deficiency. These symptoms can occur early or later in the course of B_{12} deficiency as well and their severity is inversely related to the severity of megaloblastic anemia.[70] Neurologic symptoms of cobalamin deficiency typically respond to treatment within the first 3 months, with nearly half of patients experiencing full recovery. Extent of recovery is related to the disease severity and duration of symptoms.[71]

Table 3
Neuropsychiatric symptoms of cobalamin (B_{12}) deficiency

Psychiatric	Neurologic
Depression	Sensory polyneuropathy
Anxiety/panic disorder	• Impaired vibration sense
Psychosis	• Impaired proprioception
Mania	Decreased visual acuity
Hallucinations/delusions	Dysgeusia/dysosmia
Insomnia	Urinary/fecal incontinence
	Erectile dysfunction
	Cerebellar ataxia
	Cognitive impairment
	• Memory impairment
	• Disorientation
	Obtundation
	Spasticity

Data from Stabler S, Allen R. Cecil textbook of medicine. Philadelphia: Saunders; 2004. p. 1054–5.

Calcium Disorders

Both hypocalcemia and hypercalcemia can cause neuropsychiatric manifestations. The severity of symptoms caused by hypocalcemia depends on both the acuity of change in calcium levels and the degree of hypocalcemia. Hypocalcemia can cause seizures and increased neuromuscular excitability, as well as psychiatric symptoms such as emotional lability, depression, psychosis, and anxiety. Hypercalcemia can cause confusion, lethargy, generalized weakness, and in severe cases coma and death.[70] These symptoms typically resolve with correction of the underlying electrolyte abnormality.[72]

Porphyrias

Acute porphyrias, rare disorders that result from abnormalities in heme biosynthesis, can cause neurologic and psychiatric symptoms. The porphyrias that can cause neurologic sequelae include the acute hepatic porphyrias: acute intermittent porphyria (AIP), hereditary coproporphyria, and variegate porphyria.[73] AIP is the most common of these rare, autosomal dominant disorders with incomplete penetrance, and all three can manifest similar neuropsychiatric sequelae. These acute porphyrias typically present with neurovisceral symptoms: the classic triad consists of abdominal pain, peripheral neuropathy, and altered mental status. There are isolated reports of patients presenting with neuropathy, encephalopathy, or psychosis, without associated abdominal symptoms.[74,75] The peripheral neuropathy seen with the porphyrias is usually a motor neuropathy, preferentially affecting proximal muscles. Sensory neuropathies are also common, and can follow either a stocking-glove or more central pattern of distribution. Cranial neuropathies are also a common manifestation of acute attacks.[74] Psychiatric symptoms are present in more than half of patients with symptomatic acute porphyria.[76] These psychiatric sequelae commonly include psychotic disorders, but can also include depression, anxiety, and delirium.[75] Diagnosis is made by qualitative testing for urine porphobilinogen (PBG) during an acute attack with additional second-line tests including quantitative PBG, plasma, erythrocyte, and fecal porphyrins, and enzymatic and DNA testing to confirm the diagnosis.[77,78] Prevention of acute attacks is an important aspect of long-term management and may include careful attention to diet, avoidance of medications known to exacerbate acute porphyria, and heme arginate (hemin) prophylaxis. Treatment of acute attacks typically involves symptom-directed therapies and supportive care, as well as IV hemin, and dietary loading with carbohydrates. Patients often require hospitalization for acute attacks.[78]

Wilson Disease

Wilson disease is a rare, autosomal recessive disorder of copper transport. In addition to liver failure, which is the best known manifestation of this disease, patients can also have neurologic sequelae. The prevalence estimates of neurologic symptoms attributable to Wilson disease are widely variable. Neurologic sequelae can include choreoathetosis, dysarthria, dystonia, tremor, ataxia, parkinsonism, and cognitive impairment, usually involving either the frontal lobe or a subcortical dementia. Although serum ceruloplasmin is a commonly used screening test, 24-hour urine copper quantification is more sensitive. Most patients with neurologic manifestations of Wilson disease also have Kayser-Fleischer rings present on slit-lamp ophthalmologic examination.[79,80] Wilson disease is unusual compared with some of the other medical conditions discussed here, in that early diagnosis and treatment can prevent severe neurologic symptoms and appropriately treated patients can even have a normal life span.[81]

NEOPLASTIC
Paraneoplastic Syndromes

Paraneoplastic syndromes involve organ and tissue damage distant from the site of a malignancy or metastases, are thought to be autoimmune mediated, are associated with antineuronal antibodies, and may affect the peripheral nervous system or CNS. They may affect any anatomic part of the nervous system, and any specific cell type as well, making the symptoms and signs potentially attributable to paraneoplastic disease numerous. Paraneoplastic syndromes can be seen in patients with already diagnosed neoplasms, but can sometimes precede the diagnosis of cancer, making awareness of this condition important for clinicians. Symptoms can range from peripheral neuropathies to neuropsychiatric symptoms including cognitive impairment, mood disorders, and changes in consciousness.[82] See **Table 4** for a listing of possible neurologic and psychiatric abnormalities associated with paraneoplastic syndromes.

Limbic encephalitis is one of the best described neuropsychiatric manifestations of paraneoplastic syndromes. It can be caused not only by paraneoplastic processes but also autoimmune diseases outside the setting of cancer and viral infections. Limbic encephalitis involves gray matter in the limbic area of the brain (amygdala, cingulate gyrus, and hippocampus) and patients typically present with short-term memory loss, seizures, and psychiatric symptoms[83] ranging from mood disorders (depression, irritability) and personality changes to hallucinations.[84] Treatment is directed at treatment of the underlying cancer, and immune suppression, although there are no established protocols or guidelines for treating paraneoplastic syndromes.[82]

FUTURE CONSIDERATIONS/SUMMARY

Early recognition of medical conditions underlying neuropsychiatric symptoms is critical for effective management, particularly for those patients with other signs or

Table 4	
Neuropsychiatric symptoms associated with paraneoplastic syndromes	
Psychiatric	**Neurologic**
Mood disorders • Depression • Irritability/agitation • Panic disorder • Obsessive-compulsive behavior	Seizures
Personality changes	Altered level of consciousness
Hallucinations	Cognitive impairment • Short-term memory loss • Dementia
Sleep disturbances	Chorea
Psychosis	Parkinsonism
Apathy	Ataxia Visual changes Myelopathy/myelitis Peripheral neuropathy (sensory, motor, or autonomic) Myasthenia gravis Myotonia

Data from Darnell RB, Posner JB. Paraneoplastic syndromes affecting the nervous system. Semin Oncol 2006;33(3):270–98; and Kayser MS, Kohler CG, Dalmau J. Psychiatric manifestations of paraneoplastic disorders. Am J Psychiatry 2010;167(9):1039–50.

symptoms that might suggest a non-neuropsychiatric origin of the illness and/or systemic cause. The number of medical conditions that have been associated with such symptoms is vast; thus, casting a broad differential diagnosis is imperative when such unexplained, and often acute, symptoms are present. Treatment of the underlying condition causing these symptoms is usually indicated, as is careful attention to symptom management. Certain conditions are well understood and treatments well established, such as the electrolyte abnormalities listed earlier, although knowledge of many of these complex causes continues to evolve, as does understanding of the best therapeutic interventions, particularly given that many of these diseases are rare. Through careful history taking, physical examination, and ancillary testing when indicated, these medical conditions can rapidly be identified and treated, usually resulting in symptom improvement, if not complete resolution.

REFERENCES

1. Janssen RS, Cornblath DR, Epstein LG, et al. Human immunodeficiency virus (HIV) infection and the nervous system: report from the American Academy of Neurology AIDS Task Force. Neurology 1989;39(1):119–22.
2. Grassi B, Garghentini G, Gambini O, et al. Neuropsychiatric aspects of HIV infection: a liaison psychiatry study. Eur Psychiatry 1997;12(1):16–20.
3. Gisslén M, Price RW, Nilsson S. The definition of HIV-associated neurocognitive disorders: are we overestimating the real prevalence? BMC Infect Dis 2011;11: 356.
4. Heaton RK, Franklin DR, Ellis RJ, et al. HIV-associated neurocognitive disorders before and during the era of combination antiretroviral therapy: differences in rates, nature, and predictors. J Neurovirol 2011;17(1):3–16.
5. Crum-Cianflone NF, Moore DJ, Letendre S, et al. Low prevalence of neurocognitive impairment in early diagnosed and managed HIV-infected persons. Neurology 2013;80(4):371–9.
6. Nomenclature and research case definitions for neurologic manifestations of human immunodeficiency virus-type 1 (HIV-1) infection. Report of a working group of the American Academy of Neurology AIDS Task Force. Neurology 1991;41(6): 778–85.
7. McDaniel JS, Purcell DW, Farber EW. Severe mental illness and HIV-related medical and neuropsychiatric sequelae. Clin Psychol Rev 1997;17(3):311–25.
8. Power C, Gladden JG, Halliday W, et al. AIDS- and non-AIDS-related PML association with distinct p53 polymorphism. Neurology 2000;54(3):743–6.
9. Tan CS, Koralnik IJ. Progressive multifocal leukoencephalopathy and other disorders caused by JC virus: clinical features and pathogenesis. Lancet Neurol 2010;9(4):425–37.
10. Bernal-Cano F, Joseph JT, Koralnik IJ. Spinal cord lesions of progressive multifocal leukoencephalopathy in an acquired immunodeficiency syndrome patient. J Neurovirol 2007;13(5):474–6.
11. Engsig FN, Hansen AB, Omland LH, et al. Incidence, clinical presentation, and outcome of progressive multifocal leukoencephalopathy in HIV-infected patients during the highly active antiretroviral therapy era: a nationwide cohort study. J Infect Dis 2009;199(1):77–83.
12. Hall CD, Dafni U, Simpson D, et al. Failure of cytarabine in progressive multifocal leukoencephalopathy associated with human immunodeficiency virus infection. AIDS Clinical Trials Group 243 Team. N Engl J Med 1998;338(19): 1345–51.

13. Kaplan JE, Benson C, Holmes KK, et al. Guidelines for prevention and treatment of opportunistic infections in HIV-infected adults and adolescents: recommendations from CDC, the National Institutes of Health, and the HIV Medicine Association of the Infectious Diseases Society of America. MMWR Recomm Rep 2009;58(RR-4):1–207 [quiz: CE1–4].

14. Pirskanen-Matell R, Grützmeier S, Nennesmo I, et al. Impairment of short-term memory and Korsakoff syndrome are common in AIDS patients with cytomegalovirus encephalitis. Eur J Neurol 2009;16(1):48–53.

15. Arribas JR, Clifford DB, Fichtenbaum CJ, et al. Level of cytomegalovirus (CMV) DNA in cerebrospinal fluid of subjects with AIDS and CMV infection of the central nervous system. J Infect Dis 1995;172(2):527–31.

16. Mussini C, Mongiardo N, Manicardi G, et al. Relevance of clinical and laboratory findings in the diagnosis of cytomegalovirus encephalitis in patients with AIDS. Eur J Clin Microbiol Infect Dis 1997;16(6):437–44.

17. Whitley RJ, Jacobson MA, Friedberg DN, et al. Guidelines for the treatment of cytomegalovirus diseases in patients with AIDS in the era of potent antiretroviral therapy: recommendations of an international panel. International AIDS Society-USA. Arch Intern Med 1998;158(9):957–69.

18. Anduze-Faris BM, Fillet AM, Gozlan J, et al. Induction and maintenance therapy of cytomegalovirus central nervous system infection in HIV-infected patients. AIDS 2000;14(5):517–24.

19. Cohen BA. Prognosis and response to therapy of cytomegalovirus encephalitis and meningomyelitis in AIDS. Neurology 1996;46(2):444–50.

20. Fauci AS, Isselbacher KJ, Wilson JD, et al. Harrison's principles of internal medicine. 14th edition. New York: McGraw-Hill; 1998.

21. Read PJ, Donovan B. Clinical aspects of adult syphilis. Intern Med J 2012;42(6): 614–20.

22. Mattei PL, Beachkofsky TM, Gilson RT, et al. Syphilis: a reemerging infection. Am Fam Physician 2012;86(5):433–40.

23. Workowski KA, Berman S, Centers for Disease Control and Prevention (CDC). Sexually transmitted diseases treatment guidelines, 2010. MMWR Recomm Rep 2010;59(RR-12):1–110.

24. Wormser GP, Halperin JJ. Toward a better understanding of European Lyme neuroborreliosis. Clin Infect Dis 2013;57(4):510–2.

25. Dattwyler RJ, Luft BJ. Overview of the clinical manifestations of Borrelia burgdorferi infection. Can J Infect Dis 1991;2(2):61–3.

26. Halperin J, Luft BJ, Volkman DJ, et al. Lyme neuroborreliosis. Peripheral nervous system manifestations. Brain 1990;113(Pt 4):1207–21.

27. Lakos A. CSF findings in Lyme meningitis. J Infect 1992;25(2):155–61.

28. Wormser GP, Dattwyler RJ, Shapiro ED, et al. The clinical assessment, treatment, and prevention of Lyme disease, human granulocytic anaplasmosis, and babesiosis: clinical practice guidelines by the Infectious Diseases Society of America. Clin Infect Dis 2006;43(9):1089–134.

29. Jennekens FG, Kater L. The central nervous system in systemic lupus erythematosus. Part 1. Clinical syndromes: a literature investigation. Rheumatology (Oxford) 2002;41(6):605–18.

30. Ward MM, Studenski S. The time course of acute psychiatric episodes in systemic lupus erythematosus. J Rheumatol 1991;18(4):535–9.

31. Hochberg MC. Updating the American College of Rheumatology revised criteria for the classification of systemic lupus erythematosus. Arthritis Rheum 1997; 40(9):1725.

32. Tan EM, Cohen AS, Fries JF, et al. The 1982 revised criteria for the classification of systemic lupus erythematosus. Arthritis Rheum 1982;25(11):1271–7.
33. Petri M, Orbai AM, Alarcón GS, et al. Derivation and validation of the Systemic Lupus International Collaborating Clinics classification criteria for systemic lupus erythematosus. Arthritis Rheum 2012;64(8):2677–86.
34. The American College of Rheumatology nomenclature and case definitions for neuropsychiatric lupus syndromes. Arthritis Rheum 1999;42(4):599–608.
35. Hanly JG. ACR classification criteria for systemic lupus erythematosus: limitations and revisions to neuropsychiatric variables. Lupus 2004;13(11):861–4.
36. Efthimiou P, Blanco M. Pathogenesis of neuropsychiatric systemic lupus erythematosus and potential biomarkers. Mod Rheumatol 2009;19(5):457–68.
37. Conti F, Alessandri C, Bompane D, et al. Autoantibody profile in systemic lupus erythematosus with psychiatric manifestations: a role for anti-endothelial-cell antibodies. Arthritis Res Ther 2004;6(4):R366–72.
38. Denburg JA, Behmann SA. Lymphocyte and neuronal antigens in neuropsychiatric lupus: presence of an elutable, immunoprecipitable lymphocyte/neuronal 52 kd reactivity. Ann Rheum Dis 1994;53(5):304–8.
39. Burns TM. Neurosarcoidosis. Arch Neurol 2003;60(8):1166–8.
40. Krumholz A, Stern BJ. Neurologic manifestations of sarcoidosis. Handb Clin Neurol 2014;119:305–33.
41. Rybicki BA, Popovich J Jr, Maliarik MJ, et al. Racial differences in sarcoidosis incidence: a 5-year study in a health maintenance organization. Am J Epidemiol 1997;145(3):234–41.
42. Hoitsma E, Drent M, Sharma OP. A pragmatic approach to diagnosing and treating neurosarcoidosis in the 21st century. Curr Opin Pulm Med 2010;16(5): 472–9.
43. Hoitsma E, Marziniak M, Faber CG, et al. Small fibre neuropathy in sarcoidosis. Lancet 2002;359(9323):2085–6.
44. Bihan H, Christozova V, Dumas JL, et al. Sarcoidosis: clinical, hormonal, and magnetic resonance imaging (MRI) manifestations of hypothalamic-pituitary disease in 9 patients and review of the literature. Medicine (Baltimore) 2007;86(5): 259–68.
45. Cahill DW, Salcman M. Neurosarcoidosis: a review of the rarer manifestations. Surg Neurol 1981;15(3):204–11.
46. Elfferich MD, Nelemans PJ, Ponds RW, et al. Everyday cognitive failure in sarcoidosis: the prevalence and the effect of anti-TNF-alpha treatment. Respiration 2010;80(3):212–9.
47. Leigh H, Kramer SI. The psychiatric manifestations of endocrine disease. Adv Intern Med 1984;29:413–45.
48. Constant EL, Adam S, Seron X, et al. Anxiety and depression, attention, and executive functions in hypothyroidism. J Int Neuropsychol Soc 2005;11(5):535–44.
49. Knopman DS, Petersen RC, Cha RH, et al. Incidence and causes of nondegenerative nonvascular dementia: a population-based study. Arch Neurol 2006; 63(2):218–21.
50. Haupt M, Kurz A. Reversibility of dementia in hypothyroidism. J Neurol 1993; 240(6):333–5.
51. Nickel SN, Frame B. Neurologic manifestations of myxedema. Neurology 1958; 8(7):511–7.
52. Stern RA, Robinson B, Thorner AR, et al. A survey study of neuropsychiatric complaints in patients with Graves' disease. J Neuropsychiatry Clin Neurosci 1996;8(2):181–5.

53. Martin FI, Deam DR. Hyperthyroidism in elderly hospitalised patients. Clinical features and treatment outcomes. Med J Aust 1996;164(4):200–3.
54. Duyff RF, Van den Bosch J, Laman DM, et al. Neuromuscular findings in thyroid dysfunction: a prospective clinical and electrodiagnostic study. J Neurol Neurosurg Psychiatr 2000;68(6):750–5.
55. Song TJ, Kim SJ, Kim GS, et al. The prevalence of thyrotoxicosis-related seizures. Thyroid 2010;20(9):955–8.
56. Sahni V, Gupta N, Anuradha S, et al. Thyrotoxic neuropathy- an under diagnosed condition. Med J Malaysia 2007;62(1):76–7.
57. Pereira AM, Tiemensma J, Romijn JA. Neuropsychiatric disorders in Cushing's syndrome. Neuroendocrinology 2010;92(Suppl 1):65–70.
58. Kelly WF, Kelly MJ, Faragher B. A prospective study of psychiatric and psychological aspects of Cushing's syndrome. Clin Endocrinol (Oxf) 1996;45(6):715–20.
59. Starkman MN, Schteingart DE, Schork MA. Depressed mood and other psychiatric manifestations of Cushing's syndrome: relationship to hormone levels. Psychosom Med 1981;43(1):3–18.
60. Kelly WF. Psychiatric aspects of Cushing's syndrome. QJM 1996;89(7):543–51.
61. Starkman MN. Neuropsychiatric findings in Cushing syndrome and exogenous glucocorticoid administration. Endocrinol Metab Clin North Am 2013;42(3):477–88.
62. Sharma ST, Nieman LK. Cushing's syndrome: all variants, detection, and treatment. Endocrinol Metab Clin North Am 2011;40(2):379–91, viii–ix.
63. Heald AH, Ghosh S, Bray S, et al. Long-term negative impact on quality of life in patients with successfully treated Cushing's disease. Clin Endocrinol (Oxf) 2004;61(4):458–65.
64. Gotch PM. Cushing's syndrome from the patient's perspective. Endocrinol Metab Clin North Am 1994;23(3):607–17.
65. Charmandari E, Nicolaides NC, Chrousos GP. Adrenal insufficiency. Lancet 2014. http://dx.doi.org/10.1016/S0140-6736(13)61684-0. pii:S0140-6736(13)61684-0.
66. Smith CK, Barish J, Correa J, et al. Psychiatric disturbance in endocrinologic disease. Psychosom Med 1972;34(1):69–86.
67. Hahner S, Loeffler M, Fassnacht M, et al. Impaired subjective health status in 256 patients with adrenal insufficiency on standard therapy based on cross-sectional analysis. J Clin Endocrinol Metab 2007;92(10):3912–22.
68. Victor M, Adams RD, Collins GH. The Wernicke-Korsakoff syndrome. A clinical and pathological study of 245 patients, 82 with post-mortem examinations. Contemp Neurol Ser 1971;7:1–206.
69. Lachner C, Steinle NI, Regenold WT. The neuropsychiatry of vitamin B12 deficiency in elderly patients. J Neuropsychiatry Clin Neurosci 2012;24(1):5–15.
70. Stabler S, Allen R. Cecil textbook of medicine. Philadelphia: Saunders; 2004. p. 1054–5.
71. Healton EB, Savage DG, Brust JC, et al. Neurologic aspects of cobalamin deficiency. Medicine (Baltimore) 1991;70(4):229–45.
72. Maiti A, Chatterjee S. Neuropsychiatric manifestations and their outcomes in chronic hypocalcaemia. J Indian Med Assoc 2013;111(3):174–7.
73. Tracy JA, Dyck PJ. Porphyria and its neurologic manifestations. Handb Clin Neurol 2014;120:839–49.
74. Simon NG, Herkes GK. The neurologic manifestations of the acute porphyrias. J Clin Neurosci 2011;18(9):1147–53.

75. Crimlisk HL. The little imitator–porphyria: a neuropsychiatric disorder. J Neurol Neurosurg Psychiatr 1997;62(4):319–28.
76. Walterfang M, Bonnot O, Mocellin R, et al. The neuropsychiatry of inborn errors of metabolism. J Inherit Metab Dis 2013;36(4):687–702.
77. Anderson KE, Bloomer JR, Bonkovsky HL, et al. Recommendations for the diagnosis and treatment of the acute porphyrias. Ann Intern Med 2005;142(6): 439–50.
78. Balwani M, Desnick RJ. The porphyrias: advances in diagnosis and treatment. Blood 2012;120(23):4496–504.
79. Brewer GJ, Yuzbasiyan-Gurkan V. Wilson disease. Medicine (Baltimore) 1992; 71(3):139–64.
80. Wiebers DO, Hollenhorst RW, Goldstein NP. The ophthalmologic manifestations of Wilson's disease. Mayo Clin Proc 1977;52(7):409–16.
81. Lorincz MT. Recognition and treatment of neurologic Wilson's disease. Semin Neurol 2012;32(5):538–43.
82. Darnell RB, Posner JB. Paraneoplastic syndromes affecting the nervous system. Semin Oncol 2006;33(3):270–98.
83. Tüzün E, Dalmau J. Limbic encephalitis and variants: classification, diagnosis and treatment. Neurologist 2007;13(5):261–71.
84. Kayser MS, Kohler CG, Dalmau J. Psychiatric manifestations of paraneoplastic disorders. Am J Psychiatry 2010;167(9):1039–50.

Index

Note: Page numbers of article titles are in **boldface** type.

A

Abuse, autism spectrum as victims of, 1178
Acamprosate, for alcohol withdrawal, 1106–1109
Acetylcholine inhibitors, 996
Addison disease, neuropsychiatric manifestations of, 1200–1201
Adjustment disorders, 988, 1071–1074
Adrenal insufficiency, neuropsychiatric manifestations of, 1200–1201
Adult ADHD Rating Scales, 968
Adult Self Report, for ADHD screening, 968
Advanced sleep phase syndrome, 1131
Affective dysregulation, in borderline personality disorder, 1052
Alcohol use. See Substance abuse.
Alzheimer disease, 1152–1153
Amodafinil, 1136
ANK3 gene, in bipolar disorder, 1026
Antianxiety medications, 929
Anticipatory grief, 1069–1071
Anticonvulsants, 940–942, 1105
Antidepressants, 928–931
    efficacy of, 995
    failure of, 997–998
    for bipolar disorder, 1032–1034
    for borderline personality disorder, 1055–1056
    for depression, 994–998, 1159–1161
    for grief, 1071
    for insomnia, 1127, 1131
    for multiple somatic symptoms, 1089
    for seasonal affective disorder, 1068–1069
    for sleep disorders, 1128
    mechanism of action of, 995
    medication interactions with, 997
    side effects of, 931, 995–997
Antipsychotics, 930, 943–951
    atypical, 943–944, 948–949, 1035–1036, 1128
    drug interactions with, 946
    for autism spectrum, 1185–1186
    for bipolar disorder, 1032, 1035–1036
    for borderline personality disorder, 1056
    for dementia, 950–951
    for sleep disorders, 1128
    side effects of, 945

Med Clin N Am 98 (2014) 1209–1223
http://dx.doi.org/10.1016/S0025-7125(14)00120-5
0025-7125/14/$ – see front matter

D